05/07

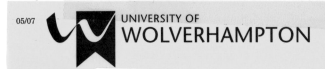

UNIVERSITY OF
WOLVERHAMPTON

ONE WEEK LOAN

D1332339

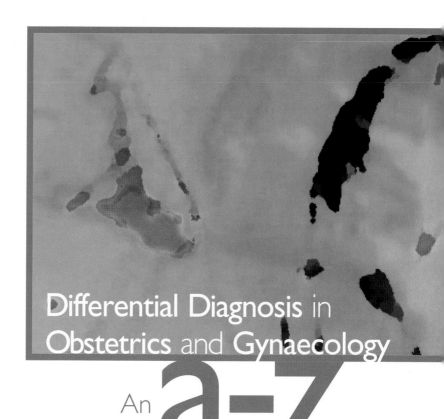

Differential Diagnosis in Obstetrics and Gynaecology

An a-z

Edited by **Tony Hollingworth**

Consultant in Obstetrics and Gynaecology
Whipps Cross University Hospital Trust, London, UK

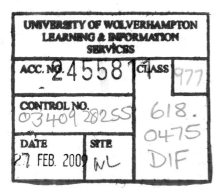
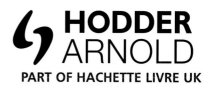

HODDER
ARNOLD

PART OF HACHETTE LIVRE UK

First published in Great Britain in 2008 by
Hodder Arnold, an imprint of Hodder Education and a member of the Hodder Headline Group,
338 Euston Road, London NW1 3BH

http://www.hoddereducation.com

British Library Cataloguing in Publication Data
A catalogue record for this book is available from the British Library

Library of Congress Cataloging-in-Publication Data
A catalog record for this book is available from the Library of Congress

ISBN-13   978-0-340-92825-7

1 2 3 4 5 6 7 8 9 10

Commissioning Editor: Gavin Jamieson
Project Editor: Francesca Naish
Production Controller: Andre Sim
Cover Design: Helen Townson

Typeset in 9/12 pt minion by Charon Tec Ltd., A Macmillan Company
Printed and bound in India

For

Ann

Vicki, Chloe and Adam

and their support!

Contents

Differential Diagnosis in
Obstetrics and Gynaecology

An a-z

Contributors

Dr Naim Akhtar
Consultant Haematologist
Whipps Cross University Hospital Trust
London
UK

Dr Mala Arora
Consultant Obstetrician and Gynaecologist,
  and Specialist in Fertility
Noble Hospital
Faridabad
India

Dr Kausik Banerjee
Consultant Paediatrician
Whipps Cross University Hospital Trust
London
UK
and
Honorary Consultant in Paediatric
  Endocrinology
Royal London Hospital
London
UK

Dr Anthony Bewley
Consultant Dermatologist
Whipps Cross University Hospital Trust &
St Bartholomew's and the Royal London NHS
  Trust
London
UK

Mr Nigel Bickerton
Consultant in Obstetrics and Gynaecology
Glan Clwyd Hospital
Bodelwyddan
Rhyl
UK

Dr Oliver Brain
Specialist Registrar in Gastroenterology
Royal Berkshire Hospital
Reading
UK

Dr Deborah Chee
Consultant in Perinatal Psychiatry
Department of Psychological Medicine
Kings College Hospital
Denmark Hill
London
UK

Dr Anne Clark
Fertility First
Hurstville
NSW
Australia

Dr Greg Davis
Consultant Obstetrician
St George Hospital and Community
  Health Service
Kogarah
NSW
Australia

Dr Rina Davison MB Bchir MRCP MD
Consultant Physician and Endocrinologist
Whipps Cross University Hospital Trust
London
UK

Professor Cynthia Farquhar
Professor of Obstetrics and Gynaecology
National Women's Hospital
Auckland
New Zealand

Dr Nicola Fattizzi MB
Honorary Senior House Officer in
  Gynaecological Oncology
St Bartholomew's and the Royal London
  NHS Trust
London
UK

Mr Peter Frecker
Consultant Surgeon
Whipps Cross University Hospital Trust
London
UK

Mr James Green
Consultant Urologist
Whipps Cross University Hospital Trust
London
UK

Dr Sandy Gupta
Consultant Cardiologist
Whipps Cross University Hospital Trust
London
UK

Mr Tony Hollingworth
Consultant in Obstetrics and Gynaecology
Whipps Cross University Hospital Trust &
St Bartholomew's and the Royal London
  NHS Trust
London
UK

Dr Ana Ignjatovic
Specialist Registrar in Gastroenterology
Royal Berkshire Hospital
Reading
UK

**Dr Urvashi Prasad Jha MD MRCOG FICS
FRCOG (UK)**
Senior Consultant Gynaecological
Laparoscopic & Onco-surgeon
Academic Co-ordinator
Department of Gynaecology and Obstetrics
Indraprastha Apollo Hospitals
New Delhi
India

Dr Alamgir Kabir
Specialist Registrar in Cardiology
St Bartholomew's and the Royal London
  NHS Trust
London
UK

Mr Ramesh Kuppusamy
Specialist Registrar in Obstetrics and
  Gynaecology
Queen's Hospital
Romford
UK

Dr Velmurugan C Kuppuswamy MBBS MRCP
Specialist Registrar
Homerton University Hospital NHS
  Foundation Trust
London
UK

Mr Richard Maplethorpe
Consultant in Obstetrics and Gynaecology
Newham University Hospital Trust
London
UK

Dr Peter Muller
Department of Obstetrics
Women's and Children's Hospital
North Adelaide
SA
Australia

Dr Margaret Myszor
Consultant Physician and Gastroenterologist
Royal Berkshire Hospital
Reading
UK

Dr Eva Lundeskov Papesch
Clinical Fellow in Otolaryngology
St Bartholomew's and the Royal London
  NHS Trust
London
UK

Mr Mike Papesch
Consultant in Otolaryngology
Whipps Cross University Hospital Trust
London
UK

Dr Simon Quantrill
Consultant Chest Physician
Whipps Cross University Hospital Trust
London
UK

Ms Karina Reynolds
Consultant Gynaecological Oncologist
St Bartholomew's and the Royal London
    NHS Trust
London
UK

Assistant Professor Jai B Sharma
All India Institute of Medical Science
New Delhi
India

Dr Nanda Shetty
Specialist Registrar in Obstetrics and
    Gynaecology
Whipps Cross University Hospital Trust
London
UK

Mr Dhammike Silva
Senior Registrar in Obstetrics and Gynaecology
Colombo South Teaching Hospital
Kalubowila
Sri Lanka

Dr Swasti MBBS DNB (Obs & Gynae)
Diploma Advanced Gynae Endoscopy
(Germany)
Clinical Assistant and Research Fellow
Department of Obstetrics & Gynaecology
Indraprastha Apollo Hospitals,
New Delhi
India

Mr Dilip Visvanathan
Consultant in Obstetrics and Gynaecology
Whipps Cross University Hospital
London
UK

Dr Sharmistha Williams
Associate Specialist
Department of Rheumatology
Queens Hospital
Romford
Essex
UK

Foreword

One of the major challenges in obstetrics and gynaecology is the need for a broad knowledge of medicine and surgery as well as the conditions specific to reproduction. The comprehensive nature of this book achieves this goal.

Differential Diagnosis in Obstetrics and Gynaecology covers everything you ever wanted to know about what can occur in pregnant and non-pregnant women. The editor has included experts in many specialties to contribute to this book which is particularly valuable as it takes the reader outside the realm of an obstetrician and gynaecologist. From minor symptoms to major symptoms the differential diagnoses are explored and offered in a way that is easy to read and leads the reader on to straightforward and practical management.

This book is suitable for all grades of healthcare professional, not only as a reference book but also for revising for any qualifying or licensing examination. Inevitably medical words are used but lay people would also find this book very useful.

The layout of the book is engaging as the text is interspersed with excellent illustrations and useful boxes highlighting important points. For the reader who would like to delve even further into each area there are up-to-date references.

Obstetrics and Gynaecology is a rewarding speciality but one that is forever confronting you with what you do not know. This book will undoubtedly help you to solve the problems and should be on the bookshelf of everyone who deals with women!

Janice Rymer MD FRCOG FRANZCOG FHEA
Professor of Obstetrics and Gynaecology
Department of Women's Health
King's College School of Medicine
London
UK

This book is based on *French's Index of Differential Diagnosis* which was first published in 1912. The aim of that book was 'to help in the differential diagnosis of any condition in medicine, surgery or any specialty that may be seen in general or hospital practice'. I was asked to edit the gynaecological sections for the most recent edition, which was published in 2005. On completion, I felt there was room for a similar type of book for obstetrics and gynaecology.

Subsequently I enlisted the help of current and former colleagues as well as friends from around the world to produce this book, which aims to cover most of the symptoms that may be commonly seen in a woman presenting to the gynaecologist or to the obstetrician during her pregnancy. I have tried to make the book as accessible as possible to all doctors regardless of specialty and grade, as well as midwives, nurses, medical students and patients alike.

In some sections management of the symptoms has been addressed but the main emphasis of this book is differential diagnosis. References and websites have been included where appropriate and a glossary of common terms and terminology used in obstetrics and gynaecology has been provided at the end.

Tony Hollingworth
June 2008

Acknowledgements

This book has taken quite a while to come to fruition and I would like to take this opportunity to express my thanks to the contributors for its publication. I would like to thank Sarah Burrows who helped to set the project in motion before moving to RSM publications and to Janice Rymer for kindly agreeing to write the Foreword.

I would like to thank all the contributors, who comprise of colleagues at Whipps Cross as well as former colleagues I have worked with in some form during my career plus some friends from medical school days. They have all risen to the challenge and have produced excellent contributions which have certainly helped with my continuing medical education!

I would like to thank Dr Barthi George and Dr Andrzej Karmolinski from the Pathology Department, Dr Rex Melville from the Department of Sexual Health, and Dr Nick Reading and the ultrasonographers from the Radiology Department at Whipps Cross for providing appropriate illustrations. There have been contributions from other local departments of the various contributors, which have been acknowledged throughout the book, and I would like to thank them for their help.

I would like to thank Dr Simon Barton, Dr Peter Greenhouse and Mr Michael Jones for allowing me to use some of their illustrations in the chapters on the cervix and vaginal discharge.

I would like to thank Kate Nardoni and Cactus Design & Illustration Ltd for their beautiful diagrams which have surpassed my expectations. I would like to say many thanks to Clare Freeman who was the copy editor and helped iron out many of the problems with the some of the text.

Finally I would like to say a big thank you to Francesca Naish who was my project editor, she has steered this project to a successful completion and I am in her debt.

Tony Hollingworth
June 2008

List of Abbreviations

ACTH	adrenocorticotrophic hormone	DHEAS	dehydroepiandrosterone sulphate
AF	atrial fibrillation		
AFE	amniotic fluid embolism	DIC	disseminated intravascular coagulation/coagulopathy
AFI	amniotic fluid index		
AFV	amniotic fluid volume	DMPA	depot medroxyprogesterone acetate
ALP	alkaline phosphatase		
ALT	alanine aminotransferase	DSD	disorders of sex development
AMH	anti-Müllerian hormone	DVT	deep venous/vein thrombosis
APCR	activated protein C resistance	ECG	electrocardiogram
APS	antiphospholipid antibody syndrome	ESPE	European Society for Paediatric Endocrinology
APTT	activated partial thromboplastin time	ESR	erythrocyte sedimentation rate
ARDS	adult respiratory distress syndrome	EUA	examination under anaesthetic
ASD	atrial septal defect	FDPs	fibrin degradation products
AST	aspartate aminotransferase	FENa	fractional excretion of sodium
ATN	acute tubular necrosis	FEP	free erythrocyte protoporphyrin
BBC	benign breast change syndrome	FEV1	forced expiratory volume in one second
BCG	bacille Calmette–Guérin	FGR	fetal growth restriction
BMI	body mass index	FSH	follicle-stimulating hormone
BPD	biparietal diameter	FT3	free tri-iodothyronine
bpm	beats per minute	FT4	free thyroxine
BUN	blood urea nitrogen	FTA–ABS	fluorescent treponemal antibody absorption (test)
CAH	congenital adrenal hyperplasia	FVC	forced vital capacity
CEE	conjugated equine oestrogens	GABA	γ-aminobutyric acid
CGIN	cervical glandular intraepithelial neoplasia	GDM	gestational diabetes
		GI	gastrointestinal
CHD	coronary heart disease	GnRH	gonadotrophin-releasing hormone
CIN	cervical intraepithelial neoplasia	GORD	gastro-oesophageal reflux disease
CMV	cytomegalovirus		
CNS	central nervous system	GTD	gestational trophoblastic disease
CRL	crown–rump length	GTT	glucose tolerance test
CTG	cardiotocograph	Hb	haemoglobin
CTPA	computerised tomographic pulmonary angiography	HbF	fetal haemoglobin
		HBV	hepatitis B virus
D&C	dilatation and curettage	HBC	hepatitis C virus
DCIS	ductal carcinoma *in situ*	HCG	human chorionic gonadotrophin

HELLP	haemolysis, elevated liver enzymes and low platelets (syndrome)
5-HIAA	5-hydroxyindoleacetic acid
HIE	hypoxic ischaemic encephalopathy
HIT	heparin-induced thrombocytopenia
HIV	human immunodeficiency virus
HMB	heavy menstrual bleeding
HOCM	hypertrophic cardiomyopathy
HPA-1a	human platelet antigen-1a
HPG	hypothalamo–pituitary–gonadal (axis)
HPV	human papillomavirus
HRCT	high-resolution computerised tomography
HRT	hormone replacement therapy
HSG	hysterosalpingogram
HSV	herpes simplex virus
HUS	haemolytic–uraemic syndrome
Hy-Co-Sy	hysterosalpingo-contrast sonography
IBD	inflammatory bowel disease
IBS	irritable bowel syndrome
ICD	implantable cardioverter defibrillator
IDA	iron-deficiency anaemia
Ig	immunoglobulin
INR	international normalised ratio
ITP	immune thrombocytopenic purpura
IUCD	intrauterine contraceptive device
IUFD	intrauterine fetal death
IUGR	intrauterine growth restriction
IV	intravenous
IVF	in vitro fertilisation
IVH	intraventricular haemorrhage
IVP	intravenous pyelogram
JVP	jugular venous pressure
LBC	liquid-based cytology
LFT	liver function test
LH	luteinising hormone
LLETZ	large loop excision of the transformation zone

LMWH	low-molecular-weight heparin
LSC	lichen simplex chronicus
LSCS	lower segment Caesarean section
LWPES	Lawson Wilkins Pediatric Endocrine Society
MAO	monoamine oxidase
MCH	mean corpuscular haemoglobin
MCHC	mean corpuscular haemoglobin concentration
MCV	mean corpuscular volume
MHA	microangiopathic haemolytic anaemia
MI	myocardial infarction
MRI	magnetic resonance imaging
MSU	mid-stream urine
NHSCSP	National Health Service Cervical Screening Programme
NICE	National Institute for Health and Clinical Excellence
NSAIDs	non-steroidal anti-inflammatory drugs
NYHA	New York Heart Association
OGTT	oral glucose tolerance test
17αOHP	17α-hydroxyprogesterone
OP	occipitoposterior
PCOS	polycystic ovarian/ovary syndrome
PCR	polymerase chain reaction
PE	pulmonary embolism
PFA	platelet function analyser
PID	pelvic inflammatory disease
PIH	pregnancy-induced hypertension
PMB	postmenopausal bleeding
PMS	premenstrual syndrome
POEMS	polyneuropathy, organomegaly, endocrinopathy, monoclonal proteinaemia and skin changes
POPQ	pelvic organ prolapse quantification
PPI	proton pump inhibitor
PPROM	preterm premature rupture of the membranes

PT	prothrombin time
PTU	propylthiouracil
PTP	pre-test probability
qid	quater in die (four times daily)
RA	rheumatoid arthritis
RBC	red blood cell
RCOG	Royal College of Obstetricians and Gynaecologists
RDS	respiratory distress syndrome
RMI	risk of malignancy index
RR	relative risks
RVOT	right ventricular outflow tract
SLE	systemic lupus erythematosus
SPD	symphysis pubis dysfunction
SPVT	septic pelvic vein thrombophlebitis
SRY	sex-determining region in the Y chromosome (gene)
SSRI	selective serotonin reuptake inhibitor
STD	sexually transmitted disease
SUI	stress urinary incontinence
SVTs	supraventricular tachycardias
TB	tuberculosis
T/E	testosterone/epitestosterone (ratio)
TGF-α	transforming growth factor α
TIBC	total iron binding capacity

TPI	treponemal immobilization (test)
TSH	thyroid-stimulating hormone
TT	thrombin time
TTP	thrombotic thrombocytopenic purpura
UH	unfractionated heparin
UI	urinary incontinence
UOsm	urine osmolality
USS	ultrasound scan
UTI	urinary tract infection
UUI	urge urinary incontinence
VDRL	Venereal Disease Research Laboratory (test)
VIN	vulval intraepithelial neoplasia
VIP	vasoactive intestinal peptide
V/Q	ventilation/perfusion
VSD	ventricular septal defect
VT	ventricular tachycardia
VTE	venous thromboembolism
vWD	von Willebrand's disease
vWF	von Willebrand's factor
WHO	World Health Organization
ZIG	zoster immune globulin

Differential Diagnosis in Obstetrics and Gynaecology: An A–Z

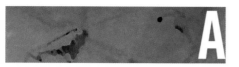

ABDOMINAL PAIN

Nigel Bickerton

Each year in the UK, hundreds of thousands of patients are seen in accident and emergency departments across the country or they are admitted on to a hospital ward following the sudden onset of abdominal pain as their main symptom. This group makes up 5–10 per cent of the total number of patients seen in UK hospitals. In the USA it has been estimated that this number is 5 million patients per year. Despite patients seeing clinicians experienced in history-taking and clinical examination, about 30 per cent of patients do not receive a specific diagnosis, despite having a series of clinical investigations.

The term *acute abdomen* is used to describe a patient with sudden onset of severe symptoms related to the abdomen and its contents. The symptoms associated with acute abdomen may be due to pathological changes that require urgent surgical intervention.

The pain may be somatic, visceral or referred, all of which have different innervations. Somatic pain, transmitted through the somatic nerve fibres from the parietal peritoneum, may be caused by physical or chemical irritation of the peritoneum. The pain feels sharp, very localised and is constant until the cause of the pain is removed. Visceral pain is transmitted through the autonomic nerves. The quality of the perceived pain is different, being dull, sometimes described as cramp-like. Women may describe the quality of visceral pain as 'like just before the start of a period'.

This section is not going to list a whole symptomatology or all the clinical signs related to specific diagnoses in women presenting with an acute abdomen. It is designed to give a broad overview with some aspects of pain being discussed in other sections of the book.

Diagnosis starts with taking a focused and precise history, which may put a lot of pieces of the diagnostic puzzle together even before examination. Quite often, the patient holds the key to the correct diagnosis, but needs to be given the chance to answer the right questions.

The history should include the timing and nature of the onset of pain, together with its site (see Box 1) and radiating features plus any aggravating or alleviating factors. People often find the nature of the pain difficult to describe, although precision in this area can be very valuable for the correct diagnosis. The doctor needs to know whether the patient has constant, intermittent or colicky pain. Colicky pain is the most difficult to describe, but a patient with this type of pain will often demonstrate the pain with a hand or finger drawing a sine wave in the air; even down to the crescendo–decrescendo representing pain intensity.

A full gynaecological history should be taken with specific reference to the possibility of pregnancy. Most units in the UK will do a urinary pregnancy test as a routine part of an emergency admission. All medicines prescribed or otherwise taken should be recorded including recreational drugs. Long-term prednisolone therapy should alert the clinician to the possibility of upper gastrointestinal perforation as a cause for acute pain. The history should include a review of all the systems with particular reference to the respiratory, cardiac, alimentary and renal systems.

One significant risk in women with abdominal pain is that the pain will very often be attributed to a gynaecological cause. This can happen whatever route the woman takes into hospital. There are several ways that a doctor can improve the outcome of a woman's admission with abdominal pain. These start with remembering that it is best to think outside of our specialty for possible causes, whilst at the same time recognising that common things happen commonly.

A woman with acute abdominal pain may require to be examined by several doctors over a short period of time, both to reach the correct diagnosis and because the patient's symptoms and signs may change as the condition causing

Box 1 Causes of abdominal pain in relation to the site of symptoms (see Fig. 1)

Epigastrium

- Stomach – dyspepsia, gastritis (alcohol/non-steroidal anti-inflammatory drugs), gastro-oesophageal reflux, gastric volvulus, ulcer, carcinoma
- Small bowel – duodenal ulcer
- Oesophagus – rupture (Boerhaave's syndrome), tear (Mallory–Weiss)
- Gallbladder – cholelithiasis, colic
- Pancreatitis – alcohol, gallbladder disease, bulimia
- Giardiasis – known in North America as beaver fever
- Vascular – visceral ischaemia, aortic aneurysm, splenic artery aneurysm
- Abdominal wall – epigastric hernia

Referred pain to the epigastrium includes:
- Myocardial ischaemia
- Inferior myocardial infarction
- Pericarditis
- Pneumonia – basal

Central/umbilical

- Bowel – irritable bowel syndrome (IBS), appendicitis, obstruction, Crohn's disease
- Pancreatitis
- Vascular – mesenteric artery thrombosis, aortic aneurysm
- Abdominal wall – umbilical hernia

Left upper quadrant/hypochondrium

- Stomach – gastritis, ulcer, carcinoma
- Pancreas – pancreatitis, carcinoma
- Large bowel – diverticulitis, perforation
- Spleen – leukaemia, lymphoma, infarct, rupture, malaria, infectious mononucleosis, kala azar
- Kidney – pyelonephritis, hydronephrosis, calculi
- Viral – herpes zoster

Referred left upper quadrant includes:
- Lung – left lower lobe pneumonia, pulmonary embolus
- Cardiac – ischaemia or infarction

Right upper quadrant/hypochondrium

- Gallbladder – biliary colic, cholecystitis, carcinoma
- Liver – right heart failure, hepatic vein obstruction, malignancy, abscess, Fitz-Hugh–Curtis syndrome, HELLP (haemolysis, elevated liver enzymes and low platelets) syndrome (in pregnancy)
- Small bowel – ulcer
- Large bowel – Crohn's disease, carcinoma
- Pancreas – pancreatitis, carcinoma
- Kidney – pyelonephritis, hydronephrosis, calculi
- Viral – herpes zoster

Referred right upper quadrant includes:
- Lung – right lower lobe pneumonia, pulmonary embolus
- Cardiac – ischaemia or infarction

Left lower quadrant/iliac fossa
- Bowel – constipation, gastroenteritis, colitis, diverticulitis, IBS, obstruction, carcinoma, carcinoma with perforation
- Reproductive – ectopic pregnancy, ovarian cyst accident, pelvic inflammatory disease (PID), mittelschmerz
- Abdominal wall – herniae: inguinal, femoral, umbilical, psoas abscess
- Urological – cystitis, ureteric colic
- Vascular – aneurysm
- Viral – herpes zoster

Right lower quadrant/iliac fossa
- Bowel – constipation, gastroenteritis, colitis, diverticulitis, IBS, appendicitis, obstruction, Crohn's, Meckel's diverticulum, carcinoma, carcinoma with perforation, caecal volvulus
- Reproductive – ectopic pregnancy, ovarian cyst accident, PID, mittelschmerz
- Abdominal wall – herniae: inguinal, femoral, umbilical, psoas abscess
- Urological – cystitis, ureteric colic
- Vascular – aneurysm
- Viral – herpes zoster

Medical causes of diffuse/generalised abdominal pain
- Pneumonia
- Diabetic ketoacidosis
- Henoch–Schönlein purpura
- Sickle cell crisis
- Acute intermittent porphyria
- Familial Mediterranean fever – paroxysmal peritonitis
- Lead poisoning
- Infections – malaria, typhoid fever, cholera, giardiasis
- Drugs – heroin withdrawal

pain develops. This should be done as carefully as possible as the examination itself can cause pain. Patients with severe pain will require analgesia, and nowadays there is no place for the view that analgesia masks clinical signs and should be withheld.

Physical examination should have commenced through observation during the history taking, noting any dyspnoea during conversation, and seeing whether the patient stays still or is unable to get comfortable in any position. Blood pressure, pulse rhythm and rate, respiratory rate and urinalysis should be recorded. The shocked patient needs resuscitation alongside the history-taking and examination.

Despite the complaint of abdominal pain, one should start with examination of the heart and lungs, otherwise pneumonia, pleurisy and atrial fibrillation leading to mesenteric artery thrombosis may be missed. The abdomen

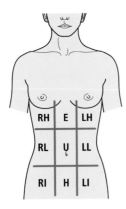

RH - Right Hypochondrum
E - Epigasrium
LH - Left Hypochondium
RL - Right Lumbar
U - Umbilical
LL - Left lumbar
RI - Right iliac fossa
H - Hypogastrium
LI - Left iliac fossa

Figure 1 Diagram of anatomical areas of the abdomen.

should be inspected in good light to avoid missing the erythematous streak of shingles before the characteristic vesicles developed. Absent abdominal wall excursion with breathing is suggestive of peritonitis.

Auscultation of the abdomen is often skimmed over by gynaecology trainees. It can give useful information. Active bowel sounds of normal pitch (compare with your own) are often suggestive of non-surgical disease, e.g. self-limiting gastroenteritis. High-frequency bowel sounds in runs or clusters suggest bowel obstruction. The totally silent abdomen is the most worrying and requires the urgent attention of a general surgical colleague.

Abdominal palpation should always commence distant to the most painful area, eventually covering all quadrants. The clinical signs of guarding and rebound tenderness are then sought. Patients find a demonstration of rebound tenderness extremely uncomfortable and it should not be serially repeated 'just to

make sure'. Recent studies have shown that severe abdominal pain induced by coughing has a comparable sensitivity and a higher specificity than a positive rebound tenderness test for the presence of peritonitis.

All patients should have the common sites for herniae examined. A bimanual examination of the pelvic organs should be followed by rectal examination to exclude blood or a local mass, if appropriate.

Investigations should be ordered logically aimed at narrowing down the differential diagnosis rather than ordering a massive 'fishing' list of expensive and very often unnecessary tests. The majority of blood investigations are not specific to a diagnosis and the results should be interpreted together with the clinical picture rather than separately.

Imaging for the acute abdomen may include an erect chest X-ray and supine abdominal X-rays looking for gas under the diaphragm or signs of bowel obstruction. In the USA, computerised tomography (CT) studies are more commonly used to assess possible cases of appendicitis; CT has a high sensitivity and specificity for this condition. CT is less reliable for pelvic organ diagnosis and ultrasound is still the modality of choice for assessing pain of possible gynaecological origin.

■ Abdominal pain in pregnancy

Assessment of the woman with abdominal pain during pregnancy requires the clinician to ask whether the pain is pregnancy related or not. In the latter case, specialist help may need to be requested, as even the diagnosis of appendicitis (Fig. 2) can be very difficult in pregnancy.

Essentially the causes can be divided into:

■ those due to pregnancy;
■ those related to the reproductive organs;
■ other causes listed in Box 1.

These topics may be dealt with elsewhere in the book in the relevant chapters.

In early pregnancy, miscarriage, ectopic pregnancy and ovarian cyst accident may cause pain.

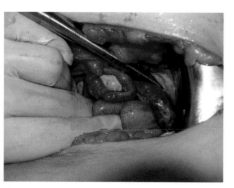

Figure 2 An acutely inflamed appendix before removal. The patient was 24 weeks pregnant. Note the position of the appendix and the relative size of the structure compared with the right uterine tube.

ABDOMINAL SWELLINGS IN PREGNANCY

Nanda Shetty and Dilip Visvanathan

Abdominal swellings may present at any stage of pregnancy. In early pregnancy the diagnosis would be similar to that of a non-pregnant female. However, as pregnancy advances, any abdominal mass may be displaced upwards and laterally, a fact that must be borne in mind when making a diagnosis. Furthermore, signs of peritonitis in abdominal swellings of an inflammatory nature can be markedly altered, resulting in a diagnosis being easily missed with potential serious consequences.

Abdominal swellings may be classified according to the anatomical layer of the abdomen (Box 1). This comprises the anterior abdominal wall, the peritoneal cavity and the retroperitoneal space.

Hyperemesis gravidarum may cause abdominal muscular pain secondary to persistent vomiting. Heartburn may be particularly severe in hyperemesis, to a degree that peptic ulceration is suspected. Later in pregnancy (second trimester), gestational trophoblastic disease may present as lower abdominal pain owing to rapid uterine distension, hyperemesis and large theca lutein cysts. Later still (late second, and third trimesters), sudden-onset polyhydramnios may cause pain in the central and upper abdomen through uterine distension, sometimes with dyspnoea.

Premature rupture of fetal membranes with ascending infection causes increasing tenderness over the uterus that may be initially localised but usually ends with generalised signs. Placental abruption causes a severe pain of sudden onset. The uterus is tender and the fundal height may increase in size with concealed bleeding; as the process continues, the uterus becomes hard and generally tender.

Other causes related to the reproductive organs in pregnancy include:

- uterus – fibroid degeneration, uterine scar dehiscence, torsion of uterus;
- vascular – spontaneous rupture of the uterine artery or infundibulopelvic vessels (rare).

> **Box 1** The layers of the abdominal wall that may give rise to abdominal wall swellings
>
> - Skin and appendages
> - Subcutaneous tissue
> - Herniation of intra-abdominal contents

■ Abdominal swellings arising from the anterior abdominal wall

Lumps can arise from the skin and its appendages. Skin swellings are diagnosed by the fact that they do not move independently of the overlying skin. A punctum may be visible in sebaceous cysts, which, if they become infected, may be tender and erythematous. Other skin lesions that may have surface elevation are malignant melanomas. While these are relatively rare, they are important as they cause the highest death rates from all skin cancers. Diagnostic confusion may occur as pigmented naevi may change during pregnancy owing to an increase in junctional activity. It is important to be aware of the ABCDE criteria (Table 1) for

Table 1 The ABCDE criteria for the early detection of melanomas

Asymmetry	Half the lesion does not match the other half
Border	The edges are ragged, notched or blurred
Colour	Pigmentation is not uniform and may display shades of tan, brown or black; white, reddish or blue discoloration is of particular concern
Diameter	A diameter greater than 6 mm is characteristic, although some melanomas may have smaller diameters; any growth in a naevus warrants an evaluation
Evolving	Changes in the lesion over time are characteristic

a changing mole, which may help in the early diagnosis of melanomas, particularly the superficial spreading type.[1,2] It is also important to remember that, with amelanotic melanomas, this may not apply but any change from other lesions or within the lesion should be promptly investigated.

The commonest subcutaneous swelling is a lipoma, which is usually a soft lobulated lump with a soft edge giving rise to the 'slipping sign'. The overlying skin can be made to move independently of a lipoma and asking the woman to tense her abdominal muscles will make the lump more prominent.

Swellings can also be due to herniation of abdominal contents through areas of potential weakness of the abdominal wall – the commonest being the umbilicus. True umbilical hernias are rare in comparison to paraumbilical herniae. Like all herniae, these masses have an expansile cough impulse and are usually reducible on lying down. As the neck of these paraumbilical herniae is usually wide, complications like irreducibility and strangulation are relatively uncommon. Herniation can also occur through previous incisions, including those made for Caesarean sections, and usually occur at the lateral edge of the Pfannensteil scar. A condition that occurs especially with repeated pregnancy is divarication of the recti. This is a defect of the median raphe, which is palpable below the level of the umbilicus.

■ Abdominal swellings arising from the abdominal cavity

Generalised abdominal distension

Swellings arising from the peritoneal cavity may cause generalised or localised abdominal swelling. The five Fs – Fluid, Faeces, Fetus, Flatus, Fat plus Large Fibroids or ovarian cysts – should be considered when there is generalised abdominal distension. In a woman who is in the later stages of pregnancy, these conditions may be suspected when the abdominal enlargement is greater than would be expected for the gestational age. If the symphysiofundal height is greater than that expected for the gestational age, then this may be due to uterine fibroids that are making the uterus larger, excess amniotic fluid, a large baby or the upward displacement of a gravid uterus by a ovarian cyst. An appropriate symphysiofundal height would be found if the generalised abdominal distension is secondary to faeces or flatus, where a history of constipation with vomiting may be elicited. Clinical examination may reveal visible peristalsis. In all these conditions, the flanks are not distended. If the flanks are distended and there is shifting dullness on percussion when turning from the prone to the lateral position, then ascites should be considered.

The advances in ultrasound allow for accurate fibroid mapping in the gravid uterus. Cervical fibroids are particularly important, as they may affect the mode of delivery. Subserous pedunculated fibroids are prone to torsion in the second trimester of pregnancy and in the puerperium. Most intramural fibroids do not change in size in pregnancy. Fibroids are, however, prone to undergo red degeneration (where the fibroid outgrows the blood supply and haemorrhagic necrosis occurs) at any time during the pregnancy or in the puerperium.

Ovarian cysts that cause generalised abdominal distension are usually mucinous cystadenomas. Ultrasound features include the presence of septae making the cyst multiloculated. If detected early in pregnancy, ovarian cystectomy may be performed laparoscopically ideally early in the second trimester of pregnancy.

Localised abdominal swellings

Localised abdominal swellings are best classified by the location in which they would usually present (see Fig. 1 in Abdominal pain). Masses that arise from the pelvis have been considered in Pelvic swellings and will not be dealt with here.

■ Mass in the right hypochondrium

The possible causes of a mass in the right hypochondrium are shown in Box 2.

Box 2 The anatomical origins of masses in the right hypochondrium

- Normal variant – Riedel's lobe
- Enlargement of the liver
- Enlargement of the gallbladder

Riedel's lobe is a normal variant and is an extension of the right lobe of the liver towards the anterior axillary line. Liver masses descend during inspiration, do not have a palpable upper limit and are dull to percussion up to the eighth rib in the anterior axillary line. Enlargement of the liver may be generalised or localised. Generalised enlargement may be due to infections, cirrhosis, chronic active hepatitis and myeloproliferative disorders. If the surface of the liver is irregular, polycystic disease and carcinoma must be excluded. Liver enlargement may be accompanied by jaundice in infective hepatitis, biliary tract obstruction secondary to carcinoma or gallstones, primary or secondary malignancy of the liver and cirrhosis.

Gallbladder enlargements present as globular swellings below the tip of the ninth rib. The upper border cannot be felt and the mass is mobile and moves downwards with inspiration.

The gallbladder may be enlarged with the accumulation of bile, mucus or pus. This occurs owing to either an obstruction of the cystic duct or the common bile duct. The common causes are calculi and carcinoma of the head of the pancreas. Courvoisier's law states that, if the gallbladder is palpable in a patient who is jaundiced, the cause of the obstruction is unlikely to be a calculus. This is based on the assumption that chronic inflammation secondary to calculi causes fibrosis of the gallbladder, thereby making it difficult to distend and present as an abdominal swelling. In acute cholecystitis, pressure at the tip of the ninth rib causes the patient to catch her breath at the end of inspiration owing to an inflamed gallbladder impinging on it (Murphy's sign).

■ Mass in the epigastrium

The possible causes of a mass in the epigastrium are given in Box 3.

Box 3 The anatomical origins of masses in the epigastrium

- Enlargement of the left lobe of the liver
- Enlargement of the stomach
- Enlargement of the pancreas

Localised enlargements of the left lobe of the liver can present with a mass in the epigastrium. Epigastric pain may be the presentation in a woman with severe pre-eclampsia and is due to tension on the liver capsule. This can rupture rarely with fatal consequences. Carcinoma of the stomach rarely presents in pregnancy and it is highly unlikely that a mass can be felt. This mass is usually hard and irregular, being pre-dated by symptoms of anorexia and weight loss. Diagnosis is made usually before a mass is palpable.

A pancreatic pseudocyst can be palpated as a mass in the epigastrium. It may occur as a consequence of acute pancreatitis. Acute pancreatitis occurs in 1 in 3333 pregnancies and is most commonly secondary to gallstone disease and hypertriglyceridaemia, which is made worse by pregnancy. There is a collection of fluid around the pancreas or in the lesser sac. Pancreatic pseudocysts are usually very difficult to feel as the stomach is anterior to it, thereby making it difficult to delineate and resonant to percussion. However, there is slight movement of the mass with respiration.

■ Masses in the left hypochondrium

The structures that can enlarge to give rise to a mass in the left hypochondrium are shown in Box 4.

Box 4 The anatomical origins of masses in the left hypochondrium

- Enlargement of the spleen
- Extension of masses from the epigastrium (stomach and pancreas)

The spleen has to enlarge considerably to become palpable below the left costal margin. Once it enlarges, it grows toward the umbilicus. Small enlargements may be felt by tilting the patient towards the examiner, lifting the lower ribs forwards and asking the patient to breathe deeply. The edge of the spleen may then be palpated at the end of inspiration. Depending on the cause of splenic enlargement, the edge may be soft or firm, and a splenic notch may be palpable.

Splenomegaly occurs in the following situations.

1 *Infection* – splenomegaly in pregnant women is common in areas that are endemic for malaria. There is an increase in size in the first trimester owing to an increase in parasitaemia. The splenomegaly can be massive in chronic malaria and, therefore, prone to rupture by blunt trauma to the upper abdomen or lower chest. Other infective causes include Epstein–Barr virus infection, leptospirosis and typhoid fever.
2 *Congestion*, usually secondary to portal vein hypertension and splenic vein thrombosis.

3 *Haemolysis*, which is usually seen in hereditary spherocytosis.
4 *Myeloproliferation* can be present both in myeloid and lymphatic leukaemia, polycythaemia rubra vera and myelosclerosis.
5 *Infiltration* – sarcoidosis and other neoplasms.

Patients with splenomegaly may also have co-existing hepatomegaly.

Hepatosplenomegaly may be due to primary liver disease or haematological disease. Ascites, jaundice, caput medusae and bilirubin in the urine are suggestive of primary liver disease, while generalised lymphadenopathy and a splenic rub are suggestive of haematological disease. Investigations that help with the differential diagnosis include a full blood count, a blood picture and thick and thin blood film for malarial parasites, and tissue biopsy of lymph nodes or the liver.

■ Masses in the right and left lumbar regions

The anatomical origins of masses in the loin are shown in Box 5.

Box 5 The anatomical origins of masses in the loin

- Enlargement of the kidney
- Extension of masses from the right hypochondrium

The characteristics of an enlarged kidney are that it is present in the loin, may be palpated bimanually, moves with respiration and is ballotable. It is not dull to percussion because of the overlying bowel.

In normal pregnancy there is dilatation of the renal pelvis and the ureter.

Hydronephrosis is thought to be due to the endocrinological changes of pregnancy and secondarily to pressure effects of pregnancy. Owing to the dextrorotation of the uterus in pregnancy, it is more common for hydronephrosis to occur in the right kidney. Women usually present with pain in the loin. In the majority of cases, however, the kidneys are not palpable, the hydronephrosis being diagnosed by ultrasonography.

Palpable kidneys in pregnancy are rare and may be due to gross hydronephrosis, large renal cysts and malignancy (hypernephroma).

■ Masses in the umbilical region

These masses may originate from the organs as shown in Box 6.

> **Box 6** The anatomical origins of masses in the umbilical region
>
> ■ Aortic enlargement
> ■ Mesenteric cyst
> ■ Moderate splenomegaly

Abdominal aortic aneurysms are typically located in the umbilical region. They have expansile pulsations and, if large, may be visible on inspection, especially in the thin patient. The upper limit of most abdominal aortic aneurysms is felt as they commonly arise below the level of the renal arteries.

Abdominal aortic aneurysms are more common in males and in patients over the age of 60. They are, therefore, extremely rare in pregnant women. The more common aneurysms that have been reported during pregnancy are thoracic aneurysms in women with Marfan's syndrome.

Mesenteric cysts are usually located in the centre of the abdomen. They are tensely cystic, may be fluctuant and have a fluid thrill. They are dull to percussion and, although freely mobile at right angles to the root of the mesentery, cannot move along the line of the mesentery. Mesenteric cysts may occur in pregnancy and are usually an incidental finding in early pregnancy.

■ Mass in the right iliac fossa

The anatomical origins of masses in the right iliac fossa are shown in Box 7.

> **Box 7** The anatomical origins of masses in the right iliac fossa
>
> ■ Distension of the caecum
> ■ Distension and enlargement of the terminal ileum
> ■ Distension of the appendix
> ■ Enlargement of ileocaecal lymph nodes
> ■ Enlargement of the iliac lymph nodes
> ■ Collection of fluid under the psoas fascia
> ■ Focal enlargement of the iliac bones

Appendicular mass

Acute appendicitis usually presents with central abdominal pain that later localises to the right iliac fossa. Nausea and vomiting is usually common. Tenderness may be elicited in the right iliac fossa typically being maximal at McBurney's point (see Fig. 1 in Abdominal pain), with signs of peritonism (guarding and rebound – see Abdominal pain).

In advancing pregnancy, owing to upward displacement of the appendix, the localising symptoms and signs are easily missed, and the signs of peritoneal irritation are often masked. An appendicular mass may, therefore, form and be found in the right lumbar region, or may even extend to the right hypochondrium. These masses are usually difficult to delineate, tender, dull to percussion and may be fixed in their posterior limit. If there is no resolution, an appendicular abscess may result, the systemic features of which include pain, swinging fever and tachycardia. The appendicular abscess has the same characteristics of the appendicular mass but is extremely tender, although the signs of peritonism may not be marked and white cell counts, although elevated, may be in the normal range for pregnancy. It is, therefore, important to bear this diagnosis in mind as the fetal loss increases from less than 2 per cent if the appendix is unruptured to almost 30 per cent if it ruptures.[3]

Inflammatory bowel disease

Inflammatory bowel disease (IBD) may present as a mass in the right iliac fossa or as gross abdominal distension. The terminal ileum swells and can be palpated as a sausage-shaped mass in the right iliac fossa. It often lies in a transverse position. Symptoms include fever, vomiting, abdominal pain, diarrhoea, rectal bleeding and/or mucous discharge and tenesmus. Complications, such as abscess, toxic megacolon and bowel obstruction, can be missed owing to the altered signs in pregnancy and also if the patient is receiving steroid therapy. Perforation of the bowel leads to a high fetal and maternal mortality rate if not diagnosed and treated early. Box 8 gives the criteria for diagnosis by Jalan et al.[4] for the diagnosis of toxic dilatation of the colon from a study of 55 cases.

Box 8 The criteria for the diagnosis of toxic megacolon

- One of the following:
  - dehydration
  - electrolyte imbalance
  - altered mental state
  - hypotension
- Three of the following:
  - fever
  - tachycardia (greater than 120 beats/min)
  - increased white cell count
  - anaemia
- X-ray findings of transverse colon diameter greater than 6 cm

---

Enlarged ileocaecal lymph nodes

Enlarged ileocaecal lymph nodes may present as a mass in the right iliac fossa. Typically they are firm, immobile and the margins are difficult to delineate. Palpation of other lymph nodes is important, as it may be part of a generalised lympadenopathy. Tuberculosis may present in this way and is becoming more common in pregnancy.[5]

Psoas abscess

A psoas abscess may be felt as a soft compressible mass in the right iliac fossa. This is due to tracking down of fluid below the psoas sheath. The lower limit of the mass would, therefore, be below the level of the inguinal ligament. Tuberculosis of the dorsal spine is one of the causes of a psoas abscess. Constitutional features like loss of appetite, loss of weight, night sweats and backache are usually present. It may lead to restriction of hip movements.

■ Mass in the suprapubic region

Masses in the suprapubic region usually arise from the pelvis. This has been discussed in Pelvic swellings.

■ Mass in the left iliac fossa

The commonest mass that presents in the left iliac fossa is the inflammatory mass of diverticulitis. It is uncommon in pregnancy. A longstanding history of altered bowel habit (mainly constipation) is usually present. Pain with nausea and vomiting is a presenting feature. Clinical examination reveals a mass, which is very tender, with indistinct margins and localised peritonitis. The mass may be palpable on bimanual examination of the pelvis in the early stages of pregnancy.

■ Abdominal swellings arising from the retroperitoneal space

Retroperitoneal tumours are ones in which there is no definite organ of origin. Therefore, even though the pancreas, kidney and adrenal gland are anatomically retroperitoneal, they are not considered here.

Retroperitoneal tumours in pregnancy are rare and restricted to case reports in the literature. Malignant tumours are more common than benign ones. The commonest malignant tumour is a liposarcoma with a lymphangioma being the commonest benign tumour. They rarely present in pregnancy as an abdominal mass and are usually discovered at Caesarean section. They can obstruct labour. They are soft to firm in consistency, immobile and may have transmitted pulsations. Diagnosis is confirmed by biopsy.

References

1. Abbasi NR, Shaw HM, Rigel DS, *et al.* Early diagnosis of cutaneous melanoma: revisiting the ABCD criteria. *JAMA* 2004; **292**: 2771–6.
2. Rigel DS, Friedman RJ, Kopf AW, Polsky D. ABCDE – an evolving concept in the early detection of melanoma. *Arch Dermatol* 2005; **141**: 1032–4.
3. Mazze RI, Kallen B. Appendectomy during pregnancy: a Swedish registry study of 778 cases. *Obstet Gynecol* 1991; **77**: 835–40.
4. Jalan KN, Sircus W, Card WI, *et al.* An experience of ulcerative colitis. I. Toxic dilation in 55 cases. *Gastroenterology* 1969; **57**: 68–82.
5. Llewelyn M, Cropley I, Wilkinson RJ, Davidson RN. Tuberculosis diagnosed during pregnancy: a prospective study from London. *Thorax* 2000; **55**: 129–32.

AMNIOTIC FLUID ABNORMALITIES

Peter Muller

Amniotic fluid volumes can be readily assessed via ultrasound, and abnormalities in amniotic fluid volumes may act as clues to various fetal abnormalities and antenatal complications. Abnormal amniotic fluid volume (AFV) has long been associated with poor perinatal outcome[1,2] and AFV measurement is vital in any antenatal fetal assessment. Amniotic fluid volumes are characterised as the following:

- normal;
- oligohydramnios (diminished amniotic fluid);
- polyhydramnios or 'hydramnios' (excessive amniotic fluid).

Measurement of amniotic fluid volume

Measurement of amniotic fluid via ultrasound may be of both subjective and objective means. The most common objective approaches are by measuring AFV via the amniotic fluid index (AFI) and the deepest vertical pocket. The AFI is performed by measuring the sum of the maximum vertical amniotic pocket (transducer held perpendicular to the maternal abdomen) in each quadrant of the abdomen (Figs 1a and b).[3] A nomogram based on gestational age has also been introduced.[4] Common nomenclature for amniotic fluid volume using AFI includes:

- low = less than 5 cm (oligohydramnios);
- borderline-low = 5–9 cm;
- normal = 10–20 cm;
- borderline-high = 20–24 cm;
- high = greater than 24 cm (polyhydramnios).

The deepest vertical pocket is also used, where normal AFV is considered, when this pocket measures >2 cm and <8 cm. The AFI, secondary to the small gravid uterus, may have limited use in measuring AFV in pregnancies prior to 24 weeks' gestation.[5] Normal sonographic reference intervals for a

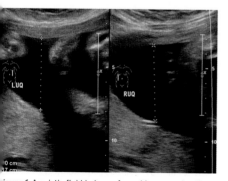
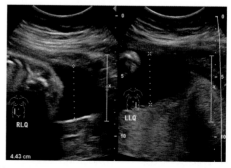

Figure 1 Amniotic fluid index performed by measuring the sum of the maximum vertical amniotic pocket in each quadrant of the abdomen: (a) upper two quadrants; (b) lower two quadrants.

single amniotic pocket have been developed for gestational ages 11–24 weeks.[6] In general, these two semi-quantitative measurements of AFV, the AFI and single deepest pocket, are equally accepted. Although there are limitations in these techniques to estimate actual AFV,[7] these ultrasound measurements have the advantage of relaying a semi-quantitative assessment of AFV to the referring clinician and comparison for follow-up ultrasound studies. It appears that operator experience has little effect on the accuracy of ultrasound estimates of AFV.[8] It is important to realise, however, that these measurements seem to be no more accurate in diagnosing abnormal AFV than subjective assessments by experienced sonographers.[9]

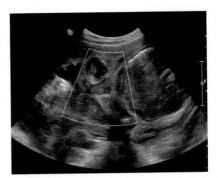

Figure 2 Severe oligohydramnios in a growth-restricted fetus. Notice that the umbilical cord fills the remaining amniotic fluid space.

Normal amniotic fluid volume

Each individual demonstrates a slight variation in AFV during the pregnancy, where the AFV increases early in pregnancy, peaks at 28–32 weeks, and starts to diminish from 33 weeks onwards. Despite this individual variation, there appears to be steady regulation of the volume between 0.5 and 2 L. It is fair to say that this regulation occurs with an adjustment of fetal production and removal of amniotic fluid during the pregnancy. Amniotic fluid transport to and from the amniotic cavity is mainly controlled by fetal renal excretion (production) and fetal swallowing (removal). The fetal respiratory tract, fetal membranes and placenta play a small part in the transport of amniotic fluid. Fetal urine production appears to begin at approximately 9 weeks' gestation, but it is not the primary source of amniotic fluid until between 14 and 18 weeks' gestation. The latter finding is important in understanding abnormalities of AFV in the early and mid second trimester. Amniotic fluid fulfils many roles in the development of the fetus, including protection from trauma, cord compression and infection (bacteriostatic properties), as well as facilitating fetal lung, musculoskeletal and gastrointestinal development.[10]

Oligohydramnios

Oligohydramnios, the finding of diminished amniotic fluid on ultrasound (Fig. 2), is relatively common. The diagnosis of oligohydramnios via ultrasound can be made subjectively by the inability

to locate obvious pools of amniotic fluid surrounding the fetus or objectively by either the AFI (<5 cm) or deepest single vertical pocket (<2 cm). Adverse pregnancy outcome is associated with the diagnosis of oligohydramnios,[11] but the severity of this outcome depends on the gestational age of the onset of this AFV abnormality. On the other hand, oligohydramnios as an isolated finding in the third trimester is commonly associated with a good outcome.[12,13] Since accurate ultrasound evaluation of AFV has its limitations,[14] one must be careful in not to misuse the diagnosis of reduced amniotic fluid with invasive pregnancy interventions such as early induction of labour. Despite this controversy, it is reasonable to evaluate ultrasound evidence of reduced amniotic fluid to ascertain whether it is truly an isolated finding.

Fetal anomalies/aneuploidy

Congenital abnormalities and fetal aneuploidy are commonly associated with oligohydramnios seen in the second trimester. The majority of fetal anomalies involve the genitourinary system, but skeletal, central nervous system and cardiovascular defects are also seen in association with oligohydramnios. It is important to remember that oligohydramnios secondary to renal anomalies may not be evident until 18 weeks' gestation, as the maternal contribution of amniotic fluid remains high until 14–18 weeks. Comprehensive fetal morphology ultrasound assessment is required particularly of the fetal kidneys and bladder. Renal agenesis, bladder outlet obstruction, multicystic dysplastic kidneys and infantile polycystic kidneys can usually be accurately diagnosed by transabdominal ultrasound. Renal agenesis can be confirmed with the inability to locate kidneys bilaterally and the absence of fluid in the fetal bladder. Further evaluation for renal agenesis includes the use of colour Doppler to locate the bilateral renal arteries and the appearance of 'lying down adrenal' glands. Multicystic dysplastic kidneys and infantile polycystic kidneys will demonstrate bilaterally enlarged hyperechoic or cystic kidneys. Bladder outlet obstruction, associated with posterior urethral valve syndrome, will demonstrate an enlarged bladder with a 'keyhole' appearance and significant renal pelvic dilation. Secondary to the severe oligohydramnios, definitive antenatal diagnosis of these fetal conditions via transabdominal ultrasound may at times be difficult.

Transvaginal ultrasound in the early second trimester may be helpful in delineating hard-to-visualise fetal anatomy. Amnioinfusion has been advocated as a way to improve the ultrasound resolution, but the advent of fetal magnetic resonance imaging (MRI) for the most part has offered a non-invasive modality to confirm the earlier ultrasound findings. Secondary to the severe oligohydramnios, fetal karyotype evaluation via amniocentesis can be difficult. However, placental biopsy is an option in these instances. Other than posterior urethral valve syndrome, where fetal interventions in selected cases may improve outcome, these conditions are considered lethal secondary to the pulmonary hypoplasia that develops in these fetuses.

Rupture of membranes

The diagnosis of rupture of membranes can readily be made based on clinical history and examination. Sterile speculum examination will be able to ascertain pooling of amniotic fluid, alkaline pH with Nitrizine and typical ferning of amniotic fluid. In those cases where the clinical history and examination are equivocal for rupture of membranes, other modalities are used to assist with the diagnosis. Amnioinfusion with indigo carmine/Ringer's solution (100–150 mL) with resultant colour staining of an inserted tampon can confirm a suspected case of preterm premature rupture of the membranes (PPROM).

Methylene blue should be avoided, secondary to its association with jejunoileal atresia.[15] Posterior fornix fetal fibronectin evaluation after 22 weeks' gestation, where its presence is uncommon in uncomplicated pregnancies, has been used as a non-invasive method for further suggesting PPROM in those cases where clinical history and examination are equivocal.[16] The earlier the PPROM, the more guarded the prognosis. PPROM with resultant severe oligohydramnios prior to 24 weeks' gestation runs the added risk of pulmonary hypoplasia, although not generally to the extent seen in bilateral fetal renal abnormalities. Amniotic leakage after amniocentesis in the second trimester, where resealing of the amnion leakage is common, has a reasonably good prognosis with over a 90 per cent survival.[17]

Fetal growth restriction

Uteroplacental insufficiency results in fetal redistribution of blood flow to vital organs such as the brain, heart and adrenal glands, and away form the kidneys, resulting in oligohydramnios. The patient's clinical history and examination may give clues to risk factors for fetal growth restriction (FGR) such as substance abuse, chronic hypertension, previous obstetric history and birth weights, and developing pre-eclampsia. Fetal biometry may demonstrate an estimated fetal weight below the 10th percentile. Asymmetric fetal biometric parameters (head circumference–abdominal circumference discordance) are commonly seen when FGR is seen in the late second and third trimester, while severe FGR in the second trimester may exhibit symmetric growth restriction.

Other findings on ultrasound may include early maturation of the placenta (i.e. early placental calcification). Maternal and fetal Doppler velocimetry may offer further clues. Abnormal uterine artery Doppler at 18–24 weeks may suggest abnormal placentation and has some predictive value in predicting adverse pregnancy outcome.[18] Umbilical artery Doppler will commonly demonstrate increased placental resistance seen in uteroplacental insufficiency. Early in the development of FGR, fetal middle cerebral artery Doppler will show 'brain sparing' consistent with fetal blood flow redistribution.[19] This is exhibited by increased diastolic flow velocity and a decreased pulsatility index. Although no single antenatal study can confirm FGR, a series of abnormal ultrasound evaluations in conjunction with clinical history allow one to make a calculated diagnosis and provide a reasonable management plan.

Perinatal morbidity and mortality are inversely proportional to the gestational age of diagnosis. In early-onset severe FGR, referring to a fetal medicine specialist for fetal surveillance should be considered.

Iatrogenic

Oligohydramnios can be secondary to numerous iatrogenic causes. These may include fetal procedures, such as chorionic villus sampling or amniocentesis, and various medications. A good clinical history will help to exclude these causes. Non-steroidal anti-inflammatory drugs and angiotensin-converting enzyme inhibitors both decrease renal perfusion and can result in oligohydramnios. Fortunately, discontinuing these medications, in a majority of cases, results in a reversible form of oligohydramnios.[20]

Postdates

The fall of amniotic fluid volume in the postdate pregnancy is a reflection of the uteroplacental insufficiency that generally occurs at these later gestations. Although monitoring amniotic fluid volume and induction of labour with evidence of oligohydramnios is commonly advocated, there is controversy concerning whether perinatal outcome is improved by such manoeuvres.[21,22]

■ Polyhydramnios

Polyhydramnios or 'hydramnios' is defined as an excessive amount of amniotic fluid. Polyhydramnios can be determined subjectively in the third trimester, if obvious pockets of amniotic fluid are present surrounding all sides of the fetal abdomen (Fig. 3). Polyhydramnios can be objectively determined by either the AFI (greater than 24 cm) or deepest vertical pocket (greater than 8 cm). Since the incidence of fetal abnormalities correlates with the severity of polyhydramnios, a deepest vertical pocket of

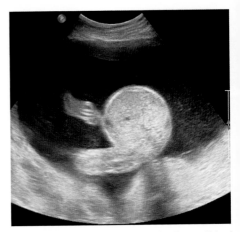

Figure 3 Polyhydramnios in a fetus with a large unilateral pleural effusion. The subsequent chest deviation inhibits normal swallowing, which produces the polyhydramnios.

12 cm and 16 cm has been used to define moderate and severe polyhydramnios respectively.[23] In general, these semi-quantitative measurements tend to underestimate the actual AFV.

Congenital abnormalities

Polyhydramnios with fetal anomalies is most likely related to an interruption of normal fetal swallowing. In general, polyhydramnios secondary to fetal anomalies does not occur prior to 25 weeks' gestation. Since a multitude of congenital abnormalities can be associated with excessive amniotic fluid, comprehensive morphology ultrasound assessment is the first line of evaluation for this condition. Sites of fetal abnormalities associated with polyhydramnios include:

■ gastrointestinal tract;
■ central nervous system;
■ respiratory and thoracic;
■ skeletal dysplasias;
■ myotonic dystrophy;
■ cardiovascular;
■ fetal and placental tumours.

Specific ultrasound findings that have been associated with polyhydramnios include:

■ stomach not seen;
■ dilated bowel loops;

- neck, chest or abdominal masses;
- diaphragmatic hernia;
- intracranial malformations;
- facial clefts;
- significantly shortened long bones with a small chest circumference;
- severe limb contractures or arthrogryposis,
- congenital heart disease;
- placental masses.

Offering karyotype evaluation with ultrasound-detected fetal anomalies or FGR is recommended, but aneuploidy is rare in isolated polyhydramnios.

Maternal diabetes

There is a clear association of polyhydramnios with macrosomia, although maternal diabetes is not always the precipitating factor. However, obtaining fetal biometry for evidence of accelerated abdominal circumference and fetal weight, often seen with poorly controlled diabetes, and testing for maternal diabetes is suggested.

Hydrops

Hydrops is defined as fluid present in two body cavities (pleural effusion, pericardial effusion, ascites or skin oedema) and is readily visible on ultrasound. Polyhydramnios accompanies approximately 30 per cent of fetuses with non-immune hydrops. Unfortunately, the aetiology of non-immune hydrops can be elusive in 20–40 per cent of cases.[24]

Twin–twin transfusion syndrome

Approximately 15 per cent of monochorionic/diamniotic twin pregnancies will develop twin–twin transfusion syndrome, thus proving the importance of early ascertainment of chorionicity of all multiple pregnancies. Twin–twin transfusion syndrome is demonstrated by amniotic fluid discordance between the recipient (deepest vertical pocket of >8 cm) and donor (deepest vertical pocket of <2 cm). Referral to a specialist experienced in the management of this condition is recommended.

Idiopathic

The amniotic fluid volume peaks in the early third trimester and this normal variant must not be confused with pathologic polyhydramnios. Commonly the AFV will be in the mild or borderline level, but will return to normal as the pregnancy progresses. However, moderate or severe polyhydramnios is rarely idiopathic, and thorough evaluation is warranted.[23]

Prognosis and management

The prognosis depends solely on the aetiology for the polyhydramnios. Preterm labour, preterm premature ruptures of the membranes and placental abruption have all been associated with moderate to severe polyhydramnios. Amnioreduction can be used to treat symptomatic polyhydramnios with an overall low risk of complications.[25] Oral indomethacin has been used to reduce fetal urine production and enhance uptake in the lungs. Although maternal side effects are small, common risks to the fetus include early constriction of the ductus arteriosus and even oligohydramnios. Because these complications are generally reversible and the risk of ductal constriction increases with gestational age, close fetal monitoring is mandatory and indomethacin is not recommended after 32 weeks' gestation. There is currently controversy in the literature on whether the antenatal use of indomethacin increases the neonatal risk of necrotising enterocolitis and intraventricular haemorrhage.

■ References

1. Chamberlain PF, Manning FA, Morrison I, Harman CR, Lange IR. Ultrasound evaluation of amniotic fluid volume. II. The relationship of increased amniotic fluid volume to perinatal outcome. *Am J Obstet Gynecol* 1984; **150:** 250–4.

2. Chamberlain PF, Manning FA, Morrison I, Harman CR, Lange IR. Ultrasound evaluation of amniotic fluid volume. I. The relationship of marginal and decreased amniotic fluid volumes to perinatal

outcome. *Am J Obstet Gynecol* 1984; **150:** 245–9.

3. Phelan JP, Ahn MO, Smith CV, Rutherford SE, Anderson E. Amniotic fluid index measurements during pregnancy. *J Reprod Med* 1987; **32:** 601–4.

4. Moore TR, Cayle JE. The amniotic fluid index in normal human pregnancy. *Am J Obstet Gynecol* 1990; **162:** 1168–73.

5. Magann EF, Whitworth NS, Klausen JH, Perry KG Jr, Martin JN Jr, Morrison JC. Accuracy of ultrasonography in evaluating amniotic fluid volume at less than 24 weeks' gestation. *J Ultrasound Med* 1995; **14:** 895–7.

6. Gramellini D, Chiaie D, Piantelli G, Sansebastiano L, Fieni S, Vadora E. Sonographic assessment of amniotic fluid volume between 11 and 24 weeks of gestation: construction of reference intervals related to gestational age. *Ultrasound Obstet Gynecol* 2001; **17:** 410–5.

7. Dildy GA III, Lira N, Moise KJ Jr, Riddle GD, Deter RL. Amniotic fluid volume assessment: comparison of ultrasonographic estimates versus direct measurements with a dye-dilution technique in human pregnancy. *Am J Obstet Gynecol* 1992; **167:** 986–94.

8. Magann EF, Perry KG Jr, Chauhan SP, Anfanger PJ, Whitworth NS, Morrison JC. The accuracy of ultrasound evaluation of amniotic fluid volume in singleton pregnancies: the effect of operator experience and ultrasound interpretative technique. *J Clin Ultrasound* 1997; **25:** 249–53.

9. Magann EF, Chauhan SP, Whitworth NS, Klausen JH, Saltzman AK, Morrison JC. Do multiple measurements employing different ultrasonic techniques improve the accuracy of amniotic fluid volume assessment? *Aust NZ J Obstet Gynaecol* 1998; **38:** 172–5.

10. *Diagnostic Imaging of Fetal Anomalies.* Baltimore: Lippincott Williams & Wilkins, 2003.

11. Chauhan SP, Sanderson M, Hendrix NW, Magann EF, Devoe LD. Perinatal outcome and amniotic fluid index in the antepartum and intrapartum periods: A meta-analysis. *Am J Obstet Gynecol* 1999; **181:** 1473–8.

12. Magann EF, Chauhan SP, Kinsella MJ, McNamara MF, Whitworth NS, Morrison JC. Antenatal testing among 1001 patients at high risk: the role of ultrasonographic estimate of amniotic fluid volume. *Am J Obstet Gynecol* 1999; **180:** 1330–6.

13. Zhang J, Troendle J, Meikle S, Klebanoff MA, Rayburn WF. Isolated oligohydramnios is not associated with adverse perinatal outcomes. *Br J Obstet Gynaecol* 2004; **111:** 220–5.

14. Magann EF, Chauhan SP, Barrilleaux PS, Whitworth NS, Martin JN. Amniotic fluid index and single deepest pocket: weak indicators of abnormal amniotic volumes. *Obstet Gynecol* 2000; **96:** 737–40.

15. Gluer S. Intestinal atresia following intraamniotic use of dyes. *Eur J Pediatr Surg* 1995; **5:** 240–2.

16. Trovo S, Brigato L, Plebani M, Brigato G, Grismondi GL. [Premature membrane rupture. Comparison of diagnostic tests]. *Minerva Ginecol* 1998; **50:** 519–22.

17. Borgida AF, Mills AA, Feldman DM, Rodis JF, Egan JF. Outcome of pregnancies complicated by ruptured membranes after genetic amniocentesis. *Am J Obstet Gynecol* 2000; **183:** 937–9.

18. Papageorghiou AT, Yu CK, Nicolaides KH. The role of uterine artery Doppler in predicting adverse pregnancy outcome. *Best Pract Res Clin Obstet Gynaecol* 2004; **18:** 383–96.

19. Baschat AA. Integrated fetal testing in growth restriction: combining multivessel Doppler and biophysical parameters. *Ultrasound Obstet Gynecol* 2003; **21:** 1–8.

20. Muller PR, James A. Pregnancy with prolonged fetal exposure to an angiotensin-converting enzyme inhibitor. *J Perinatol* 2002; **22:** 582–4.
21. Alfirevic Z, Luckas M, Walkinshaw SA, McFarlane M, Curran R. A randomised comparison between amniotic fluid index and maximum pool depth in the monitoring of post-term pregnancy. *Br J Obstet Gynaecol* 1997; **104:** 207–11.
22. Magann EF, Chauhan SP, Doherty DA, Barrilleaux PS, Martin JN Jr, Morrison JC. Predictability of intrapartum and neonatal outcomes with the amniotic fluid volume distribution: a reassessment using the amniotic fluid index, single deepest pocket, and a dye-determined amniotic fluid volume. *Am J Obstet Gynecol* 2003; **188:** 1523–7.
23. Hill LM, Breckle R, Thomas ML, Fries JK. Polyhydramnios: ultrasonically detected prevalence and neonatal outcome. *Obstet Gynecol* 1987; **69:** 21–5.
24. McCoy MC, Katz VL, Gould N, Kuller JA. Non-immune hydrops after 20 weeks' gestation: review of 10 years' experience with suggestions for management. *Obstet Gynecol* 1995; **85:** 578–82.
25. Leung WC, Jouannic JM, Hyett J, Rodeck C, Jauniaux E. Procedure-related complications of rapid amniodrainage in the treatment of polyhydramnios. *Ultrasound Obstet Gynecol* 2004; **23:** 154–8.

ANAEMIA IN PREGNANCY

Jai B Sharma

Anaemia is the commonest medical disorder during pregnancy. The World Health Organization (WHO) definition for diagnosis of anaemia in pregnancy is a haemoglobin (Hb) concentration of $<11\,g/dL$ ($7.45\,mmol/L$) and a haematocrit of <0.33. The overall prevalence of anaemia varies in different countries, affecting approximately 18 per cent of pregnant women in industrialised countries but about 56 per cent (35–75 per cent) of pregnant women in developing countries. It is responsible for significant maternal and perinatal mortality and morbidity throughout the world, but more so in developing nations.

The classification of anaemia is given in Box 1. Hereditary anaemias are less common and are seen more often in particular geographical areas. Thus thalassaemias are seen more frequently in Asia, while sickle cell haemoglobinopathies are common in Africa in areas where *falciparum* malaria is prevalent.

Box 1 Types of anaemia during pregnancy

I Hereditary causes
- Thalassaemias
- Sickle cell haemoglobinopathies
- Other haemoglobinopathies
- Hereditary haemolytic anaemias

II Acquired causes
1 Nutritional
   - Iron-deficiency anaemia (microcytic hypochromic anaemia)
   - Folate-deficiency anaemia (megaloblastic anaemia)
   - Cyanocobalamin-deficiency anaemia (megaloblastic anaemia)
2 Anaemia due to marrow failure (aplastic or hypoplastic anaemia)
3 Anaemia due to inflammation, chronic disease or malignancy
4 Anaemia due to acute blood loss
5 Acquired haemolytic anaemias

■ Haemoglobinopathies

Structure of normal haemoglobin

Normal Hb is composed of four subunits, with a single haem group (which binds to and later releases oxygen) and four species-specific globin chains. The haem group is an iron molecule with four pyrrole rings attached to it. Two pairs of globin chains (two alpha and two beta) are attached to the pyrrole rings to make up normal Hb. The integrity of the haem moiety and the amino-acid sequence of the globin chains determine the structure of the globin chains and the interaction between the four subunits of the Hb.

Thalassaemias

Thalassaemias are characterised by impaired production of one or more of the globin chains and are called alpha thalassaemias (if both alpha chains are impaired), alpha thalassaemia trait (if one chain is defective), beta thalassaemia (if both beta chains are impaired) and beta thalassaemia trait (if one beta chain is impaired). Children with beta thalassaemia usually die before reaching reproductive age. However, with repeated blood transfusions and chelation therapy, pregnancies have been reported. More important and common, however, is thalassaemia minor (trait), which is an important differential diagnosis of iron-deficiency anaemia; it can be differentiated by blood indices and HbF and HbA$_2$ levels (Table 1). If the mother has the thalassaemia trait, the father should be tested for the trait. If both are positive for the trait, then prenatal diagnosis of the fetus is indicated as there is a 1:4 chance of the fetus having thalassaemia major. Termination of the pregnancy may be offered in this situation.

Sickle cell haemoglobinopathies

Sickle Hb results from a single beta-chain substitution of glutamic acid by valine at codon 6 of the beta globin chain. It may have serious implications in pregnancy and women may manifest with sickle cell crises, an acute emergency with infarction in various organs due to intense sequestration of sickled erythrocytes causing severe pains, especially in the bones. It can happen in pregnancy, during labour or the puerperium, especially in oxygen-deficient conditions, e.g. general anaesthesia. Treatment is by intravenous hydration, oxygen administration

Table 1 Differential diagnosis of iron-deficiency anaemia (IDA) and thalassaemia

Characteristics	Normal range	IDA	Thalassaemia
Mean corpuscular volume (MCV, fL)	75–96	Reduced	Very reduced
Mean corpuscular Hb (MCH, pg)	27–33	Reduced	Very reduced
Mean corpuscular Hb concentration (MCHC, g/dL)	32–35	Reduced	Normal
Fetal Hb (HbF)	<2%	Normal	Raised
HbA2	2–3%	Normal	Raised
Red cell width		High	Normal

and red-cell transfusions. Prenatal diagnosis is indicated in sickle-cell trait women with sickle-cell trait husbands, with advice of termination of an affected pregnancy.

■ Nutritional anaemias

The sources of various nutrients required for erythropoiesis are given in Table 2.

Iron-deficiency anaemia (IDA)

This is the commonest type of anaemia and is classically described as a microcytic hypochromic anaemia. It is much more common in developing countries owing to poor dietary habits (intake of low-bioavailability diet, poor in iron and proteins, and with an excess of inhibitors of iron absorption such as phytates), defective iron absorption owing to intestinal infestations with hookworm and other worms. Schistosomiasis, chronic malaria, frequent pregnancies at short intervals, menorrhagia and blood loss from haemorrhoids are other causes of IDA. Multiple pregnancy is also an important cause of anaemia owing to increased iron and folic acid requirements.

Clinical features of IDA in pregnancy

The various symptoms and signs that can occur in anaemia during pregnancy are shown in Box 2. However, it must be noted that these symptoms or signs may be absent, especially in mild to moderate anaemia.

Table 2 Sources of various nutrients required for erythropoiesis

Nutrients	Sources
Iron	Haem iron: animal blood, flesh, viscera (liver, kidney), red meat, poultry and fish (including mussels) Non-haem iron: green leafy vegetables, cereals, seeds, vegetables (peas, baked beans), eggs, roots and tubers
Folic acid	Green vegetables (spinach and broccoli), fruits, liver, kidney
Cyanocobalamin	Meat, fish, eggs, milk
Ascorbic acid	Citrus fruits like orange, lemon, amla (Indian gooseberry)
Other B vitamins	Green leafy vegetables and fruits

Box 2 Clinical features of anaemia during pregnancy

Symptoms	Signs
Weakness	Pallor
Lassitude/tiredness/exhaustion	Glossitis
Indigestion	Stomatitis
Loss of appetite	Oedema
Palpitations	Hypoproteinemia
Dyspnoea (breathlessness)	Soft systolic murmur in mitral area owing to
Giddiness/dizziness	hyperdynamic circulation
Swelling (peripheral)	Fine crepitations at bases of lungs owing to congestion
Generalised anasarca (generalised fluid collection	(severe cases)
in peritoneal and thoracic cavity)	
Congestive cardiac failure (in severe cases)	

Effects of anaemia on pregnancy

These are shown in Box 3. There may be no maternal or fetal effects, especially in mild or moderate anaemia.

Diagnosis of IDA in pregnancy

Although Hb estimation is the most practical method of diagnosis, being cost effective and easy to perform, blood indices and other diagnostic modalities are required for diagnosis as shown in Table 3. Not all investigations are required for all cases. Hb, blood indices and peripheral blood film may be adequate in majority of cases of IDA. In developing countries, stool examination for ova and cysts should be undertaken consecutively for 3 days in all cases as well as peripheral blood film for malaria parasite in endemic areas. Other specific tests may be performed in the presence of other clinical signs. Bone marrow examination is not usually required except in cases of kala-azar or suspected aplastic anaemia.

Treatment of IDA in pregnancy

In an average pregnancy, the requirements are:

- basal iron, 280 mg;
- expansion of red cell mass, 570 mg;
- fetal transfer, 200–350 mg;
- placental, 50–150 mg;
- blood loss at delivery, 100–250 mg.

After deducting iron conserved by amenorrhoea (240–480 mg), an additional 500–600 mg of iron is required in pregnancy. It can be fulfilled by 4–6 mg/day of absorbed iron. The

Box 3 Effects of anaemia on pregnancy

Maternal effects	Fetal effects
Weakness	Preterm babies
Lack of energy	Small for gestation babies
Fatigue	Increased perinatal mortality
Poor work performance	Low iron stores in newborns
Palpitations	Iron-deficiency anaemia
Tachycardia	Cognitive and affective dysfunction in the infant
Breathlessness	Increased incidence of diabetes and cardiac
Increased cardiac output	disease in later life
Cardiac decompensation	
Cardiac failure	
Increased incidence of preterm labour	
Pre-eclampsia	
Sepsis	

Table 3 Diagnosis of iron-deficiency anaemia (IDA) in pregnancy

Characteristic	Calculation	Normal range	IDA
Haemoglobin (Hb, g/dL)	Sahli's method	11–15	<11
Mean corpuscular volume (fL)	PCV/RBC	75–96	<75
Mean corpuscular Hb (pg)	Hb/RBC	27–33	<27
Mean corpuscular Hb concentration (g/dL)	Hb/PCV	32–35	<32
Peripheral blood film		Normocytic normochromic picture	Microcytic hypochromic picture
Serum iron (μg/dL)		60–120	<60
Total iron binding capacity (TIBC, μg/dL)		300–400	>350
Transferrin saturation			<15%
Serum ferritin (mcg/dl)		13–27	<12
Free erythrocyte protoporphyrin (FEP, μg/dL)		<35	>50
Serum transferrin receptor			Increased

PCV, packed cell volume; RBC, red blood cells.

requirements are 4 mg/day (2.5 mg/day in early pregnancy, 5.5 mg/day for weeks 20–32 and 6–8 mg/day from week 32 onwards).

Prophylaxis Prevention of iron deficiency is usually possible with a good balanced diet in the absence of ongoing blood loss. Health education by the midwife or obstetrician regarding diet is important. Pregnant women should be encouraged to eat iron-rich foods like green and leafy vegetables, spinach, mustard, turnip green, cereals and sprouted pulses. They should avoid tea or coffee, which contain tannins – known inhibitors of iron absorption.

Considerable research has been published on the role of routine iron supplementation in pregnancy, including a Cochrane review. The meta-analysis of trials has concluded that there is a clear evidence of improvement in haematological indices in women receiving iron supplements during pregnancy, but no conclusions could be drawn regarding either harmful or beneficial effects for the mother or the baby. The reviewers felt that there was no evidence to advise against a policy of routine iron supplementation in pregnancy and that such a policy should be implemented in high prevalence areas. However, there is no doubt that routine iron supplementation should be given to all pregnant ladies in non-industrialised countries. WHO has recommended universal oral iron supplementation for pregnant women (60 mg elemental iron and 25 μg folic acid once or twice daily) through the primary health care system for 6 months in pregnancy in countries with a prevalence of <40 per cent and for an additional 3 months postpartum in countries where the prevalence is >40 per cent. In India, the government has recommended a daily intake of 100 mg elemental iron with 500 μg of folic acid in the second half of pregnancy for a period of at least 100 days. Twice weekly or weekly iron supplements have also given equally good results in some studies, but it is still not universally accepted. In addition, treatment of hookworm with 400 mg single-dose albendazole or 100 mg twice daily for 3 days of mebendazole is recommended in the second half of pregnancy.

Treatment   The treatment for IDA is oral iron therapy in therapeutic dosage (200 mg elemental iron with 5 mg folic acid per day). On average, there is an increase in Hb of 0.8 g/dL per week. Reticulocyte count starts to increase within 5–10 days of oral therapy. Side effects are common (10–40 per cent) and are mainly gastrointestinal, such as nausea, vomiting, constipation, abdominal cramps and diarrhoea, and are dose related. There is no scientific evidence that any particular brand is superior to any others. Slow-release preparations are often associated with a decrease in side effects but this is mainly due to decreased absorption of iron. It can be taken with ascorbic acid (orange juice). Patients who do not tolerate standard iron preparations may be given carbonyl iron. Indications of response to therapy are feeling of well-being, improved appearance, better appetite and haematological response.

There is no advantage in using parenteral iron over oral iron, if the latter is well tolerated, but it can be used for patients who cannot tolerate oral iron. The iron requirement is calculated as follows:

Elemental iron (mg) = [Normal Hb − patient's Hb (g/dL)] × weight (kg) × 2.21 + 1000

Iron sorbitol injection, which allows rapid absorption owing to its low molecular weight, can be given by deep intramuscular injection after sensitivity testing, but is associated with pain and staining at the injection site. It is administered by repeat injections over a 2-week period.

Iron dextran can be given by the intramuscular or intravenous route. Highly fractionated low-molecular-weight iron dextran can be used with minimum side effects. Newer preparations of iron sucrose can be given as single infusion or repeat intravenous injections. These should be given between 30 and 34 weeks' gestation as they will take 6–8 weeks to achieve their optimal effect.

Recombinant erythropoietin can be used with parenteral iron for renal disease patients during pregnancy, but can also be used as a blood substitute in Jehovah's witness patients and for iron-deficiency anaemia that is unresponsive to oral or parenteral iron.

Blood transfusion is required for obstetric haemorrhage or for severe anaemia in later pregnancy.

Folate-deficiency anaemia

Folate (folic acid) is needed in higher dosage during pregnancy because of the increased cell replication that is taking place in the fetus, uterus and bone marrow. The recommended daily intake is 800 μg. Its deficiency is common during pregnancy, especially in developing nations, and is mainly due to inadequate dietary intake but can be due to the malabsorption syndrome and gastrointestinal diseases. It is more common in women with multiple pregnancy, hookworm infestations, bleeding haemorrhoids, haemolytic conditions (chronic malaria) and other infections. Antifolate medications, such as antiepileptic drugs (phenytoin, primidone), pyrimethamine and trimethoprim can cause its

Table 4 Diagnosis of folate-deficiency anaemia

Characteristic	Normal range	Folate deficiency
Haemoglobin (Hb, g/dL)	11–15	<11
Mean corpuscular volume (fL)	75–96	>96
Mean corpuscular Hb (pg)	27–33	>33
Mean corpuscular Hb concentration (g/dL)	32–35	Normal
Peripheral blood film	Normocytic normochromic picture	Megaloblastic picture with hypersegmentation of neutrophils, neutropenia and thrombocytopenia
Serum folate (ng/mL)	>3	<3
Red cell folate (ng/mL)	>150	<150
Serum iron (μg/dL)	60–120	Normal
Serum lactate dehydrogenase		Increased
Homocysteine		Increased

deficiency. In developing countries, deficiency of both iron and folic acid are common.

The patient may be asymptomatic or may be unwell with loss of appetite, vomiting, diarrhoea or unexplained fever. There may be pallor, bleeding spots in the skin, enlarged spleen and liver, and neuropathy.

Folate deficiency may cause neural tube defects, abortions, growth retardation, abruptio placentae and pre-eclampsia. There is some evidence that the incidence of abortion, premature babies, small-for-dates babies and poor folate levels in neonates are higher in babies born to mothers with folate deficiency.

Diagnosis

This is made by Hb concentration and blood tests as shown in Table 4.

Treatment

The WHO recommends a daily folate consumption of 800 μg in the antenatal period and 600 μg during the lactation period. To meet this requirement, pregnant women should be encouraged to eat more green vegetables (spinach and broccoli) and offal (liver and kidneys).

Treatment of established folic acid deficiency is by giving 5 mg oral folic acid per day, which should be continued for at least 4 weeks in puerperium. Response is indicated by a fall in lactate dehydrogenase levels within 3–4 days and an increase in reticulocyte count in 5–8 days.

Cyanocobalamin (vitamin B12)-deficiency anaemia

This is a rare cause of megaloblastic anaemia in pregnancy, as the daily requirement of 3 μg/day is easily met with a normal diet. Pernicious anaemia caused by lack of intrinsic factor resulting in lack of absorption of vitamin B12 is rare during pregnancy, as it usually causes infertility. Findings are the same as in folate deficiency. Vitamin B12 levels are lower in the blood (<90 μg/L). The deoxyuridine suppression test can differentiate between B12 and folate deficiency. Treatment is with parenteral cyanocobalamin (250 μg) every month.

Key points

1 Anaemias, especially nutritional anaemias, are very common during pregnancy and are a major health problem, being more common in non-industrialised nations, and are a significant cause of maternal and perinatal mortality and morbidity.
2 Iron-deficiency anaemia continues to be the commonest anaemia during pregnancy owing to dietary habits, and can be treated by oral or parenteral iron therapy.
3 Folate-deficiency anaemia is also common but can be easily treated by oral folate supplementation.
4 Thalassaemias and sickle cell haemoglobinopathies are seen in certain geographic areas, and are associated with significant morbidity.

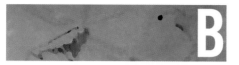

BACK PAIN IN PREGNANCY

Nigel Bickerton

Outside of pregnancy, the lifetime incidence of low back pain ranges from 50 to 70 per cent. Sciatica is less common fortunately, with a lifetime incidence of 10–40 per cent. All structures of the lower spine and pelvis, i.e. the muscles, ligament, joints, intervertebral discs and nerve root can cause back pain.

Back pain is very common during pregnancy; often women will ignore it and not report it to their carer. However, the discomfort and disability owing to backache often worsens as the pregnancy progresses, which results in a high proportion of women eventually reporting symptoms. Between 50 and 80 per cent of women admit to some degree of back pain during pregnancy. The pain may be associated with certain activities only, or it may be so severe that the woman has such limited mobility as to be at risk of venous thrombosis.

Back pain most frequently presents between the fifth and seventh months (20–28 weeks) of pregnancy. It may present earlier, especially in women with pre-pregnancy pain. The two commonest types of back pain are lumbar and sacral/pelvic.

Lumbar pain tends to be central over the lower lumbar vertebrae but may be associated with radiation of pain into the legs. The symptoms are similar to those experienced by the non-pregnant back-pain sufferer. It is usually aggravated by prolonged maintenance of the same position, be it sitting at a desk or standing up. Sacral/pelvic pain in pregnancy is approximately four times commoner than lumbar pain. Women describe pain over the sacrum that may be symmetrical or unilateral. It may radiate into the pubis and down the buttocks into the back of the thighs. The pain is not usually eased by short periods of rest. Rolling over in bed, rising from a seat and climbing stairs tends to make the pain worse.

The majority of pregnancy-related back pain is caused by a combination of the hormonal effects on joint laxity, postural changes and a change in the centre of gravity. Imaging has shown that the lordosis of the lumbar vertebrae in reality decreases during the latter half of pregnancy.

There is evidence to suggest that women who are overweight or who smoke cigarettes have a higher chance of developing back pain in pregnancy. Undertaking physical activity and maintaining fitness before pregnancy reduces the risk of back pain during pregnancy. Most pregnancy-related back pain tends to resolve quickly in the postpartum period. One third of sufferers will continue to have back pain for 4 weeks after delivery and one sixth 9 weeks postpartum.

In the majority of cases of back pain in pregnancy, the origin is mechanical. However, on closer questioning, pre-pregnancy symptoms may be elicited. Most mechanical back pain is of sudden onset after lifting or straining. In contrast, pregnancy-related back pain tends to be of a more gradual onset. The woman should be asked about any previous physical injury. In areas of the world affected by civil conflict, it is often women and children who suffer injuries that will cause them problems in later life.

The causes of back pain are myriad and fortunately rare in pregnancy; in fact, many of these causes are likely to affect fertility and result in difficulties in becoming pregnant. However, a list of causes is included for completeness (Box 1).

The management of mechanical back pain in the absence of any evidence of prolapsed intervertebral disc consists of:

- avoidance of aggravating factors;
- wearing shoes with a low heel or no heel;
- bed rest
- analgesia – but not non-steroidal anti-inflammatory drugs;
- exercise to strengthen the back, e.g. swimming.

In an increasing litigious world, the subject of back pain has become linked with litigation related to misdiagnosis and failure of diagnosis

Box 1 Causes of back pain

Mechanical
- Muscle pain
- Prolapse of intervertebral disc
- Spondylolisthesis
- Lumbar spondylosis
- Fibromyalgia
- Osteoarthritis
- Spinal stenosis

Traumatic
- Fracture of vertebra
- Soft tissue injury
- Foreign body migration including shot pellets and/or shrapnel

Inflammatory
- Rheumatoid arthritis
- Ankylosing spondylitis
- Reiter's syndrome
- Psoriatic arthritis

Infective
- Osteomyelitis
- Tuberculosis

Metabolic
- Osteomalacia
- Paget's disease of bone
- Osteoporosis and vertebral collapse

Tumours
- Primary of bone – benign or malignant
- Secondary of bone
- Multiple myeloma

Haematological
- Sickle cell disease

Referred from other organs
- Gastric ulcer
- Duodenal ulcer
- Gallbladder disease
- Pancreatitis
- Renal: infection, stones or tumour

Vascular
- Aneurysm

of more serious problems. The two diagnoses that should not be missed are:

- acute lumbar disc herniation;
- cauda equina syndrome.

The intervertebral discs are made up of a fibrous outer part that in health surrounds a central area of gel. In disc prolapse, the gel extrudes through a weakness in the fibrous wall of the disc. The weakest part of the disc is posterolateral (Fig. 1) and, when gel extrudes through at this point, it may press on spinal nerve roots emerging from the spinal canal. The onset of pain is usually both sudden and severe, with nerve root pain that follows the dermatome involved, usually extending below the knee. In addition, there may be radiation of pain to the sacroiliac region and to the buttocks. In general, though not always, the pain is worse in the leg than in the back. The majority of disc herniations are unilateral.

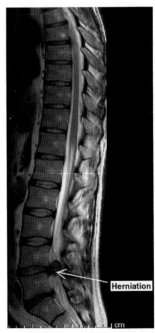

Figure 1 Magnetic resonance scan showing a posterolateral intervertebral disc prolapse at the L4/5 level. This was associated with neurological symptoms. Image courtesy of Dr Carl Wright, FRCR, Ysbyty Glan Clwyd, Bodelwyddan.

The nerve root affected will determine the site of the pain. For example, unilateral disc herniation at the L4–5 level will compress the L5 nerve root, giving pain in that dermatome; L5–S1 herniation will affect the S1 nerve root.

Midline rather than posterolateral disc herniation causes the cauda equina syndrome. The pressure effect is on several roots of the cauda equina. The disc lesion causing this is usually at the L4–5 level. In addition to back and buttock pain, the patient may note perianal pain (S2–4 dermatomes). The patient may develop urinary symptoms including difficulty in voiding urine, increased frequency or even overflow incontinence. In addition, foot numbness and difficulty in walking may develop either slowly or rapidly.

Patients with suspected disc prolapse should be assessed and managed as a matter of urgency by an orthopaedic surgeon or neurosurgeon, according to local practice. Patients with bladder symptoms or anal sphincter tone deficit become a neurosurgical emergency as delay in decompression may lead to permanent disability.

Examination of these patients may reveal a limited straight leg raise, and loss of power and sensation in the lower limb corresponding to the root affected. If imaging is needed, then magnetic resonance imaging can safely be undertaken during pregnancy.

BIRTH INJURIES, MATERNAL

Jai B Sharma

Perineal trauma is common, especially after the birth of a first child, and is responsible for considerable long-term maternal morbidity, such as complete perineal tear, relaxed perineum, genital prolapse, stress urinary incontinence and faecal incontinence.

◼ Anatomy of the pelvic floor

The perineum is the diamond-shaped area of pelvic outlet caudal to the pelvic diaphragm with boundaries formed by the inferior pubic rami anteriorly and by the sacrotuberous ligament posteriorly and is further divided into the urogenital triangle anteriorly and the anal triangle

posteriorly by a transverse line joining the anterior parts of the ischial tuberosities (Fig. 1).

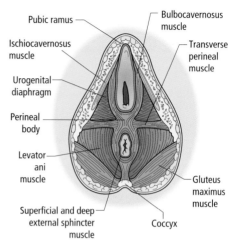

Figure 1 Transverse view of the perineal muscles.

The urogenital triangle has three superficial muscles: the bulbospongiosus, which encircles the vagina and inserts anteriorly into corpus cavernosus clitoridis: the superficial transverse perineal muscle, which lies transversely; and the ischiocavernosus muscle, which lies laterally in the labia. Deep muscles include the deep transverse perineal muscles and the levator ani (Fig. 1).

The anal triangle is posterior, and includes the anal sphincter and ischiorectal fossae. The perineal body is a fibromuscular area between the vagina and the anal canal in which there is interlacing of muscle fibres from the bulbospongiosus, the superficial transverse perineal muscle and the external anal sphincter muscle.

The anorectum consists of the lower 3.5 cm of the anal canal and the rectum. The external anal sphincter is composed of three parts: subcutaneous, superficial and deep. The internal anal sphincter comprises the circular muscles of the rectum separated from the external anal sphincter by longitudinal muscles, which are a continuation of the longitudinal muscle of the rectum (Fig. 2).

◼ Definition of genital trauma

Genital trauma is the injury to genital organs during childbirth and can involve one or more genital organs as shown in Table 1.

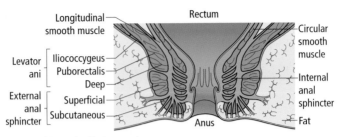

Figure 2 Longitudinal view of the anal sphincter muscles.

Table 1 Genital tract injuries

Type of injury	Class
Tears or lacerations in the perineum	Perineal tears
Tears in the cervix	Cervical tears
Haematomas in the vagina/perineum	Genital haematomas
Tears or rupture in the uterus	Uterine rupture

■ Perineal tears

The various types of perineal tear are shown in Table 2.

Table 2 Classification of perineal tears

Grade of tear (class)	Features
First degree	Laceration (tear) involving the vaginal epithelium or perineal skin only
Second degree	Involvement (tear) of the perineal muscles but not the anal sphincter
Third degree	Involvement of anal sphincter
Grade 3a	Tear of <50% thickness of the external sphincter
Grade 3b	Tear of >50% thickness of the external sphincter
Grade 3c	Tear of the internal sphincter
Fourth degree	Third-degree tear with involvement of anal epithelium

Risk factors

The various risk factors for perineal floor trauma are as follows:

■ big baby;
■ prolonged labour;
■ precipitate labour;
■ difficult labour;
■ shoulder dystocia;
■ occipitoposterior delivery;
■ breech delivery;
■ instrumental delivery.

Prevention of perineal tears

Role of episiotomy

Liberal use of episiotomy does not reduce the incidence of third-degree tears. Midline episiotomy increases the risk of third-degree tears by 4.5–6 times. Episiotomy should only be used judiciously for large babies, forceps delivery or where a tear is imminent, breech delivery, manipulations for shoulder dystocia and other intrauterine manipulations.

Perineal massage

The use of perineal massage in the weeks leading up to delivery has been associated with slightly lower rates of episiotomy; the prevalence of perineal trauma was equal in the two groups studied.

Mode of delivery

This has a great impact on the rate of perineal trauma. Elective Caesarean section prevents damage to perineum from labour-related events. Ventouse delivery is associated with less perineal trauma than forceps delivery. Use of both instruments is associated with a higher rate of severe perineal damage than single instrument. Episiotomy is recommended before instrumental delivery, especially forceps delivery. Ventouse may sometimes be applied without episiotomy if there is no imminent tear.

Duration of second stage

Prolonged second stage is associated with perineal trauma. It is also associated with increased risk of instrumental delivery, which itself is a factor for increased perineal damage.

Epidural analgesia

This is associated with an increased risk of instrumental delivery with associated perineal damage. However, epidural analgesia has been shown to allow a passive second stage in nulliparous women, which may reduce the incidence of difficult instrumental delivery and thus reduce the prevalence of perineal trauma.

Position for delivery

This is not related to perineal trauma.

■ Management of first- and second-degree perineal tears

Minor first-degree lacerations may not need suturing provided they are not bleeding. However, all first- and second-degree tears should be meticulously sutured for optimum outcome.

Prerequisites for suturing of perineal tears are:

- proper lighting;
- good analgesia, preferably epidural analgesia;
- good assistance;
- good exposure and proper examination to avoid missing the apex or other lacerations, especially of the anal sphincter, are important for proper suturing.

Technique

It is important to secure the apex of a vaginal tear to avoid formation of a paravaginal haematoma. All tears that are bleeding should be identified and ligated separately. The suturing is started from the apex of the vagina with polyglycolic acid (vicryl) 1-0 suture with continuous or interrupted sutures. The muscles are then stitched using same suture (vicryl 1-0) as interrupted sutures, taking full-thickness muscle and achieving complete haemostasis. The skin is stitched with interrupted mattress sutures using 1-0 vicryl or even as a subcuticular suture by starting from the last muscle suture and tying the last knot to the last suture in the vaginal epithelium

to avoid any knots in the skin, for least perineal discomfort in the postpartum period. Complete haemostasis must be achieved to avoid any vulval haematoma.

When the suturing is complete, ensure any vaginal packs or tampons used for aiding visualization are removed. All the swabs and needles must be counted and disposed of safely. A rectal examination is important to ensure the anal sphincter is intact and that no sutures have breached the rectal mucosa.

It is advisable to prescribe analgesics but antibiotics are not usually required. However, in developing countries, most hospitals use a course of ampicillin or amoxycillin for 4–5 days in cases of episiotomy and perineal tears.

Patients can be discharged on the second or third day, if they are asymptomatic. Most first-degree and second-degree perineal repairs heal quite well without any problems. However, they should be followed up in the clinic for any problems, especially any anal incontinence, in which case the patient should be referred to a dedicated perineal dysfunction clinic, as it is usually the failure on the part of the attending obstetrician to detect anal sphincter damage.

Third-degree and fourth-degree perineal tears

Any damage to internal or external anal sphincter causes faecal incontinence or faecal urgency, and is a serious condition if not repaired well at the time of delivery. The prevalence is 2.8 per cent in primigravidae and 0.4 per cent in multigravidae.

Risk factors are as follows:

- nulliparity;
- big baby;
- prolonged second stage of labour;
- persistent occipitoposterior position and face to pubes delivery;
- instrumental delivery;
- midline episiotomy;
- epidural analgesia;
- previous third-degree tear;
- shoulder dystocia.

A classification of perineal tears is given in Table 2.

Repair of third- and fourth-degree perineal tears

Prerequisites are:

- written consent;
- spinal or effective epidural analgesia;
- repair must be performed in an operating theatre;
- repair must be performed by a trained obstetrician (at least a registrar);
- good lighting and adequate exposure;
- good assistance;
- proper instruments and sutures.

Repair procedure

1 The full extent of the injury should be evaluated by a meticulous vaginal and rectal examination in the lithotomy position in an operating theatre under good analgesia.
2 The type of tear must be classified and included in the notes.
3 The torn anal epithelium should be repaired with interrupted polyglycolic acid (vicryl) 3-0 sutures with the knots tied towards the anal canal.
4 The internal anal sphincter tear is then repaired separately using interrupted 3-0 polydioxanone sutures (PDSs) by end-to-end approximation. Being monofilamentous, PDSs are less likely to cause infection and are thus preferred. However, vicryl 3-0 can also be used if PDS is not available.
5 If the external anal sphincter is torn by <50 per cent (Grade 3a tear), an end-to-end repair should be performed with 3-0 vicryl mattress sutures by approximating the muscle ends.
6 If the external anal sphincter is torn by >50 per cent (Grade 3b tear), one should identify the torn muscles and grasp them with Allis forceps. The muscle should be mobilized and pulled across to overlap before suturing it with 3-0 PDS *stitches* in a double breast fashion, which enables overlapping of the sphincter muscles for better results. If the attending obstetrician is not familiar with the over-lapping technique, end-to-end mattress sutures can be used for the external anal sphincter.
7 The rest of the suturing is similar to that for the repair of a second-degree tear or episiotomy repair using vicryl 3-0 sutures. It is very important to suture the vagina, perineal muscles and perineal skin properly to avoid any tension on the sphincter

repair. The knots and suture ends of PDSs should be properly buried with overlying tissue to prevent suture migration.

Postoperative care

1 Adequate analgesia should be given by prescribing anti-inflammatory and analgesic agents.
2 Continuous bladder drainage should be ensured for at least 24 hours using a Foley catheter, as many patients tend to have urinary retention after a severe perineal tear.
3 Parenteral antibiotics must be given to all patients after repair using intravenous cephalosporins (cefuroxime) and metronidazole during the repair followed by oral treatment for a week.
4 After the repair, all women should be given lactulose (15 mL twice a day) as a stool softener and fybogel (1 satchet twice a day) as a bulking agent for 2 weeks to avoid any hard stool damaging the repair.
5 Proper counselling of all women with severe tears is mandatory to avoid any medicolegal problems.
6 A proper follow-up of patients must be arranged, preferably in a perineal clinic, to ensure optimal outcome. In the case of residual deficit, an anal scan may be required.

Future delivery after third- and fourth-degree tears

All such patients should be followed up and managed in perineal clinics by an obstetrician with special interest in the subject. They should have anal ultrasound and manometry for any residual deficit in the sphincter. Women without any symptoms and any deficit in the sphincter can have vaginal delivery under the observation of an obstetrician or a senior midwife. However, women with anal incontinence or residual sphincter damage should be counselled to have an elective Caesarean section in their next delivery. There is no evidence that prophylactic episiotomy prevents sphincter damage in future deliveries, hence episiotomy should be used only if indicated for obstetric reasons.

■ Injuries to cervix

Small (<0.5 cm) cervical tears are common in obstetric practice; however, deep cervical tears are less common but are more dangerous. They may extend to the upper third of the vagina, and may cause partial or complete avulsion of the cervix from the vagina. Cervical tears usually occur in difficult and obstructed labour, delivery through an incompletely dilated cervix, or as a part of extensive genital injuries involving the perineum, the vagina and sometimes the lower segment of the uterus.

Repair of cervical tears

1 Proper visualization under adequate analgesia is important for proper identification of the tear and to rule out additional genital trauma.
2 Deep cervical lacerations involving the vaginal vault should be repaired in the operating theatre.
3 Blood should be arranged.
4 A cervical tear is exposed using four sponge-holding forceps applied at various sites on the cervix and after retracting the posterior vaginal wall with Sim's speculum. Any bleeding area or laceration on the cervix is repaired using 1-0 vicryl suture starting from the apex, which is best seen by pulling out the margins of the tear with two sponge-holding forceps. If after making the suture , the apex is still not reached, one can pull the suture for better visualization of the apex for proper suturing. Care must be taken to avoid injury to the bladder in anterior tears or the ureter in lateral cervical tears.
5 If the tear is going into the uterus or uterine vessels are involved in the tear or there is a broad ligament haematoma, it is better to perform a laparotomy for haemostasis.
6 Complete haemostasis must be achieved. All other genital tears, such as vaginal lacerations and perineal tears, must be sutured properly for optimum results.
7 Antibiotics and analgesics should be prescribed to all patients who then should be carefully monitored in the postoperative period.

Genital haematomas

Acute puerperal haematomas are seen 1 in 1000 to 1 in 4000 deliveries. They are caused by complications of episiotomy in 85–90 per cent of cases, especially in difficult deliveries where complete haemostasis could not be achieved during suturing. Other causes include instrumental vaginal delivery, primiparity, pre-eclampsia, multiple pregnancy, big babies, prolonged second stage of labour and vulval varicosities. Prevention is by adequate suturing of perineal and vaginal tears and episiotomy, and by achieving complete haemostasis at the time of repair.

Types of genital haematomas
Infralevator haematomas
Infralevator haematomas are usually associated with vaginal delivery and are limited by the levator ani muscles superiorly, perineal body medially, and by the Colles fascia and fascia lata laterally, and may extend into ischiorectal fossa. They are caused by injury to small labial or vulvar vessels, the inferior vesical or vaginal branch of the uterine arteries, or branches of the inferior rectal arteries. They usually present as vulval or perineal pain out of proportion to the episiotomy, and local swelling in the perineum, vulva or vagina, with ischiorectal mass with discoloration. There may be associated continuous vaginal bleeding or urinary retention. Small non-expanding haematomas of less than 3 cm can be managed expectantly.

Expanding or large haematomas require surgical management to prevent pressure necrosis, septicaemia, bleeding and even death. Adequate rehydration and resuscitation is mandatory before their evacuation under adequate analgesia, good assistance and proper lighting for adequate exposure. All blood clots must be evacuated after opening the haematoma. All bleeding vessels must be secured tightly using 1-0 vicryl sutures, and complete haemostasis must be achieved and the dead space should be obliterated using vicryl sutures.

All patients should be given antibiotics and analgesics in the postoperative period. Foley's catheter should be used for 24 hours. The patient should be followed up for any recurrence of the haematoma.

Supralevator haematoma
Supralevator haematomas are serious haematomas that have no fibrous boundaries and arise

from branches of the uterine artery, pudendal artery or the inferior vesical artery. Bleeding can extend into the broad ligament, the presacral space and the retroperitoneal space. They may present as rectal pain and pressure. They can also manifest as enlarging vaginal or rectal masses with signs and symptoms of shock. There may be continued vaginal bleeding or even cardiovascular collapse. Broad ligament haematomas may cause upward and lateral displacement of the uterus, which feels well retracted. The revealed vaginal bleeding may not be significant. They may occur as an extension of a cervical tear into the fornices or into the uterus, or may appear in the presence of uterine rupture.

The management of supralevator haematomas requires laparotomy after resuscitating the patient. This will require a general anaesthetic as opposed to a regional block. Blood will need to be available and the patient will require antibiotic cover. In the case of broad ligament haematoma, care must be exercised to avoid injury to the ureters. Complete haemostasis must be achieved by securing all bleeding vessels. In the case of rupture of the uterus, hysterectomy may be required. Sometimes angiographic embolisation of the vessels may be required. Postoperatively, all patients must be monitored carefully for vital signs, any recurrence of haematomas, and adequate blood, antibiotics and analgesics should be administered.

■ **Uterine injuries**

Uterine injuries can form part of other genital injuries extending into the uterus, such as cervical lacerations extending into the lower uterine segment, injury to the uterine vessels, the rupture of a previous scar or the rupture of an unscarred uterus in cases of obstructed labour. Rupture of the uterus is a serious condition with high maternal and perinatal mortality and morbidity. The patient presents with features of obstructed labour followed by features of shock, vaginal bleeding, abdominal distension and tenderness. There may be haematuria. Fetal heart beat is usually absent.

Management includes immediate resuscitation with adequate hydration, blood transfusion, intravenous antibiotics and urgent laparotomy under general anaesthesia. The uterus can be salvaged in case of a clean cut in the uterus in the case of scar rupture; however, in the majority of cases of rupture of the uterus in obstructed labour, the margins are ragged. Caesarean hysterectomy is usually required for such cases. Complete haemostasis must be achieved, which may need ligation of anterior division of internal iliac artery. One has to be careful to avoid injury to the bladder and ureters in such cases. Postoperatively, patients need careful monitoring, bladder drainage by Foley's catheter, intravenous antibiotics, analgesics, and adequate blood and hydration.

BIRTH INJURIES, NEONATAL

Kausik Banerjee

The term 'birth injury' refers to avoidable and unavoidable mechanical and hypoxic–ischaemic injury incurred by an infant during labour and delivery. The definition does not include injury from amniocentesis, intrauterine transfusion, scalp blood sampling or resuscitation procedures.

■ **Incidence and mortality**

Incidence of birth injuries has been estimated at 2–7 per 1000 live births. Prolonged labour, macrosomia, cephalopelvic disproportion, dystocia, prematurity, breech presentation predispose to birth injury. Birth injuries account for 2–3 per cent of neonatal deaths. The technologic advances which enable today's obstetrician to recognise birth trauma risk factors by ultrasonography and fetal monitoring prior to attempting vaginal delivery are partly responsible for this low rate. Even transient injuries in babies can cause significant parental anxiety. This demands supportive and informative counselling.

The different types of birth injuries are listed in Box 1.

Box 1 Different types of birth injuries

- Cranial injuries
- Intraventricular haemorrhage
- Spinal injuries
- Peripheral nerve injuries
- Visceral injury
- Fractures
- Hypoxia–ischaemia

Cranial injuries

Caput succedaneum is a diffuse subcutaneous, extraperiosteal fluid collection with poorly defined margins. It may extend across the suture lines and across the midline (Fig. 1). It is caused by the pressure of the presenting part against the dilating cervix. Caput succedaneum does not usually cause complications and tends to resolve within the first few days after birth. If this is associated with extensive ecchymosis, phototherapy for hyperbilirubinaemia may be indicated.

Cephalohaematoma is a subperiosteal haemorrhage, which is always limited to the surface of one cranial bone (Fig. 2). Usually, the swelling is not visible at birth and there is no discoloration of the overlying scalp. Occasionally it could be associated with underlying skull fracture. Most cephalohaematomas are resorbed within 2–12 weeks. Sometimes they may be calcified. Palpation of an organised cephalohaematoma gives an impression of 'scalloping' at the margins. A massive haematoma may rarely result in blood loss severe enough to require a transfusion.

Erythema, ecchymosis, abrasions and subcutaneous fat necrosis of the scalp or face may occur following instrumental deliveries. Ecchymosis (subcutaneous collection of blood following rupture of small blood vessels) is common in premature babies. Subcutaneous fat necrosis is not usually detected at birth and may take several weeks before it is visible. An irregular, hard, non-pitting subcutaneous plaque with purple discoloration is the typical finding. Usually no treatment is required but occasionally this may cause hypercalcaemia, which demands intervention.

Subconjunctival and retinal haemorrhages are frequent and petechial spots over the face and neck are also common. These are secondary to sudden rise in intrathoracic pressure during passage of the chest through the birth canal. No treatment is required apart from parental reassurance.

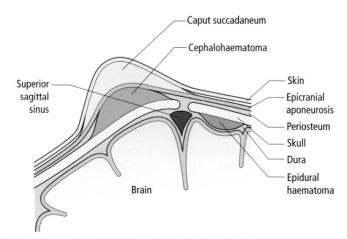

Figure 1 Schematic diagram showing different types of cranial injuries related to birth trauma.

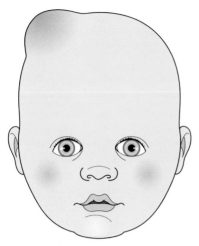

Figure 2 Cephalohaematoma.

Fractures of the skull may occur as a result of pressure from forceps or from maternal pelvic bones. Linear fractures are the commonest and require no treatment. Depressed fractures are usually secondary to forceps delivery. Fracture of the occipital bone poses a significant danger of potentially fatal haemorrhage owing to disruption of vascular sinuses. This may result during breech deliveries.

■ Intracranial–intraventricular haemorrhage

Intracranial haemorrhage may result from trauma or asphyxia and, rarely, from a primary bleeding diathesis. Cephalopelvic disproportion, breech or precipitate deliveries, or mechanical assistance with delivery are predisposing factors. Massive subdural haemorrhages are rare but are encountered more often in term neonates. Intracranial bleeding may be associated with neonatal vitamin K deficiency, isoimmune thrombocytopenia and disseminated intravascular coagulopathy.

Intraventricular haemorrhage (IVH) in premature infants may occur without any apparent trauma. Incidence of IVH increases with decreasing birth weight. Two-thirds of premature babies with birth weight below 750 g may be affected by this. This is rarely present at birth but 50 per cent occur in the first 24 hours. Bleeding occurs in the subependymal germinal matrix.

Immature blood vessels in this highly vascular periventricular area may be subjected to various forces, which, together with poor vascular support, predispose the premature infants to IVH.

The most common symptoms are diminished or absent Moro reflex, poor muscle tone, lethargy, apnoea and pallor. Premature infants with IVH often have a sudden deterioration on day 2 or day 3 of life. Severe IVH may cause significant neurological deterioration but milder forms may remain asymptomatic.

Diagnosis is on the basis of history and clinical manifestations. Cranial ultrasound scan (USS) is the standard mode of imaging for confirmation of the diagnosis. Large babies born at term with subdural haemorrhage may not show any sign for up to a month. Term neonates with suspected intracranial haemorrhage should be considered for magnetic resonance imaging (MRI) or computerised tomography (CT) scan of brain, as USS may not pick up the intraparenchymal bleed or infarction.

The incidence of traumatic intracranial haemorrhage may be reduced by proactive management of cephalopelvic disproportion and operative delivery. The incidence of IVH in premature neonates can be reduced by antenatal steroids and meticulous management of ventilation. Vitamin K should be given to all infants to prevent bleeding secondary to vitamin K deficiency.

Prognosis

Neonates with massive haemorrhage deteriorate rapidly and often die. Most neonates with small IVH do not develop post-haemorrhagic hydrocephalus. Progressive hydrocephalus will require intervention with ventriculoperitoneal shunt.

■ Spine and spinal cord

A neonate may sustain injury to the spinal cord during delivery when the spine is hyperextended (traction) or rotated. Traction is more significant in breech deliveries and causes injury to the lower cervical–upper thoracic vertebrae. Rotation or torsion is significant in vertex deliveries causing damage to the fourth cervical vertebra.

Major neuropathological changes consist of acute lesions, e.g. haemorrhages, oedema and, rarely, vertebral fractures or dislocations may occur. Haemorrhagic events may be associated with varying degrees of laceration, disruption or total transection of the cord.

Absence of reflexes, loss of sensation and complete lack of spontaneous movement occur below the level of the injury. If the injury is severe, the neonate is at risk of dying rapidly from respiratory depression, shock and hypothermia. Alternatively, the clinical course may be protracted with gradual evolution of symptoms and signs. Severe respiratory failure may be obscured by mechanical ventilation and may cause an ethical dilemma later. Apnoea on day 1 and poor motor recovery by 3 months are poor prognostic signs.

Prevention is the most important aspect of perinatal care and management of labour must be appropriate. Occasionally, the injury may be sustained *in utero*.

The diagnosis is confirmed by MRI or CT myelography. Differential diagnosis includes amyotonia congenita and myelodysplasia with spina bifida occulta.

■ Peripheral nerve injury
Brachial palsy

Brachial plexus injury occurs most commonly in large babies, often with shoulder dystocia or breech delivery. Incidence is 0.5–2.0 per 1000 live births. The majority of cases are Erb's palsy.

In *Erb–Duchenne* palsy, the injury is limited to the fifth and sixth cervical nerves. The infant loses the power to abduct the arm from the shoulder, to rotate the arm externally and to supinate the forearm. The characteristic position consists of adduction and internal rotation of the arm with pronation of the forearm (waiter's tip). The Moro and biceps reflexes are absent, but the grasp reflex is usually retained. Five per cent of patients with Erb's palsy may have ipsilateral phrenic nerve palsy.

Klumpke's paralysis is a rarer form of brachial palsy which affects seventh and eighth cervical and first thoracic nerve. It results in weakness of the intrinsic muscles of the hand; the grasp reflex is absent. If the first thoracic spinal nerve is involved, Horner's syndrome (ipsilateral ptosis and myosis) is present.

The prognosis depends on whether the nerve was merely injured or lacerated. Involvement of deltoid muscle is usually the most serious problem and may result in shoulder drop. In general, paralysis of the upper arm has a better prognosis than paralysis of the lower arm.

Treatment consists of prevention of contractures by partial immobilisation and appropriate positioning. In upper arm paralysis, the arm is abducted 90 degrees, with external rotation at the shoulder and with full supination of the forearm with the palm turned toward the face. Immobilisation should be intermittent through the day and between feedings. In lower arm or hand paralysis, the wrist is splinted in neutral position with padding placed in the fist. If the paralysis persists beyond 3–6 months, neurosurgical opinion should be sought.

Phrenic nerve palsy

The presence of cyanosis and irregular, laboured breathing in a neonate raises the suspicion of phrenic nerve (third, fourth and fifth cervical) palsy. Often such injuries are associated with brachial palsy. The diagnosis is established by fluoroscopy or ultrasonography. There is no specific treatment. Oxygen delivery is optimised and feeding is supported. Nursing on the involved side (splinting the affected diaphragm) is recommended. Usually spontaneous recovery occurs by 3 months.

Facial nerve palsy

Facial nerve palsy is usually peripheral in nature. It often results from pressure over the facial nerve. This can occur whilst *in utero*, from efforts during labour, from forceps during assisted delivery or, rarely, secondary to nuclear agenesis. Peripheral palsy is flaccid and often involves the whole side of the face, including the forehead. When the infant cries, there is movement only on the unaffected side of the face and hence the mouth is drawn to that side. The forehead is smooth on the affected side and the eye cannot be closed. In central facial palsy, the forehead remains unaffected.

Most infants begin to recover within a few weeks in peripheral palsy. Care of the affected eye is essential. Consultation with a paediatric neurologist or neurosurgeon is indicated if no improvement is observed within 2 weeks. Neuroplasty is indicated for permanent palsy.

Differential diagnoses include nuclear agenesis, congenital absence of facial muscles, unilateral absence of the orbicularis oris muscle and intracranial haemorrhage.

■ Viscera

The liver is the only internal organ apart from brain that is vulnerable to injury during birth. Large baby, intrauterine asphyxia, bleeding disorders, extreme prematurity, breech presentation and hepatomegaly are all predisposing factors. The most common lesion is subcapsular haematoma. Symptoms of shock may be delayed. Lacerations are less common. Early detection by means of ultrasonographic diagnosis and institution of prompt supportive therapy may be life saving.

Splenic rupture may rarely occur alone or in association with liver rupture.

Although adrenal haemorrhage occurs in some cases, especially after breech deliveries, its cause is undetermined. Trauma, stress, anoxia or severe sepsis may be contributory; 90 per cent are unilateral. Presenting features are profound shock and cyanosis though not all adrenal haemorrhages are fatal.

■ Fractures

These are most often observed following breech delivery and/or shoulder dystocia in macrosomic babies.

The clavicle is the most frequently fractured bone in the neonate during birth, and sometimes is an unpredictable and unavoidable complication of normal birth. The infant may present with pseudo paralysis; X-rays confirm the fracture. The prognosis is excellent with healing occurring by 10 days. Arm motion may

be limited by pinning the infant's sleeve to the shirt.

Loss of spontaneous movement of the limbs is regarded as an early sign of fracture. The Moro reflex is also absent in the involved upper limb. Associated nerve injury may also be present. The obstetrician may hear or feel a 'snap' suggestive of fracture at the time of delivery. X-rays of the limbs confirm the diagnosis.

Humeral shaft fracture is usually treated with a splint and the arm is strapped to the chest. Healing occurs within 2–4 weeks. For femoral fractures, good results can be obtained with traction–suspension of both the lower extremities, even if the fracture is unilateral. Healing is usually accompanied by excess callus formation. Fractures in preterm babies may be related to osteopenia. Orthopaedic consultation is recommended.

■ Dislocations and epiphyseal separations

These injuries rarely result from birth trauma. The upper femoral epiphysis may be separated during breech extraction. The affected leg shows swelling, limitation of active movement and painful passive movement. Prognosis is usually good.

■ Hypoxia–ischaemia

Hypoxic ischaemic encephalopathy (HIE) is an important cause of permanent damage to the central nervous system, which may result in neonatal death or may manifest later as cerebral palsy. A total of 15–20 per cent of neonates with HIE die in the neonatal period and 25–30 per cent of the survivors develop permanent neurodevelopmental abnormalities. Its prevention and treatment are those of the primary causative conditions. Disability and death can be reduced by optimising ventilation, oxygenation and correction of associated multiorgan dysfunction. A fetal pH of less than 7, a 5-minute Apgar score of 0–3 and clinical features of multiorgan dysfunction are suggestive of asphyxia.

Further reading

Fanaroff AA, Martin RJ, eds. *Neonatal Perinatal Medicine: diseases of the fetus and infant*. St Louis, MO: Mosby, 1996.

Hearle M, Gilbert A. Management of complete obstetric brachial plexus lesions. *J Pediatr Orthop* 2004; **24:** 194–200.

Patel PR, Murphy DJ. Forceps delivery in modern obstetric practice. *BMJ* 2004; **328:** 1302–5.

Stoll BJ, Kliegman RM. The fetus and the neonatal infant. In: *Nelson Textbook of Pediatrics*, 16th edn. Philadelphia: WB Saunders, 2000: 488–92.

Volpe JJ. Injuries of extracranial, cranial, intracranial, spinal cord and peripheral nervous system structures. *Neurology of the Newborn*, 3rd edn. Philadelphia: WB Saunders, 1995: 769–92.

BLEEDING DISORDERS IN PREGNANCY, INCLUDING THROMBOCYTOPENIA

Naim Akhtar

The fine physiological haemostatic balance between haemostasis and fibrinolysis is shifted in pregnancy to favour pro-coagulation (Box 1).

Box 1 Physiological coagulation changes in pregnancy

- Predominantly pro-haemostatic changes (shortened clotting times)
  - increased fibrinogen concentration
  - increased factor VIII and other coagulation factors
- Increased plasminogen activator inhibitor concentration (reduced systemic fibrinolytic capacity)
- Reduced protein S concentration
- Increased protein C concentration

As a consequence, Virchow's triad of coagulation, vessel wall damage and flow rate are affected, making venous thromboembolic disease a potential problem. Bleeding may result from the resulting disequilibrium and subsequent anticoagulation therapy.

Bleeding in pregnancy may result predominantly from a coagulation defect or deficiency (coagulopathy), or a reduction or functional defect in platelets (thrombocytopathies). Both may arise from inherent tendencies or may be acquired (Box 2).

Coagulation disorders

The inherited coagulation bleeding disorders are all relatively uncommon and can be classified as follows.

Common (20 – 100 cases per million):

- haemophilia A, an X-linked Factor VIII-deficient or defective condition;
- haemophilia B, an X-linked Factor IX-deficient or defective condition;
- Von Willebrand's disease (vWD), an autosomal dominant or recessive condition resulting in deficient or defective von Willebrand factor (vWF).

Rare (up to 1 case per million):

- haemophilia C, an autosomal dominant or recessive condition resulting in Factor XI deficiency, common in Ashkenazi Jews;
- autosomal recessive conditions resulting in deficiencies of Factors X, V, VII, II, XIII, combined V + VIII, afibrinogenaemia and dysfibrinogenaemia.

In haemophilia A, females are carriers and 50 per cent will have sufficiently by low levels of Factor VIII to require replacement therapy to cover surgery, including Caesarean section. True haemophilia A is rare (in a child of a carrier and an affected male, or in Turner's syndrome).

However, the most common reason for a female to have Factor VIII deficiency is vWD. vWD is easily distinguished by the demonstration of reduction in vWF antigen immunologically, and a prolonged bleeding time (failure of

Box 2 Bleeding disorders in pregnancy

Coagulation disorders
Congenital and inherited

- Haemophilia A (Factor VIII deficiency)
- Haemophilia B (Factor IX deficiency)
- Haemophilia C (Factor XI deficiency)
- Von Willebrand's disease
- Rarer factor deficiencies (Factors XIII, X)

Acquired

- Disseminated intravascular coagulopathy (DIC)
- Coagulopathy associated with severe sepsis
- Coagulopathy associated with acute pro-myelocytic leukaemia
- Coagulopathy associated with massive blood loss
- Coagulopathy associated with renal and hepatic disease
- Acquired inhibitors of coagulation – antiphospholipid syndromes
- Acquired inhibitors of coagulation – Factor VIII antibodies
- Thrombotic thrombocytopenic purpura (TTP)
- Other thrombotic microangiopathies

Thrombocytopathies (platelet disorders)
Congenital and inherited

- Inherited thrombocytopenia and functional defects
- Drugs/chemicals (ethanol, thiazides, oestrogens)
- Isoimmune (neonatal alloimmune thrombocytopenia)
- Bone marrow infiltration (mucopolysaccharidosis)
- Congenital infections (cytomegalovirus, toxoplasmosis, rubella)

Acquired

- Gestational thrombocytopenia
- Immune thrombocytopenia
- Associated with pregnancy-induced hypertension
- Drug induced (heparin, quinine, zidovudine, sulphonamides)
- Antiphospholipid syndromes
- Associated with human immunodeficiency virus infection
- Other secondary causes (DIC, TTP, hypersplenism)

vWF in assisting platelets to adhere to cut surfaces). Up to 20 per cent of women with menorrhagia have undiagnosed vWD. However, during pregnancy, vWF rises to normal or low normal range, except in the rare severe type 3 disease.

The rarer congenital bleeding disorders have a higher incidence where consanguineous marriages are frequent (Muslims, India). These conditions are generally heterogeneous and have a relatively mild presentation.

Factor XI deficiency is prevalent in Ashkenazi Jews, with a heterozygosity as high as 8 per cent, but they are mildly affected. In studies with Iranian non-Jews, no correlation was found between clinical bleeding and moderate/severe deficiency (Factor XI <5 per cent), and mild deficiency (6–30 per cent). Both groups had a mild bleeding diathesis, with 25 per cent having muscle haematomas and haemarthrosis, and 50 per cent oral or postoperative bleeding. Women requiring Caesarean section should be covered with Factor XI concentrate or fresh-frozen plasma.

Factor XIII deficiency is associated with a severe bleeding tendency, affecting mucosal and skeletal surfaces (mouth bleeding, epistaxis, haematomas, haemarthrosis). Up to 20 per cent of women of reproductive age will have an intraperitoneal bleed, with some requiring hysterectomy. A total of 50 per cent of pregnant women will have had at least one miscarriage.

Factor X deficiency is associated with haematomas and haemarthrosis in two-thirds of patients, and some with gastrointestinal bleeding.

The acquired coagulopathies are more common in pregnancy and may complicate many high-risk pregnancies, particularly associated with obstetric calamities such as amniotic fluid embolism or abruptio placentae. The coagulopathy is defined on the basis of prolonged coagulation times, consumptive thrombocytopenia and increased fibrinolysis (Table 1). This helps to differentiate other causes of a thrombotic microangiopathy (Table 2).

Clinical assessment of a patient reveals continual oozing from sites of venous access and mucosal surfaces (bleeding from gums, epistaxis). The main causes are:

- disseminated intravascular coagulopathy;
- coagulopathy associated with severe sepsis;
- massive blood loss;
- hepatic dysfunction or disease;
- renal disease;
- acquired inhibitors of coagulation.

Disseminated intravascular coagulopathy (DIC) is common in obstetrical practice, with multifactorial contributing factors (Box 3). Direct activation of coagulation causes DIC in amniotic fluid embolism and via leakage of thromboplastin into the maternal circulation in placental abruption.

Table 1 Simple laboratory screening tests in acquired coagulation disorders

Test	Description
Coagulation	
Prothrombin time (PT)	Prolonged PT, APTT (perform 50:50 mix with normal plasma to correct for factor deficiencies)
Activated partial thromboplastin time (APTT)	
Thrombin time (TT)	Prolonged TT (perform Reptilase to exclude heparin effect)
Fibrinogen assay	Reduced fibrinogen
Platelets	
Absolute count	Blood film inspection for clumps, confirm reduction and morphology
Function	Bleeding time (skin template or PFA 100)
Fibrinolysis	
Fibrin degradation products (FDPs)	Increased FDPs
Accelerated clot lysis	Enhanced euglobulin clot lysis time

PFA, platelet function analyser.

Table 2 Differential diagnosis of thrombotic microangiopathies

Condition	Specific tests
Disseminated intravascular coagulopathy	Raised fibrin degradation products, D-dimers, reduced fibrinogen, prolonged PT/APTT
Pre-eclampsia/HELLP	Raised transaminases
SLE/scleroderma/vasculitis/APS	Positive ANA, anticardiolipin antibodies, lupus anticoagulant
Evans' syndrome (haemolysis and ITP)	Positive direct Coombs' test
Haemagglutinin inhibition test	Platelet-associated and heparin antibodies
TTP/HUS	ADAMTS-13 absent

ADAMTS-13, a disintegrin and metalloproteinase with thrombospondin motif 13; ANA, antibody to nuclear antigen; APS, antiphospholipid antibody syndrome; APTT, activated partial thromboplastin time; FDPs, fibrin degradation products; HELLP, haemolysis, elevated liver enzymes, low platelets; HUS, haemolytic–uraemic syndrome; ITP, immune thrombocytopenic purpura; PT, prothrombin time; SLE, systemic lupus erythematosus; TTP, thrombotic thrombocytopenic purpura.

Box 3 Contributing factors of disseminated intravascular coagulopathy in obstetrical practice

- Sepsis/severe infection
- Birth trauma/surgical intervention
- Obstetrical calamities (amniotic fluid embolism, abruptio placentae)
- Toxic/immunological reactions (transfusion reactions, recreational drugs)
- Massive blood loss with inadequate replacement therapy
- Co-morbidities (diabetes, heart failure, renal/liver disease, sickle cell disease, underlying malignancy)

In patients with a thrombotic microangiopathy, the haematologist should be asked to help differentiate several related causes on the basis of simple coagulation tests, blood film examination and specific confirmatory tests. The differential diagnosis and important distinguishing features are enumerated in Table 2.

Thrombotic thrombocytopenic purpura (TTP) is an uncommon but potentially devastating condition, which may arise in pregnancy and the postpartum period. The consistent features are thrombocytopenia, microangiopathic haemolytic anaemia and ischaemic symptoms due to widespread formation of thrombi in the terminal circulation of several organs resulting in neurological and renal manifestations.

Thrombotic thrombocytopenic purpura is rare (2–10 per million); however, had a high mortality (80–90 per cent) until the introduction of plasma exchange but is still around 10–20 per cent. The condition is now known to be due to ADAMTS-13 deficiency. ADAMTS-13 (a disintegrin and metalloprotease with thrombospondin-13 repeats) is a plasma ion-dependent plasma metalloproteinase (which cleaves endothelial-bound ultralarge vWF multimers). Failure to cleave vWF multimers leads to persistence in plasma and endothelial cells of ultralarge multimers, which tend to aggregate platelets. ADAMTS-13 is, therefore, absent in TTP, but mild to moderate deficiency of ADAMTS-13 has been found in pregnancy, liver disease, HELLP (haemolysis, elevated liver enzymes, low platelets) syndrome, inflammatory states, the postoperative period and autoimmune diseases.

■ The thrombocytopathies (platelet disorders)

The clinical manifestations of a reduction in platelets or functional abnormality are characterised by:

- spontaneous or immediate bleeding after trauma;
- mucosal bleeding;
- petechiae or purpura;
- haemarthrosis or deep haematomas (rarely occur).

The congenital and inherited thrombocytopathies are uncommon (Box 4) but worthy of exclusion.

In neonatal alloimmune thrombocytopenia the maternal platelet count is normal, complicating 1:1000 to 2000 live births, with half of the cases presenting in primigravids. Haemorrhagic manifestations (petechiae, ecchymoses) are common but 10–20 per cent of infants will have an intracranial haemorrhage *in utero*. Half of the cases are due to sensitisation and the development of alloantibody to the paternal human platelet antigen-1a (HPA-1a), also known as platelet antigen 1 (Pl-A1), present on the infant's platelets but lacking in the mother. The infant will be born severely haemorrhagic and thrombocytopenic (50 per cent cases with a platelet count <20), and the treatment is to infuse HPA-1a-negative platelets or, if unavailable, the mother's harvested platelets to the infant. The recurrence rate is high: up to 100 per cent depending on the zygosity of the father. Infants in subsequent pregnancies will be equally or more severely affected.

Thrombocytopenia in pregnancy is relatively common, but it is important to be clear about

Box 4 Congenital and inherited platelet disorders

Congenital
Drugs/chemicals
- Maternal ingestion of ethanol, thiazides, oestrogens

Isoimmune
- Neonatal alloimmune thrombocytopenia (NATN)

Bone marrow infiltration
- Congenital leukaemia, mucopolysaccharidosis

Infections
- Maternal toxoplasmosis, cytomegalovirus, rubella, herpes simplex virus, hepatitis

Inherited
Thrombocytopenia with:
- Reduced platelet size (Wiskott–Aldrich syndrome)
- Normal platelet size [TAR (thrombocytopenia, absent radii), amegakaryocytosis]
- Increased platelet size (May–Hegglin anomaly)

Thrombocytopathies
Disorders of:
- Platelet adhesion (Bernard–Soulier syndrome)
- Platelet aggregation (Glanzmann's thrombasthenia)

Box 5 Thrombocytopenia in pregnancy

Definition and terminology
- Mild thrombocytopenia (100–150)
- Moderate (50–100)
- Severe (<50)

Differential diagnosis
- Increased platelet destruction – immune, abnormal platelet activation, consumption
- Decreased platelet production – leukaemia, aplastic anaemia, folate deficiency

Box 6 Causes of thrombocytopenia in pregnancy

- Gestational thrombocytopenia
- Pregnancy-induced hypertension
- HELLP (haemolysis, elevated liver enzymes, low platelets) syndrome
- Pseudothrombocytopenia
- Human immunodeficiency virus infection
- Immune thrombocytopenic purpura
- Antiphospholipid syndromes
- Hypersplenism
- Disseminated intravascular coagulation
- Thrombotic thrombocytopenic purpura
- Haemolytic–uraemic syndrome
- Congenital thrombocytopenia
- Drug-induced (heparin, quinine, quinidine, zidovudine, sulphonamides)

definitions and terminology (Box 5). The main causes are listed in Box 6. Blood film examination will exclude pseudothrombocytopenia due to consumption, platelet clumps or *in vitro* aggregation. However, the common differential diagnosis is between the following:

- gestational thrombocytopenia;
- immune thrombocytopenia (ITP);
- associated with pregnancy-induced hypertension (PIH).

Gestational thrombocytopenia is common (8 per cent of pregnancies) and mild (invariably with a platelet count over 70, usually over 100). There are no clinical manifestations or bleeding, and it is usually picked up incidentally on routine full blood count. The platelet count returns to normal 2–12 weeks after delivery. There is therefore an extremely low risk of fetal or neonatal thrombocytopenia. The aetiology remains uncertain, but is perhaps related to accelerated platelet consumption.

Immune thrombocytopenia complicated between 1:1000 and 10 000 pregnancies, resulting from the presence of an immunoglobulin G (IgG) antiplatelet antibody and immune-mediated platelet destruction. However, with the variable detection of the platelet-associated antibody, the diagnosis remains one of exclusion, namely:

- persistent thrombocytopenia <100;
- normal or increased megakaryocytes on bone marrow examination;
- exclusion of other systemic disorders or splenomegaly.

The symptoms are usually mild both for the mother (easy bruising, gingival bleeding) and infant (minor bleeding associated with thrombocytopenia, approximately 10 per cent will have platelets <50). Serious bleeding occurs in about 3 per cent of affected infants, with intracranial haemorrhage in less than 1 per cent. The infant platelet count nadir will be several days after delivery.

There is incomplete correlation between maternal and fetal thrombocytopenia and outcome. However, the maternal platelet count is used as a surrogate marker and corticosteroid therapy is indicated (1 mg/kg per day) when the platelet count is below 80 or falling rapidly. Nearer term, intravenous immunoglobulin is used (0.4 g/kg per day) for a more rapid response. The exact mechanism of action of these therapies is unknown, but involves immune suppression and blockade to some degree.

Pregnancy-induced hypertension accounts for approximately 1:5 of maternal thrombocytopenia in pregnancy (21 per cent), is usually moderate and rarely below 20. In 10 per cent of cases, it is associated with a microangiopathic blood picture and haemolysis, and elevated liver enzymes – the so-called HELLP (haemolysis, elevated liver enzymes, low platelets) syndrome. The cause is unknown but is likely to be multi-factorial; the management is expectant with replacement therapy of blood products and early delivery, where indicated.

BLEEDING IN CHILDHOOD (VAGINAL)

Kausik Banerjee

The main causes of vaginal bleeding in children are listed in Box 1.

Box 1 Common causes of vaginal bleeding in childhood

- Foreign body
- Vulvovaginitis
- Trauma, which may or may not be associated with sexual abuse
- Precocious puberty
- Haemorrhagic cystitis
- Bleeding diathesis
- Neoplasms
- Urethral prolapse
- Exposure to exogenous sex steroids

A *foreign body* is commonly responsible for vaginal bleeding in paediatric patients. Bleeding in the presence of a foul-smelling discharge is suggestive of foreign body in the vagina. Ultrasonography is often helpful. Examination under anaesthesia often using a small hysteroscope placed in the vagina confirms the diagnosis; the irrigating fluid can often flush out the foreign body and resolve the problem.

Poor hygiene often contributes to recurrent *vulvovaginitis* and appropriate advice is necessary regarding personal hygiene.

Most injuries to the genital area are accidental. However, the possibility of sexual *abuse* should be considered in every case where vaginal trauma is suspected. Blunt injury may cause formation of a haematoma. A small vulvar haematoma can be managed by local pressure. Analgesics are recommended.

Penetrating vaginal injury warrants very careful examination and child sexual abuse needs to be seriously considered. Urgent communication with the hospital's paediatric team is of paramount importance if sexual abuse is suspected. It may be necessary to involve other agencies (police and social services). A good clinical practice is to organise a joint examination by a paediatrician trained in child sexual abuse and by a forensic specialist for suspected sexual abuse so that maximum information can be gathered with minimum discomfort to the child.

Vaginal bleeding could be the first manifestation of *precocious puberty* in a young girl. This is discussed in detail in Puberty, precocious.

Adenovirus infection or drug toxicity (cyclophosphamide) are two common causes of *haemorrhagic cystitis*. It usually presents with sterile haematuria, dysuria, frequency and urgency. Viral infection is self-limiting while the drug toxicity resolves after withdrawal of treatment.

Blood dyscrasias responsible for vaginal bleeding in a child are listed in Table 1. A detailed history and systemic examination followed by a full blood count and coagulation screen are diagnostic. Treatment depends on the primary cause.

Table 1 Bleeding disorders responsible for vaginal bleeding in childhood

Underlying pathology	Clinical entity
Low platelets	Idiopathic thrombocytopenic purpura, leukaemia, aplastic anaemia, chemotherapy-related bone marrow depression, hypersplenism
Platelet dysfunction	Glanzmann's thrombasthenia, Bernard–Soulier's disease
Clotting disorders	Von Willebrand's disease, liver dysfunction

Urethral prolapse, although uncommon, is a known cause of vaginal bleeding. This is characterised by the urethral mucosa protruding through the meatus and forming a haemorrhagic vulvar mass. A big 'mass' is often responsible for dysuria. Often this responds to topical oestrogen.

Benign and malignant *tumours* of the vulva may present as vaginal bleeding. Sarcoma botryoides

is a vaginal carcinoma that occurs primarily in girls under the age of 2 years (90 per cent are under the age of 5). Mesonephric carcinoma commonly affects girls above the age of 3 years. Clear cell adenocarcinoma is often associated with antenatal exposure to diethyl stilbestrol. Suspicion of any of these conditions warrants urgent referral to a paediatric oncologist for confirmation of diagnosis, treatment and counselling.

Capillary venous malformation of the labia majora has been reported as a cause of vaginal bleeding in children. The differential diagnoses include capillary haemangioma and other vascular malformation. The malformation can be locally excised.

■ **Further reading**

Daniels RV, McCuskey C. Abnormal vaginal bleeding in the nonpregnant patient. *Emerg Med Clin North Am* 2003; **21:** 751–72.

Ellis MH, Byeth Y. Abnormal vaginal bleeding in adolescence as the presenting symptom of a bleeding diathesis. *J Pediatr Adolesc Gynecol* 1999; **12:** 127–31.

Minjarez DA. Abnormal bleeding in adolescents. *Semin Reprod Med* 2003; **21:** 363–3.

Sanfilippo JS. Gynecologic problems of childhood. In: Behrman RE, Kliegman R, Jenson WE, eds. *Nelson Textbook of Pediatrics*, 16th edn. Philadelphia: WB Saunders, 2000: 1663–4.

BLEEDING DURING EARLY PREGNANCY

Mala Arora

Bleeding in the first trimester of pregnancy may occur in one-fifth of all pregnancies and nearly half of them miscarry.[1] The incidence of spontaneous abortion is estimated at 15–22 per cent of all pregnancies. It is thus a commonly encountered problem that can be due to a variety of causes classifiable as obstetric, i.e. related to pregnancy, and non-obstetric, i.e. not related to pregnancy, of which the former are more common.

■ Obstetric causes

Bleeding with viable embryo

This can only be ascertained by performing an ultrasound scan.

It is generally believed that bleeding from the uterine cavity in early pregnancy is associated with fetal demise.

- However, in some patients, there may bleeding at the time of the missed menstrual period for the first couple of months of pregnancy owing to shedding of the decidua parietalis.
- It has also been clinically observed that embryos with karyotypical abnormalities like trisomies, monosomies or Robertsonian translocations can present with threatened abortion in early pregnancy. The pregnancy, however, continues but there is an increased incidence of intrauterine growth restriction, hydrops fetalis and stillbirth.
- In rare instances of bicornuate uterus, there may cyclical bleeding from the non-pregnant horn.

Low implantation of the gestational sac

The implantation occurs in the fundus or body of the uterus in the majority of pregnancies. However, sometimes it may implant in the lower segment and, as the lower uterine segment stretches to accommodate the growing sac, there may be bleeding. In this case the pregnancy may develop a placenta praevia and subsequent haemorrhage may occur later in the pregnancy.

Retrochorionic bleeding

In patients with early pregnancy bleeding there may be ultrasound evidence of retrochorionic collection of blood (Fig. 1) This is analogous to abruptio placentae in late pregnancy. This bleeding may vary in amount but may resolve spontaneously in many instances allowing the pregnancy to proceed normally thereafter.

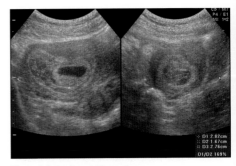

Figure 1 Retroplacental haematoma.

Multifetal gestation

In pregnancies induced by artificial reproductive techniques there may be multifetal gestation of the higher order, such as quintuplets or sextuplets. This may result in bleeding due to distension of the lower segment.

Bleeding with a non viable embryo

This can be due to a variety of causes as listed below.

Missed miscarriage

This occurs when fetal growth is arrested in early pregnancy but the products have not been expelled. The cause of fetal demise could be intrinsic to the embryo, such as karyotypical abnormalities or extrinsic in its environment. The first manifestation of this condition is bleeding or discharge in early pregnancy. The bleeding may be painless initially but is later accompanied with uterine cramps.

Occasionally, a routine ultrasound scan will diagnose a missed miscarriage before the bleeding becomes obvious.

Ectopic pregnancy

The main symptom of an ectopic or tubal pregnancy is pain, but this is accompanied by vaginal bleeding in many cases. The bleeding is due to shedding of the decidua formed in the uterine cavity. In women with irregular bleeding where the periods have previously been normal and regular, it is worth considering whether the woman is pregnant and, if so, exactly where the pregnancy is located.

Gestational trophoblastic disease (GTD)

Molar pregnancy is the commonest form of GTD, which manifests classically as bleeding in early pregnancy. The bleeding in this case may be heavy and persistent, often painless. The uterus is larger than the period of amenorrhea would indicate and has a soft boggy feel. Ultrasound scan may show an absence of gestational sac and the interior of the uterus has a 'snowstorm' appearance. Occasionally, a viable embryo may be present with gestational trophoblastic disease (Fig. 2).

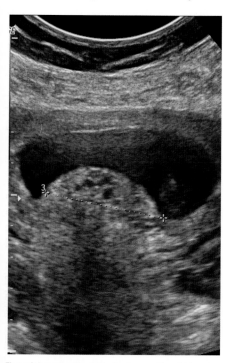

Figure 2 Gestational trophoblastic disease with a viable embryo.

The cause is genetic. At the time of fertilization the genetic component of the oocyte is lost and both genetic components are derived from the paternal germ line. The chromosomal composition is 46XX.

Vanishing twin syndrome

Pregnancy may start as a twin gestation but, for some reason, one of the twins may stop growing at an early stage. The non-viable sac is then absorbed gradually but may result in bleeding during this period. In this case the bleeding consists of altered brown blood, and may or may not be accompanied by cramps.

Vasa praevia

The presence of a blood vessel on the underside of the gestational sac will lead to bleeding from that vessel as the gestational sac grows. This bleeding is more commonly seen in the second and third trimester, but occasionally can occur in the first trimester.

■ Non-obstetric causes

These are listed in Box 1.

> **Box 1** Non-obstetric causes of bleeding per vaginam
>
> **Cervical**
> - Cervical polyps
> - Cervical ectropion
> - Cervical pregnancy
> - Cervical cancer
>
> **Vaginal**
> - Trichomonas vaginitis
> - Bacterial vaginosis
> - Foreign bodies in the vagina
> - Vaginal tumours
>
> **Bleeding disorders**
> - Thrombocytopenia
> - Haemophilia
> - Von Willebrand's disease
>
> **Drug induced**
> - Heparin
> - Aspirin
> - Warfarin

Cervical

Bleeding from the cervix can be due to the following.

Cervical polyps

These are benign lesions that can be fibrous or myomatous in nature. They may be small or large, and are seen protruding through the cervical os. Very often they can be easily avulsed in the outpatient setting and sent for histopathological examination.

Cervical ectropion

Prior to puberty the squamocolumnar junction is within the endocervical canal. As a result of puberty, the pill or pregnancy, the columnar epithelium everts and comes to face the vagina. This will cause metaplasia in that the columnar epithelium will change to squamous cells. The area can become inflamed and develop cervicitis. The cervix appears reddened as the columnar epithelium is one-cell-thick and thus translucent, giving the impression of vascularity beneath. Likewise it can be easily traumatised and can develop contact bleeding (smear or coitus). If significant, it can be treated with cautery or cryotherapy. This should probably be avoided in pregnancy unless absolutely essential.

Cervical pregnancy

The cervix is a rare site for ectopic pregnancy. This can be a cause of bleeding and may also be difficult to treat or remove surgically owing to the possibility of considerable haemorrhage.

Cervical cancer

This may be a squamous cell carcinoma or adenocarcinoma. The age of presentation of cervical cancer is often in the reproductive age group. Hence it can occasionally present for the first time in pregnancy (see Cervical swelling).

Vaginal

Bleeding from the vagina can be due to the following:

- vaginitis most commonly due to vaginal thrush, which is common in early pregnancy;
- *Trichomonas vaginalis* may cause vaginitis, which presents as bleeding;
- bacterial vaginosis, which is a mixed infection of the vagina by organisms of low virulence, such as *Peptostreptococcus, Ureaplasma urealyticum*, etc.;
- foreign bodies in the vagina, the commonest being forgotton tampons, may also present with a blood-mixed discharge;
- vaginal tumours, such as polyps, may cause bleeding, but are uncommon, as are any malignant tumours in the vagina.

Bleeding disorders

Bleeding disorders, such as thrombocytopenia, haemophilia and von Willebrand's disease, may cause problems, although haemophilia is rare in women. However, Christmas disease does occur in women.

Drug induced

The use of heparin, aspirin or warfarin during pregnancy may lead to spontaneous bleeding.

Bleeding from other sites

Bleeding haemorrhoids are often confused with vaginal bleeding. Similarly, lesions on the vulva, such as haemangiomas that bleed, may be confused with vaginal bleeding.

■ Diagnosis and investigations

Bleeding in early pregnancy is most often from the uterus in the form of threatened miscarriage; however a careful history of the amount of bleeding and any accompanying pain should be elicited. Prior to the advent of ultrasound, a prediction of viability was made, based on signs and symptoms.[2] Today, an ultrasound scan should be performed in all cases. It has been elucidated that clinical judgement is not a valid substitution for ultrasonographic assessment;[3] hence a transvaginal scan is the gold standard for diagnosing the cause of early pregnancy bleeding. It will diagnose all obstetric causes of bleeding. However, it is not able to predict an abnormal karyotype in early pregnancy,[4] and will only give a snapshot in time and may have limited predictive value.

Gentle per speculum examination should be performed if the cause is suspected to be local.

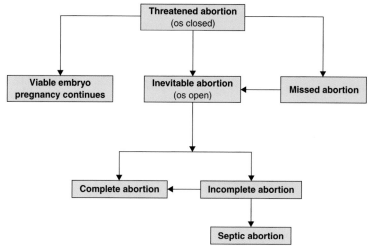

Figure 3 Bleeding in pregnancy.

Cervical (Pap) smears are usually avoided in pregnancy, but can be performed opportunistically if the woman has a poor attendance record. If no local cause is found, the patient should be investigated for bleeding disorders by tests such as platelet count, bleeding time, clotting time and prothrombin time.

In all cases, a blood group should be obtained and consideration given to administering anti-D, if the bleeding is excessive or if any operative procedure needs to be undertaken, e.g. evacuation of retained productions of conception.

■ Explanation of terminology of miscarriages (abortions; Fig. 3)

■ *Threatened miscarriage* is defined as the presence of bleeding with an intrauterine gestational sac when the cervical os is closed. The embryo may be viable, in which case the pregnancy will continue, or it may be non-viable as in a missed abortion.

■ *Inevitable miscarriage* is defined as bleeding in early pregnancy with an intrauterine gestational sac and an open cervical os. In this case, the pregnancy will abort and there may be associated pain.

■ *Incomplete miscarriage* is defined as bleeding with the presence of retained products of conception within the uterine cavity.

■ *Spontaneous miscarriage:* complete expulsion of the products of conception from the uterine

cavity is defined as 'spontaneous complete abortion'.

■ *Induced medical miscarriage:* when growth of a pregnancy is disrupted by administration of tablets of mifepristone (antiprogesterone) or misoprostol (prostaglandin).

■ *Induced surgical miscarriage:* when pregnancy is terminated by dilatation and curettage or suction evacuation.

■ *Medical termination of pregnancy* is synonymous with induced medical termination and may occur at up to 9 weeks' gestation.

■ *Septic miscarriage* is defined as incomplete abortion with intrauterine infection of retained products of conception.

■ References

1. Everet C. Incidence and outcome of bleeding before 20th week of pregnancy: prospective study from general practice. *BMJ* 1997; **315:** 32–7.

2. Chung TK, Sahota DS, Lau TK, et al. Threatened abortion, prediction of viability based on signs and symptoms. *Aust N Z J Obstet Gynecol* 1999; **39:** 443–7.

3. Wieringa de Waard M, Bonsel GJ, Ankum WM, Vos Jeroen, Bindels PJE. Threatened miscarriage in general practice: diagnostic value of history-taking and physical

examination. *Br J Gen Pract* 2002; **52:** 825–9.

4. Coulam CB, Goodman C, Dorfmann A. Comparison of ultrasonographic findings in spontaneous abortions with normal and abnormal karyotypes. *Hum Reprod* 1997; **12:** 823–6.

BLEEDING IN LATE PREGNANCY (ANTEPARTUM HAEMORRHAGE)

Nigel Bickerton

Bleeding in late pregnancy is defined as any bleeding per vaginam after 24 weeks of pregnancy and before the onset of labour. It remains a significant cause of maternal mortality and morbidity; therefore, all cases of bleeding should be taken seriously and assessed for degree of bleeding and the cause. Women who live in rural areas with a poor transport infrastructure or in areas of conflict are at greater risk of direct morbidity, as acute heavy bleeding in late pregnancy requires timely intervention. Severe bleeding can lead to impaired placental perfusion, resulting in signs of fetal distress due to hypoxia, which may cause severe neurological injury or stillbirth.

A woman with vaginal bleeding will be anxious about the cause and may be fearful for her wellbeing and that of her baby. The carer needs to be supportive and confident whilst assessing the clinical state of the woman and ascertaining the most likely cause of the bleed. It is important to remember that most bleeding arises from the maternal circulation rather than from that of the baby. Estimation of the volume of blood loss can be notoriously unreliable.

The measured incidence of antepartum haemorrhage in Europe is 3–5 per cent of pregnancies. The true incidence may be higher as some women do not report minor episodes of bleeding. The majority of patients with bleeding will fall into the following groups:

■ those with abruption of the placenta;
■ those with placenta praevia;
■ those with local causes coincidental to the pregnancy;
■ those in whom the cause is not identified.

The history usually helps to identify the cause of bleeding. The woman's clinical condition needs to be assessed whilst the history is taken rather than as a separate and later activity. The vital signs (pulse and blood pressure) should be checked to exclude clinical shock. Sometimes when there is only a small amount of external bleeding there may be extensive concealed blood loss, e.g. in abruption of the placenta. Pallor and peripheral skin clamminess often antecede hypotension and tachycardia. Healthy pregnant women may lose in excess of a unit of blood before pulse and blood pressure changes are demonstrable.

The commonest causes are usually related to placental bleeding. Ultrasound scanning performed at 20 weeks will usually rule out the diagnosis of placenta praevia, if it is away from the os at that stage. A low-lying placenta at that scan may appear to move in later pregnancy, as the lower uterine segment develops beneath it from 30 weeks onwards. Usually a repeat scan would be arranged from 34 weeks onwards to assess whether the placenta is likely to cause problems. Placenta praevia may be confirmed by scan, but abruption cannot be ruled out.

The nature and amount of bleeding may give some clue to the underlying diagnosis. Bright-red, sudden-onset, painless bleeding suggests placenta praevia, whilst darker blood loss associated with uterine pain, often constant in nature, suggests abruption. This is not invariable. A sudden loss of fetal movements may be suggestive of abruption. If labour has started there may be a 'show' of mucus and fetal membrane rupture with uterine contractions, which may present as blood loss.

■ Placental causes
Placenta praevia (Fig. 1)

The incidence is 2–5 per cent of pregnancies after 24 weeks and 1 per cent at term. The placenta implants into the lower uterine segment

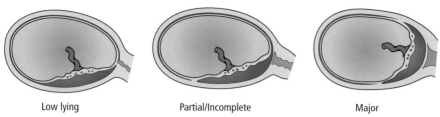

Low lying   Partial/Incomplete   Major

Figure 1 Diagram of placenta praevia.

either in whole or in part. This will account for 30 per cent of cases of bleeding in late pregnancy.

Placental abruption (Fig. 2)

The incidence is 1 per cent of pregnancies. Abruption is premature separation of the placenta due to bleeding. Women with a previously affected pregnancy have a 10 per cent chance of recurrence. This will account for about 20 per cent of cases of bleeding in late pregnancy

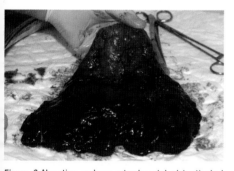

Figure 2 Abruption: a large retroplacental clot attached found at emergency Caesarean section at 30 weeks' gestation.

Marginal bleed

This will account for about 30 per cent of cases of bleeding in late pregnancy. The majority of cases in the group where no cause is identified have small episodes of bleeding that most often are due to repeated minor abruptions. The incidence of preterm delivery is increased significantly in this group.

An abdominal examination should be performed once the general clinical state of the woman has been assessed. A hard uterus due to a tonic contraction or rapid contractions is suggestive of abruption. The uterus is markedly tender over its whole surface or over a quadrant where the abruption has happened. The uterus may increase in size due to concealed bleeding. A high fetal presenting part or a malpresentation with a soft non-tender uterus suggests placenta praevia.

A speculum examination of the vagina and cervix should not be made until the woman has been scanned to exclude placenta praevia. To do so may cause profound bleeding, which could put the woman at risk. A cautious speculum examination following the exclusion of placenta praevia and after the bleeding has settled may help to find any local cause for the bleeding.

There is an association between placental abruption and pre-eclampsia. This needs to be remembered, as a woman may have signs of shock with a normal blood pressure. Despite this, such patients must have active resuscitation. After successful resuscitation patients can become hypertensive, showing the true level of their pre-eclampsia.

Urine testing for proteinuria may require the introduction of a urinary catheter.

The following possible causes for bleeding in late pregnancy should be considered when assessing the patient. The author notes that additional information may be provided during or after the examination that helps in identifying the true cause of bleeding. These causes can be considered anatomically.

■ Vulval causes

These are:

- vulval varices;
- trauma to vulva at the site of jewellery/piercings;
- vulval abscess;
- trauma to rapidly growing warts.

■ Anal causes

These are:

- haemorrhoids;
- anorectal carcinoma;
- ulcerative colitis.

■ Urethral causes

These are:

- urethral polyp;
- urethral wart;
- paraurethral abscess rupture;
- urethral trauma, e.g. with self-catheterizing.

■ Vaginal causes

These are:

- infections;
- trichomoniasis;
- candidiasis.

■ Cervical causes

These are:

- ectopy can cause bleeding, especially in labour;
- infected Nabothian follicle;
- passage of mucus operculum with blood;
- polyp;
- warts;
- carcinoma – both squamous and adenocarcinoma.

■ Uterine causes (uterine rupture)

Uterine rupture is extremely rare, usually occurring during labour (Fig. 3). It is classically described as a triad of pain, stopped contractions and abnormal cardiotocograph. Previous uterine surgery, such as Caesarean section or myomectomy, can increase this risk. Spontaneous rupture of the uterus adjacent to a fibroid has also been recorded.

■ Traumatic causes

The genital tract increases in vascularity during pregnancy, and trauma can cause significant

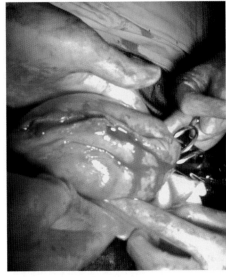

Figure 3 Spontaneous uterine rupture, in this case in an *in vitro* fertilization twin pregnancy at 35 weeks' gestation.

bleeding and is included for completeness. Causes include:

- lacerations following a fall;
- sexual assault – the woman may give no indication from the initial history that an assault has occurred;
- foreign bodies inserted and forgotten;
- incautious use of sex toys – from a circumferential tear injury at the vaginal introitus to a tear at the vaginal fornices due to a deep penetration injury. The latter may cause profound bleeding.

■ Fetal causes (vasa praevia)

As already stated most of the causes of bleeding are maternal in origin. In vasa praevia (Fig. 4), the blood vessels that converge to form the umbilical cord pass lateral to the placenta on the surface of the fetal membranes. Velamentous insertion, where the cord is inserted into the edge of the placenta, or a succenturiate lobe placenta with the vessels lying over the internal cervical os predispose to this state (Fig. 5). The incidence is 1 in 2000–3000 pregnancies.

The vessel wall may tear spontaneously during labour or due to direct trauma at amniotomy. Bleeding is bright red, sudden and profuse. Fetal tachycardia is followed rapidly by fetal shock and then death. The signs may follow artificial rupture

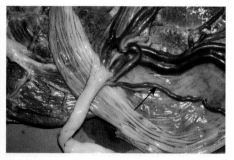

Figure 4 Blood vessel in the membranes of the amniotic sac. If this occurred over the cervix, it would be a vasa praevia.

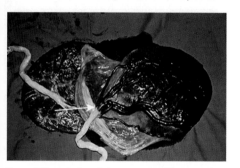

Figure 5 Placenta from twin pregnancy with velamentous insertion of cord on the right hand placenta.

of the membranes and are of rapid onset. Bleeding from vasa praevia carries a high fetal mortality due to rapid exsanguination.

BLEEDING, POSTMENOPAUSAL

Urvashi Prasad Jha and Swasti

■ Definition

Postmenopausal bleeding (PMB) is defined as any vaginal bleeding that occurs after a 12-month duration of amenorrhoea that has occurred due to menopause (which by definition is a retrospective diagnosis of amenorrhoea of 1 year duration due to failure of ovarian function and confirmed by raised follicle-stimulating hormone levels >30 U/mL). However, any vaginal bleeding that occurs after 6 months of amenorrhea from presumed menopause should be treated as 'suspect' and the cause of bleeding investigated and identified.

A single episode of postmenopausal bleeding of any amount – ranging from mere spotting of brownish discharge to heavy bleeding is abnormal and should be assessed. Both postmenopausal bleeding and discharge are common symptoms, and malignancy needs to be excluded, although most cases prove to be benign or inconsequential.

■ Common causes of postmenopausal vaginal bleeding

These are summarised in Box 1 and considered in more detail below.

> **Box 1** Common causes of postmenopausal vaginal bleeding
>
> - Atrophic vaginitis
> - Atrophic endometritis
> - Uterine polyp – endometrial/fibroid
> - Endometrial hyperplasia
> - Endometrial neoplasia/carcinoma
> - Intake of exogenous unopposed oestrogens
> - Miscellaneous causes from the genital tract, such as:
>   - cervical neoplasia/dysplasia
>   - cervical polyp
>   - adnexal masses – benign or malignant
>   - trauma – vulvovaginal, perineal, pelvic
>   - chronic endometritis, e.g. tubercular
>   - uterine sarcoma
>   - pregnancy-associated bleeding, if within the first year of menopause
> - Systemic bleeding disorders and anticoagulation usage
> - Non-vaginal causes often mistaken for vaginal bleeding, including:
>   - urethral caruncle
>   - cystitis
>   - urinary bladder polyp
>   - urinary bladder neoplasia
>   - anal haemorrhoids
>   - anal fissure
>   - rectal polyp
>   - carcinoma of rectum or anus

Atrophic vaginitis

'Senile vaginitis', a somewhat politically incorrect term is often used in place of 'atrophic vaginitis'. It is due to non-specific vaginal inflammation and extreme thinning of vaginal epithelium as a result of oestrogen deficiency. Even the slightest of trauma from intercourse or dabbing oneself dry may result in bleeding due to atrophic changes. This condition is easily treated and prevented by local application of oestrogen creams or oral oestrogens. All precautions taken with hormone replacement therapy (HRT) prescriptions must be followed.

Vaginal oestrogens are absorbed systemically to some extent. If used continuously for long durations, say beyond 8–12 weeks, by women with a uterus, the effect on the uterus is considered akin to taking prolonged systemic low doses of unopposed oestrogen HRT. This could result in prolonged unopposed oestrogenic stimulation of the endometrium, placing the woman at risk of endometrial hyperplasia and neoplasia. Hence, if continuous use of vaginal oestrogens is planned, the woman should be advised to have an intermittent progestogenic withdrawal bleed every 8–12 weeks.

Of the various types of oestrogens available for application, oestriol creams are effective and the safest of all the oestrogen types, as it is the 'weakest' oestrogen available with minimal systemic effects despite a good therapeutic effect on the vagina and the uterus.

Atrophic endometritis

Endometrial inflammation and thinning that occurs as a result of oestrogen deficiency is known as atrophic endometritis (Fig. 1). It may result in postmenopausal spotting or even bleeding, particularly in hypertensive women.

This is a diagnosis of exclusion after more sinister pathological causes of postmenopausal bleeding within the uterus are excluded by a hysteroscopy and biopsy. Other causes of bleeding from the genital tract may be due to adnexal masses or cervical lesions, and must be excluded before treatment is started for

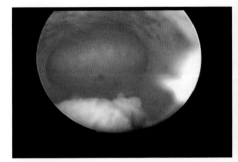

Figure 1 Hysteroscopic view of atrophic endometrial cavity.

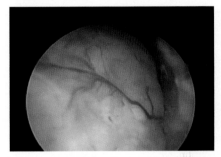

Figure 2 Hysteroscopic view of benign endometrial polyp.

atrophic endometritis. The treatment is HRT, which again should be advised using principles of HRT prescription. Any associated uncontrolled hypertension, if present, should also be controlled.

Uterine polyps

Uterine polyps are a common cause of postmenopausal bleeding. Endometrial polyps are usually inflammatory, but may occasionally have hyperplastic or neoplastic changes of the covering endometrium (Fig. 2). The uterine polyps can be of fibroid origin and are much more common if other fibroids are present, although they rarely display sarcomatous changes.

Intrauterine polyps may be identified as polyps on transvaginal ultrasound or seen just as thickened endometrium. Saline sonohysterography is a particularly useful diagnostic tool to identify intrauterine polyps. However, not only can hysteroscopy confirm the presence of polyps but it can also be used simultaneously to excise and remove them. A blind dilatation and curettage (D&C) can easily miss removing a polyp, especially if it is mobile.

Endometrial hyperplasia

The term 'hyperplasia' means thickened lining. The classification of endometrial hyperplasia has been simplified as follows:

- simple hyperplasia (risk of malignancy 1 per cent);
- complex hyperplasia (risk of malignancy 3 per cent);
- simple hyperplasia with atypia (risk of malignancy 8 per cent);
- complex hyperplasia with atypia (risk of malignancy 22–30 per cent).

These hyperplasias can be treated with progestogen therapy for 3 months followed by a repeat D&C. If by then the hyperplasia has reverted to normal, the progestogen therapy can be continued for further 9 months. If the hyperplasia without atypia persists despite progestogen therapy, the patient should be offered a hysterectomy. If the hyperplasia has atypia, the patient should also be offered hysterectomy because of its malignant potential. As a general rule, one would usually have a low threshold for surgical management as the condition may well recur. Factors aiding the decision to undertake a hysterectomy will be the presence or absence of symptoms, and the age and general medical condition of the woman.

It should be borne in mind that, in postmenopausal women, levels of circulating oestrogens are really low. The development of hyperplasia may be reflective of continuous oestrogen stimulation with either exogenous or endogenous oestrogens. In patients with unexplained endogenous oestrogen production (e.g. non-obese patients), the possibility of a small undetected ovarian granulosa cell tumor must be kept in mind and investigated by assessing oestradiol and inhibin-A levels. A hysterectomy may be warranted in such patients with even simple hyperplasias without atypia after adequate counselling.

Endometrial neoplasia

Endometrial neoplasia (Fig. 3) and its grade is diagnosed on histopathological examination of endometrial tissue. It has to be managed after appropriately investigating and assessing the extent of disease. (See Uterine swellings for details.)

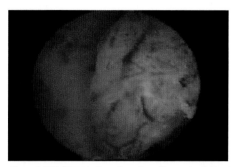

Figure 3 Hysteroscopic view of a polyp with prominent blood vessels. Histology revealed a well-differentiated endometrial cancer within the polyp.

Intake of exogenous oestrogens

After 2003, with the release of the 'Women's Health Initiative' and the 'Million Women Study' results, the use of hormone replacement therapy decreased significantly. Prior to this, one of the commonest causes of postmenopausal bleeding was from problems with exogenous oestrogen use. Missed doses of medication and failure to follow the schedule of advised HRT often results in bleeding episodes. In women on low-dose HRT, associated gastrointestinal problems, either acute or chronic, may result in partial failure of absorption of HRT, leading to waxing and waning oestrogen levels, and episodes of breakthrough postmenopausal spotting. In developing countries, with rampant problems of chronic giardiasis or amoebiasis, this is a very relevant consideration.

In women on treatment with a continuous combined HRT regimen, if irregular bleeding persists after the initial 3–6 months or irregular spotting or bleeding develops after the first 3 months of no bleeding, the woman should be investigated and assessed for another cause of postmenopausal bleeding. Additionally, if withdrawal bleeding occurs after sequential cyclic oestrogen–progestogen therapy beyond the expected time of withdrawal, the patient should be investigated as for postmenopausal bleeding.

Patients on tamoxifen therapy, with its paradoxic oestrogen-like action on the endometrium, behave similarly to patients on unopposed oestrogen therapy. They are thus at risk of developing endometrial hyperplasia, polyps or even neoplasia, and need to be managed accordingly with a low threshold to undertake hysteroscopy/D&C depending on symptoms.

Miscellaneous causes of bleeding from the genital tract

Cervical lesions, such as infected everted cervices, severe cervicitis, cervical polyps and carcinoma (squamous or adenomatous) of the cervix may also result in postmenopausal bleeding, which is usually postcoital but may also occur spontaneously without evident history of local trauma. These lesions are usually visible on a careful speculum examination, which must always be performed in women who present with postmenopausal bleeding. It is only in patients with endocervical lesions that inspection of the cervix fails to reveal the problem. A Pap smear should always be considered (NHSCSP guidelines) if there is no active bleeding. Obvious infection and contact bleeding in the absence of a cervical lesion should first be treated by local antibiotic/antifungal creams or pessaries, as appropriate, and a Pap smear taken thereafter. In the confirmed absence of endometrial malignancy, the Pap smear may need to be repeated after a 2–4-week course of local oestrogen therapy.

Adnexal tumours of ovarian and fallopian tube origin – benign or malignant – may also present with postmenopausal bleeding by virtue of functional ovarian tumours producing oestrogens, or the association of the pelvic congestion and increased vascularity with non-functional tumours.

Chronic endometritis of tuberculosis has also been known to cause postmenopausal spotting or bleeding. This is of particular relevance in countries with a high incidence of tuberculosis, such as the Indian subcontinent.

Rarely, a uterine sarcoma and other uterine tumours (mixed mullerian types) may present with postmenopausal bleeding.

Local perineal or genital tract trauma of any origin may sometimes result in significant vaginal blood loss. It is not unknown in countries like India for older women, who are unable to make hasty retreats from attacking and chasing bulls and cattle, to end up with resultant trauma to any part of their body, including damage to the pelvis and perineum from cattle horns. An intriguing cause indeed of PMB!

Systemic bleeding disorders

Rarely, even postmenopausal women may have a systemic cause of vaginal bleeding superimposed against a backdrop of severe atrophic endometritis. The common causes of these may be:

- thrombocytopenia;
- leukaemia;
- pancytopenia from immunosuppression, chemotherapy or bone marrow suppression;
- anticoagulation (iatrogenic), especially when a high international normalised ratio (INR) is a therapeutic requirement;
- secondary coagulopathy from liver disease.

Other congenital bleeding disorders, such as haemophilia and von Willebrand's disease, are usually diagnosed well before the menopause.

A high index of suspicion is required to diagnose these conditions as a cause of PMB. Diagnosis and treatment are directed at the cause.

Non-vaginal bleeding

Non-vaginal bleeding could often be mistaken by women to be vaginal in origin. Surrounding structures and problems that need to be considered from the urogenital part of the perineum are a bleeding urethral caruncle, haematuria from acute or chronic cystitis, bladder polyp or even neoplasia. This bleeding is usually painless, although occasionally associated with local perineal or pelvic pain.

Similarly, rectal bleeding can be mistaken for bleeding of vaginal origin. Anorectal piles, fissure *in ano* and malignancy may be other offending causes to be considered as the source of bleeding from the posterior part of the perineum.

■ Initial evaluation and stabilization

Assessment of blood loss

In some situations, the bleeding may be excessive, acute and possibly life threatening. In these circumstances, it is mandatory to make a rapid initial assessment of the general condition first and initiate resuscitative measures as for any patient with haemodynamically significant bleeding. After assessment of vital signs and local examination reveal whether the source of bleeding is the vulva, vagina, cervix or uterus, appropriate fluid replacement should be commenced. Tears need to be sutured; heavy bleeding from cervical malignancy requires tight vaginal packing, and intractable intrauterine bleeding requires a D&C after a quick, portable, bedside, sonographic assessment where available. It is remarkable how some patients can tolerate significant anaemia and are well compensated.

Haemostatic agents, such as extracts of micronised flavonoids, tranexemic acid or antiprostaglandin agents (e.g. mefenamic acid) should be initiated. Under certain circumstances, large doses of androgenic progestogens may be required if the intrauterine bleeding is not controllable. Under special circumstances, an intrauterine tamponade may be provided to the uterus by introducing a Foley's catheter and blowing up the balloon to a size that is appropriate.

Uncontrolled life-threatening bleeding unresponsive to the above may require heroic measures involving uterine artery embolisation, or a laparotomy with an emergency hysterectomy or bilateral internal iliac artery ligation.

It is well to remember in these situations that there is a risk of disseminated intravascular coagulation (DIC) from consumption and baseline tests should be obtained for a DIC profile. Blood and blood products may be required (see Collapse in the puerperium and Bleeding disorders in pregnancy for details).

■ Diagnostic approach to a patient with postmenopausal bleeding (Fig. 4)

History

A good history should elucidate details of the pattern, amount and type of bleeding, and discern whether it is postcoital or from other precipitating causes, if any. The premenopausal menstrual history of the patient is useful background information. Of particular relevance is history of oral intake of drugs/HRT/tamoxifen or local vaginal application. It is also important to establish whether the bleeding site is indeed vaginal, and not rectal or urethral, and whether there is an associated recent history of easy bruising and bleeding from other sites.

Examination

A general physical examination assesses whether the patient is stable with chronic loss or is having an acute haemorrhage requiring immediate resuscitation.

An abdominal examination may reveal a pelvic mass. A pelvic examination starts with inspection in good light. A Pap smear may be taken, followed by colposcopy and cervical biopsy, if appropriate. A polyp arising from the ectocervix or from within the cervical canal or endometrial cavity may be visualised.

On bimanual examination, uterine fibroids and adnexal masses may be palpable. With increasing passage of time, uteri decrease in size. A bulky uterus without fibroids or adenomyosis is not normal after menopause and should alert the physician to the possibility of endometrial neoplasia.

Investigations

A vaginal ultrasound should always measure the endometrial thickness and comment on the

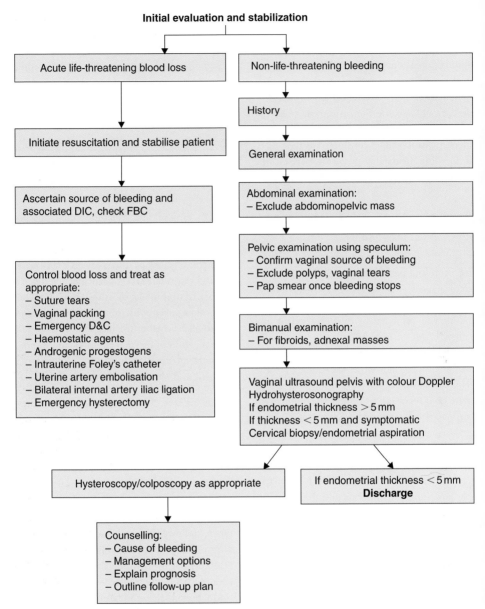

Figure 4 Management of postmenopausal bleeding. DIC, disseminated intravascular coagulation.

presence or absence of homogeneity in it. Polyps, submucus fibroids and adnexal masses, if identified, provide useful clues to the possible causes of bleeding.

A hydrohysterosonography, also known as saline infusion sonography, is particularly useful, if polyps or submucous fibroids are

suspected. The presence of endometrial calcification should alert the physician to the rare presence of tubercular endometritis, which is not unlikely in many parts of the developing world.

Colour Doppler studies of the uterine and ovarian vessels may support but not exclude a neoplastic aetiology.

These radiological investigations are sharp indicators of the likely aetiology. However, the diagnosis needs to be backed and confirmed by a tissue diagnosis.

A full blood count will be necessary to assess blood loss and if operative intervention will be required.

Cytology

A Pap smear provides information about cervical disease but may be falsely negative in up to 40–50 per cent of patients with cervical malignancy. The National Health Service Cervical Screening Programme recommends discontinuing cervical cytology after the age of 65 years.

Endometrial aspiration cytology is a cost effective and an almost non-invasive procedure that can be easily be performed in the outpatient setting. A positive report is specifically indicative of disease. However, a negative report, particularly in the presence of other suspicious features must be confirmed by a hysteroscopic assessment of the cervicoendometrial cavity.

Endometrial biopsy

Endometrial biopsy has become the standard of care in a patient with PMB. If inadequate or no sample is obtained owing to patient discomfort, cervical stenosis or inadequate tissue, a hysteroscopic assessment with a biopsy under vision, and a D&C must be performed.

Hysteroscopic assessment and directed biopsy

The gold standard of assessment of the endocervical canal and uterine cavity is a diagnostic hysteroscopy with a directed biopsy under vision of any suspicious area in the endocervical canal followed by endocervical curettage. Thereafter, the cervical os is dilated, the endometrial cavity is visualised and directed biopsy performed of any suspicious part of the endometrium. A hysteroscopic polypectomy is performed, if there are any polyps. This is followed by a uterine curettage.

In postmenopausal patients with a homogenous endometrium <4 mm thick without any abnormal vascularity in the absence of HRT, the chances of malignancy are extremely unlikely. Many clinicians use 5–6 mm as the cut-off point for normal postmenopausal endometrial thickness. The acceptable thickness of the endometrium is 5.5 mm in the presence of continuous combined HRT or tibolone, 4.0 mm if the woman is on raloxifene or sequential HRT on day 5 of the cycle and 8 mm if the woman is on tamoxifen. However, hysteroscopy should be undertaken regardless of endometrial thickness if the woman's symptoms persist.

Colposcopy with cervical biopsy

If the cervix or the cervical Pap smear is suspicious, a colposcopic assessment of the cervix must be performed and directed punch biopsies performed where indicated.

■ Further management

After the initial assessment of a woman with postmenopausal bleeding, it is imperative that the woman is appropriately counselled. Counselling is directed at allaying unnecessary fears, providing insight into possible causes, outlining the management plan, explaining the prognosis and helping women take informed decisions about their health. It should be an ongoing process that gradually narrows down the cause of the bleeding with each investigation and thereafter helps women decide whether the advised appropriate treatment is acceptable to them or not. It helps greatly to ensure acceptance of continued long-term treatment, where indicated and may prevent recurrences and unnecessary repeat investigations and heartache. In those women faced with malignancy, it forms the basis of future support and formulation of treatment plans as suitable to the individual woman.

In those circumstances where the woman is incapable of making decisions, as may happen in elderly postmenopausal women or in these social situations where family involvement is significant, counselling must involve the family or those caring for these women. If compliance with medical management is poor, the patient could be exposed repeatedly to major haemodynamic insults in some circumstances.

A therapeutic plan should be made out and clearly explained to the woman and her caregivers.

BLEEDING, RECTAL, DURING PREGNANCY

Dilip Visvanathan

Rectal bleeding usually occurs from diseases involving the colon, rectum and anus (Box 1). Bleeding from the upper gastrointestinal tract, like the oesophagus, stomach and small intestine, can present with dark-red blood loss per rectum because of a rapid transit time,[1] but usually presents as melaena (see Haematemesis in pregnancy). Rectal bleeding may be obvious as a result of acute/sudden blood loss. Patients with a more chronic blood loss may present with iron-deficiency anaemia and be found to have blood only on faecal occult blood testing. This section will consider rectal bleeding secondary to acute haemorrhage from the lower gastrointestinal tract.

Box 1 Causes of rectal bleeding in pregnancy

Anorectal conditions
- Haemorrhoids
- Anal fissure
- Solitary rectal ulcer syndrome (mucosal prolapse)

Large bowel conditions
- Inflammatory bowel disease
- Adenomatous polyps
- Carcinoma
- Arteriovenous malformation
- Meckel's diverticulum

■ History and evaluation

A detailed history from the patient may give clues to the underlying cause of the colorectal bleeding.

Bright-red blood separate from the stool suggests an anorectal cause. Diarrhoea and mucus mixed with darker blood suggests colitis or a neoplasm. A history of alteration in bowel habits, namely constipation and diarrhoea, with abdominal discomfort may suggest malignancy, whereas faecal urgency, acute bleeding and abdominal pain are more suggestive of colitis. A digital examination and proctosigmoidos copy can help diagnose an anorectal condition. A colonoscopy, although difficult in the bleeding patient, will help at least to identify the segment involved. Mesenteric angiography can help in diagnosis if radiological expertise is present. In the event of a woman who presents with acute rectal bleeding and haemodynamic compromise, surgical evaluation at the time of emergency treatment may be required. If a lower gastrointestinal cause cannot be found, then investigation of the upper gastrointestinal (GI) tract by upper GI endoscopy is recommended.[1]

■ Anorectal disease

Haemorrhoids and anal fissures are the commonest anorectal conditions that present during pregnancy, and may cause significant distress. The real incidence of these lesions is unknown.[2] They tend to be inadequately investigated and treated until after the pregnancy.

Haemorrhoids

Haemorrhoids in pregnancy are due to an increased circulating volume, increased venous congestion caused by compression of the superior rectal veins by the pregnant uterus, as well as the relaxing effect of progesterone on the smooth muscle in the walls of the veins.[3] Haemorrhoids may present with bleeding, prolapse, mucoid discharge, pruritus and rectal discomfort. It is important to exclude other causes of these symptoms, such as inflammatory bowel disease, anal fissure, and carcinoma of the colon, rectum or anus. However, the diagnosis may be obvious from simple inspection of the anus. Sigmoidoscopy and colonoscopy can be done safely in pregnancy.

Treatment during pregnancy is mainly directed to the relief of symptoms, especially pain control. The conservative management includes dietary modifications, increased fluid intake, stool softeners and analgesics. For many women, symptoms will resolve spontaneously soon after birth. Definitive treatments are, therefore, deferred until after delivery.

Rubber-band ligation can be safely performed in pregnancy for internal haemorrhoids. If the haemorrhoids are severely prolapsed or have associated ulceration, severe bleeding, fissure, or fistula and symptoms fail to respond to conservative measures, haemorrhoidectomy may need to be considered.[4,5]

Anal fissure

Anal fissure is a painful condition that affects a sizable majority of the population. It is usually caused by the passing of hard stools that damage the lining of the anus and cause a breach in its integrity. This leads to pain on defaecation with blood on the motion or after wiping the anus. Pregnant women are susceptible to this problem as a result of the increased incidence of constipation during the pregnancy. An increase in progesterone production in pregnancy results in relaxation of involuntary muscle and hence slowing of the bowel. A further contributing factor may be the prophylactic and therapeutic use of iron supplements during pregnancy, which can also have a constipating action.

Selecting a method of treating the condition that could achieve optimal clinical results, and the least pain and inconvenience to the patient, has always posed a challenge to the surgeons. While acute fissures could be managed with medical therapy alone, chronic fissures do need some form of manipulation or surgery to relieve internal sphincter spasm.[6]

Inflammatory bowel disease

Most pregnant women with a history of inflammatory bowel disease have uneventful pregnancies and exacerbations of disease can be controlled with medical therapy. It is rare for inflammatory bowel disease to present for the first time in pregnancy. When relapses of Crohn's disease do occur during pregnancy, they usually present during the first trimester. Most patients are already on some form of medical therapy. Surgery in pregnancy should be carried out depending on the mother's condition and especially in the presence of a suspected abscess causing peritonism.[7,8]

Many patients with a history of ulcerative colitis managed with ileal pouch anal anastomosis will become pregnant. Long-term outcomes of pregnancy and vaginal delivery in such patients are good.[9]

Colorectal cancer

Colon cancer during pregnancy is very rare and the majority of cases of colorectal carcinomas in pregnant women arise from the rectum. The diagnosis frequently is delayed because symptoms of colorectal cancer, such as rectal bleeding, nausea and vomiting, and constipation, are usually attributed to normal pregnancy or minor complications of pregnancy. Digital rectal examination, tests for occult blood, and flexible sigmoidoscopy followed by colonoscopy should be performed for complaints consistent with colonic disease.[1,10]

Treatment of colorectal cancer follows the same general guidelines as for non-pregnant patients. Primary surgical treatment should be performed whenever it is indicated. Later in pregnancy, it is preferable to delay surgery to allow fetal maturation and delivery. With respect to colon cancer, many authors recommend primary surgical treatment during the first half of the pregnancy because delaying treatment until after delivery may result in tumour spread. Therefore, in the first half of pregnancy, primary resection and anastomosis are advised.[11] Rectal cancer presenting in pregnancy is managed somewhat differently from colon cancer. During the first 20 weeks of pregnancy, patients wishing to carry their pregnancies to term may elect to have primary resection followed by chemotherapy after delivery. If the patient chooses to terminate the pregnancy, she may be managed as a non-pregnant patient after therapeutic abortion.[12]

During pregnancy, a variety of colorectal conditions merit special consideration for reasons related to the safety and timeliness of operation while preserving fetal viability and fertility. In benign conditions, there is more latitude to adopt a conservative approach. In the patient with malignancy, delaying surgical, chemotherapy or radiation therapy carries an unknown risk to the patient.[1] The patient's personal views regarding future fertility would also need to be addressed. A multidisciplinary team approach is recommended with close collaboration between the obstetrician, surgeon, oncologist, neonatologist and paediatrician.

■ References

1. Warrell D, Cox TM, Firth JD, Benz EJ. Oxford Textbook of Medicine, 4th edn. Oxford: Oxford University Press, 2004.
2. Simmons SC. Anorectal disorders in pregnancy. *Proc R Soc Med* 1972; **65**: 286.
3. Holschneider CH. Surgical diseases and disorders in pregnancy. In: DeCherney AH, Murphy Goodwin T, Nathan L, eds. *Current Obstetric and Gynecologic Diagnosis and Treatment*, 9th edn. New York: McGraw-Hill, 2003.
4. Cappell MS. The safety and efficacy of gastrointestinal endoscopy during pregnancy, *Gastroenterol Clin North Am* 1998; **27**: 37–71 (Abstract).
5. Abramowitz L, Sobhani I, Benifla JL, *et al.* Anal fissure and thrombosed external haemorrhoids before and after delivery. *Dis Colon Rectum* 2002; **45**: 650–5.
6. Medich DS, Fazio VW. Haemorrhoids, anal fissure, and carcinoma of the colon, rectum, and anus during pregnancy. *Surg Clin North Am* 1995; **75**: 77.
7. Hill JCA, Scott NA. Surgical treatment of acute manifestations of Crohn's disease during pregnancy. *J R Soc Med* 1997; **90**: 64–6.
8. Goetler CE, Stellato TA. Initial presentation of Crohn's disease in pregnancy: report of a case. *Dis Colon Rectum* 2003; **46**: 406–10.
9. Hahnloser D, Pemberton JH, Wolff BG, *et al.* Pregnancy and delivery before and after ileal pouch-anal anastomosis for inflammatory bowel disease: immediate and long-term consequences and outcomes. *Dis Colon Rectum* 2004; **47**: 1127–35.
10. Skilling JS. Colorectal cancer complicating pregnancy, *Obstet Gynecol Clin North Am* 1998; **25**: 417–21 (Abstract).
11. Cunningham F, Gant NF, Leveno KJ. *Williams Obstetrics.* New York: McGraw-Hill, 2001.
12. Ochshorn Y, Kupferminc MJ, Lessing JB, *et al.* Rectal carcinoma during pregnancy: a reminder and updated treatment protocols. *Eur J Obstet Gynecol Reprod Biol* 2000; **91**: 201–2.

BLOCKED NOSE IN PREGNANCY

Eva Lunderskov Papesch and Mike Papesch

Nasal obstruction in pregnancy can be due to all the usual causes (Box 1). In addition, nasal obstruction during pregnancy or 'rhinitis of pregnancy' occurs in up to 30 per cent of pregnant women.[1–3] It commonly occurs at the end of the third month of pregnancy and may persist for 1–2 months after delivery.[4] Symptoms include blocked nose, sneezing, rhinorrhoea and nasal itch. Nasal congestion is caused by oedema and increased blood volume in the nasal mucosa. Women who already have nasal obstruction prior to becoming pregnant may suffer considerable exacerbation of their blocked nose. Conversely the rhinitis of pregnancy itself leaves women more susceptible to obstruction and infection from common 'cold' viruses, and resultant bacterial sinusitis. Sinusitis has been

Box 1 Nasal obstruction: causes

Congenital
- Choanal atresia, septal deviation

Traumatic
- Septal deviation

Infection
- Acute/chronic viral/bacterial/fungal rhinitis/sinusitis

Neoplastic
- Benign: nasal polyps, inverted papilloma, pyogenic granuloma
- Malignant: adenocarcinoma

Allergy
- Allergic rhinitis

Autoimmune
- Wegener's granulomatosis, sarcoidosis, atrophic rhinitis

Iatrogenic
- Surgical, drug induced

Foreign body

Hormonal
- Rhinitis of pregnancy

Pharmacological
- Rhinitis medica mentosa

Vasomotor[6]
- Secondary to odours, alcohol, emotion, temperature change, pressure change, bright light, spicy food, gastro-oesophageal reflux disease

Occupational

Aetiology

Nasal obstruction during pregnancy is related to endocrine factors and is similarly seen in nasal blockage associated with the menstrual cycle. Topically applied oestrogens have produced congestion of the nasal mucosa and increased nasal resistance. However, increased levels of oestradiol and progesterone were not found in a study of pregnant women with nasal congestion compared to a control group of women without nasal congestion.[2] The regular use of the combined oral contraceptive pill has not been associated with increasing symptoms.[7]

Animal models have shown that vasoactive intestinal peptide (VIP), stimulated by progesterone and oxytocin, leads to increased nasal congestion.

The allergic manifestations in some pregnant women may be due to oestrogen deficiency, which results in low cortisone blood levels and a shorter hydrocortisone half-life than that present in normal pregnancy.

Electron micrographic and histochemical studies performed on the inferior turbinates of pregnant women have showed hyperactive tunical, goblet and seromucinous glands. There was also increased enzymic activity, particularly in the symptomatic group of women, indicating increased vascularity and metabolic activity. Increased cholinesterase activity suggested an overactivity of the parasympathetic system leading to increased glandular secretion and vascular congestion. This overactivity of the parasympathetic system may be an allergic response to placental or fetal proteins.[7]

The generalised increase in interstitial fluid volume, most marked in the third trimester of pregnancy, also directly affects the nasal mucosa, contributing to congestion.[3]

reported to be six times more common in pregnant than non-pregnant women.[5]

Interestingly, however, there are some women who experience nasal allergy symptom relief during pregnancy, possibly due to elevated cortisol levels.

Management

History

The relevant points include the length of history, the side of obstruction, any previous injury/surgery, exacerbating and relieving factors, associated symptoms consistent with sinusitis, history of atopy and response to previous treatments.

Examination

Anterior rhinoscopy allows assessment of the anterior nasal septum and the turbinates, and excludes any anterior nasal polyps. Prominent turbinates are often confused for nasal polyps. However, they are different in colour, and the easiest differentiating feature is that polyps are insensate to touch, whereas turbinates are not.

Rigid nasendoscopy allows complete examination of the nasal cavity as well as assessment of the postnasal space.

Investigation

RAST (radioallergosorbent test) testing for common environmental allergens as well as pets, animal dander and, if suspected, specific food allergy, may be useful.

Nasal rhinometry assesses airflow and is particularly used in research. Nitric oxide levels in the nose are measured to assess nasal blood flow indirectly. Levels are elevated in conditions such as rhinitis and are decreased with nasal polyps. Assessment of smell is performed by 'scratch and sniff' cards (University of Pennsylvania Smell Identification Test) cards or 'Sniffin' sticks' (University of Erlangen Smell Test).[8,9]

Computerised tomography (CT) scanning is used to assess the anatomy of the nose and sinuses, and also to assess the degree of sinusitis and/or polyposis. Ideally unnecessary radiological imaging is to be avoided, especially in the first trimester of pregnancy unless it is urgent or acute. In practice, diagnostic radiography during pregnancy not involving direct abdominal/pelvic high dosage is not associated with any significant adverse events.[10–13]

■ Treatment

General

Allergen avoidance remains important in known allergic rhinitis.[14] Tumble-drying

clothes, showering after returning home and closing windows on high pollen-count days can achieve avoidance of pollens. Mould allergens can be avoided by limiting indoor plants, frequent emptying of kitchen waste, good ventilation in the bathroom and laundering of bedlinen and clothes. House dust mite exposure and animal dander can be reduced by frequent hoovering, the use of antiallergenic bed covers and removal of pets.

Exercise appropriate for physical condition and gestational age may reduce symptoms.[15]

Medical treatment[16]

Topical saline preparations (e.g. Sterimar saline spray) can offer symptomatic relief and are completely safe.[15,17,18] Topical sodium cromoglycate also has an excellent safety profile and is useful for rhinitis control,[14,15] although it does require qds dosage.

Topical steroids

Intranasal steroids (e.g. fluticasone, mometasone, budesonide and beclomethasone) can be used for more severe nasal obstruction. There are no documented epidemiological studies of the use of intranasal corticosteroids (e.g. budesonide, fluticasone propionate, mometasone) during pregnancy. However, inhaled corticosteroids (beclomethasone and fluticasone) are not teratogenic and are commonly used by pregnant women who have asthma.[19–21] Fluticasone and mometasone have the lowest systemic absorption and are favoured by most rhinologists. They are effective in the control of rhinitis but may require a few weeks to achieve maximal benefit.

Topical ipratropium bromide is useful for symptomatic control of water rhinorrhoea. It is safe to use for acute asthma in pregnancy.[22,23]

Decongestants

Topical preparations such as xylometazoline are readily available 'over the counter'. They cause direct vasoconstriction and shrinkage of the nasal mucosa. However, the hormonal vasodilatation of nasal mucosa is relatively resistant to topical vasoconstrictors and overuse is common. This leads to downregulation of sympathomimetic receptors and a resultant rebound nasal congestion (rhinitis medica mentosa). They are also rapidly absorbed systemically and there is concern (although not established) that local vasoconstriction may cause placental insufficiency and/or exacerbate hypertension of pregnancy. They should be used sparingly.

Oral decongestants should be avoided in the first trimester as case-control studies have linked their use with the development of gastroschisis. Following the first trimester, pseudoephedrine could be used.[15]

Corticosteroids

Systemic use in rhinitis is rare; however, steroids can be used when medically indicated (e.g. acute asthma attack) and steroids given to prevent infant respiratory distress syndrome have not resulted in drug-related abnormalities.[16]

Antihistamines

These are used to treat allergic rhinitis. There has been argument for and against the safety of these drugs in pregnancy. Even though these drugs have been used safely in pregnancy, there remain concerns (that have not been substantiated), regarding teratogenicity. Chlorpheniramine and tripelenamine are preferred.[15] As always, the relative risk versus benefits must be considered.

Antibiotics

These should be used for specific infections associated with nasal obstruction, such as acute bacterial sinusitis. Penicillins (amoxicillin), cephalosporins and marcolides (erythromycin) are commonly used and are safe. Renal and liver function as well as serum drug levels can be monitored if there are concerns.

The following should be avoided:

- sulphonamides – may lead to: haemolytic anaemia and hyperbilirubinaemia;
- tetracycline – may lead to: teeth discoloration and impaired bone growth;

- trimethoprim – may lead to: hyperbilirubinaemia;
- aminoglycosides – may lead to: renal and neural arch anomalies (first trimester), ototoxicity and nephrotoxicity (third trimester);
- chloramphenicol – may lead to: grey baby syndrome in pregnancy; owing to lack of the necessary liver enzymes to metabolize this drug; chloramphenicol accumulates in the baby, causing hypotension, cyanosis and often death.

Surgical treatment

Ideally, surgery is postponed until after delivery or later in the pregnancy. Surgical options include the following:

Inferior turbinate reduction

The reduction of inferior turbinates can be performed with diathermy, fracturing, resection or a combination of these. Direct injection of steroids (triamcinolone) into the turbinates is described in the literature, it is not commonly practised in the UK. Topical steroids provide similar symptomatic relief. There is also the risk of embolisation into the retinal circulation, with resultant blindness. This is particularly so with the increased nasal mucosa vascularity of pregnancy.

Nasal polypectomy

Intranasal polypectomy under local anaesthetic can be considered if severe nasal symptoms are present.

Endoscopic sinus surgery

This can be undertaken for more extensive polypectomy and sinus clearance. However, the relative risk of a general anaesthetic needs to be considered.

■ Conclusion

Nasal blockage in pregnancy is common. The usual causes of nasal obstruction as well as 'rhinitis of pregnancy' need to be considered. Rhinitis of pregnancy is common and can occur in up to 30 per cent of women. It is thought to be due to elevated VIP levels as well as perhaps allergy to placental or fetal proteins. In some women, allergic rhinitis can improve with pregnancy due to elevated levels of serum cortisol.

The mainstay of treatment is a topical nasal steroid. Sodium cromoglycate is a safe alternative. Decongestants are often overused but they should only be used sparingly, as they commonly lead to rebound nasal congestion. Further investigation and treatment, such as CT scanning and surgery, are ideally delayed till after delivery.

■ References

1. Mabry RL. The management of nasal obstruction during pregnancy. *Ear Nose Throat J* 1983; **62:** 28–33.
2. Bende M, Hallgarde U, Sjogren C, Uvnas-Moberg K. Nasal congestion during pregnancy. *Clin Otolaryngol* 1989; **14:** 385–7.
3. Torsiglieri AJ Jr, Tom LW, Keane WM, Atkins JP Jr. Otolaryngologic manifestations of pregnancy. *Otolaryngol Head Neck Surg* 1990; **102:** 293–7.
4. Derkay CS. Eustachian tube and nasal function during pregnancy: a prospective study. *Otolaryngol Head Neck Surg* 1988; **99:** 558–66.
5. Sorri M, Bortikanen-Sorri AI, Karja J. Rhinitis during pregnancy. *Rhinology* 1980; **18:** 83–6.
6. Wheeler PW, Wheeler SF. Vasomotor rhinitis. Am Fam Physician 2005; **72:** 1057.
7. Toppozada H, Michaels L, Toppozada M, El-Ghazzawi I, Talaat M, Elwany S. The human respiratory nasal mucosa in pregnancy. An electron microscopic and histochemical study. *J Laryngol Otol* 1982; **96:** 613–26.
8. Kobal G. A new extension to the University of Erlangen Smell Test. *Chem Senses* **30**(Suppl 1): 210–11.
9. Hummel T, Konnerth CG, Rosenheim K, Kobal G. Screening of olfactory function with a four-minute odor identification test: reliability, normative data, and investigations in patients with olfactory loss. *Ann Otol Rhinol Laryngol* 2001; **110:** 976–81.
10. Toppenberg KS, Hill DA, Miller DP. Safety of radiographic imaging during pregnancy. *Am Fam Physician* 1999; **59:** 1813–18.
11. Thompson SK, Goldman SM, Shah KB, *et al.* Acute non-traumatic maternal illnesses in pregnancy: imaging approaches. *Emerg Radiol* 2005; **11:** 199–212.
12. Kusama T, Ota K. Radiological protection for diagnostic examination of pregnant women. *Congenit Anom* 2002; **42:** 10–14.
13. Lowe SA. Diagnostic radiography in pregnancy: risks and reality. *Aust NZ J Obstet Gynaecol* 2004; **44:** 191–6.
14. Keles N. Treatment of allergic rhinitis during pregnancy. *Am J Rhinol* 2004; **18:** 23–8.
15. Dykewicz MS, Fineman S, Skoner DP, *et al.* Diagnosis and management of rhinitis: complete guidelines of the Joint Task Force on Practice Parameters in Allergy, Asthma and Immunology. *Ann Allergy Asthma Immunol* 1998; **81:** 478–518.
16. Holt GR, Mabry RL. ENT medications in pregnancy. *Otolaryngol Head Neck Surg* 1983; **91:** 338–41.
17. Lekas MD. Rhinitis during pregnancy and rhinitis medicamentosa. *Otolaryngol Head Neck Surg* 1992; **107:** 845–9.
18. Shatz M, Zeiger RS. Diagnosis and management of rhinitis during pregnancy. *Allergy Proc* 1988; **9:** 545–54.
19. Clifton VL, Rennie N, Murphy VE. Effect of inhaled glucocorticoid treatment on placental 11beta-hydroxysteroid dehydrogenase type 2 activity and neonatal birth weight in pregnancies complicated by asthma. *Aust NZ J Obstet Gynaecol* 2006; **46:** 136–40.
20. Mazzotta P, Loebstein R, Koren G. Treating allergic rhinitis in pregnancy.

Safety considerations. *Drug Safety* 1999; **20:** 361–75.

21. Lemiere C, Blais L. Are inhaled corticosteroids taken during pregnancy harmless? *J Allergy Clin Immunol* 2005; **116:** 501–2. [Erratum appears in *J Allergy Clin Immunol* 2005; **116:** 1212.]

22. The American College of Obstetricians and Gynecologists (ACOG) and The American College of Allergy, Asthma and Immunology (ACAAI). The use of newer asthma and allergy medications during pregnancy. Ann Allergy Asthma Immunol 2000; 84: 475–80.

23. Schatz M. Asthma treatment during pregnancy. What can be safely taken? *Drug Safety* 1997; **16:** 342–50.

BLOOD PRESSURE PROBLEMS IN PREGNANCY

Peter Muller

Hypertensive disorders in pregnancy account for the second leading cause of maternal mortality, after embolic disease, and occur in 12–22 per cent of pregnancies.[1] Hypertension in pregnancy is a major cause of perinatal mortality and morbidity. Hypertensive disorders in pregnancy are classified as follows:

- gestational hypertension;
- pre-eclampsia/eclampsia;
- chronic hypertension;
- pre-eclampsia superimposed on chronic hypertension.

■ Blood pressure measurement

Gestational-age dependent

Blood pressure in pregnancy starts to decrease as early as the seventh week of pregnancy[2] and reaches its nadir in the second trimester.[3] Maternal blood pressure returns to the pre-pregnancy level in the third trimester. This fact emphasises the importance of obtaining a maternal blood pressure either pre-pregnancy or in early pregnancy when deciphering any change in blood pressure during the pregnancy.

Position

Blood pressure readings should not be taken in the supine position. In the outpatient setting, the patient should be sitting upright or at 45 degrees. In a hospital setting, blood pressure may be taken in the left arm while in the lateral recumbent position ensuring that the arm is at the level of the heart.

Cuff size

The appropriate size cuff can be determined by using a cuff length at least 1.5 times the upper arm circumference or the cuff bladder encircling 80 per cent or more of the arm.[4] Others suggest using a large cuff when the upper arm circumference is greater than 33 cm.[5]

Korotkoff sounds

The diastolic pressure recorded is the level at which the sound disappears (Korotkoff phase V).[4,5]

Measurement device

Although automated blood pressure devices have been used in pregnancy, the current consensus is that manual sphygmomanometry is regarded as the gold standard.[4,5] (In the UK, mercury has been removed from all hospitals.)

Other

The blood pressure measurement should be taken after a 3–10-minute rest period and no sooner than 30 minutes after smoking or intake of caffeine.[4,5]

■ Hypertensive disorders in pregnancy

Pre-eclampsia/eclampsia

- *Pre-eclampsia* is defined as hypertension occurring after 20 weeks' gestation plus proteinuria.[4]

■ *Eclampsia* is defined as the occurrence of a new-onset, grand mal seizure in a woman with pre-eclampsia that cannot be attributed to other causes.[1,4]

Hypertension

Hypertension in pregnancy is diagnosed when systolic blood pressure is ⩾140 mmHg or diastolic blood pressure is ⩾90 mmHg measured on at least two separate occasions. Several follow-up blood pressure readings should be performed to confirm the diagnosis.

Previously a rise in blood pressure during the pregnancy of 30 mmHg systolic and/or 15 mmHg diastolic had been used as diagnostic criteria. However, no trials have confirmed this definition relating to adverse pregnancy outcome. Recent consensus suggests these criteria should not be used for the diagnosis of hypertensive disease in pregnancy[1,4] but may be taken into consideration when deciding on increased patient surveillance.

Proteinuria

Significant proteinuria is defined as ⩾300 mg/24 h or a spot protein/creatinine ratio ⩾30 mg/mmol. A protein random urine dipstick of 1+ or greater (urinary dipstick of 1+, 2+, 3+ and 4+ compares to 0.3 g/dL, 1 g/dL, 3 g/dL and ⩾20 g/dL, respectively) with no evidence of urinary tract infection can been used on initial screen but, owing to the discrepancy of random urine dipstick with the other methods, a 24-h urine protein analysis or protein/creatinine ratio should be performed for all suspected cases of hypertensive disease.[6] While the 24-h urinary protein analysis has been the gold standard for the diagnosis of significant proteinuria, spot protein/creatinine ratio has shown reasonable correlation to the 24-h study[7,8] and can be used to obtain timely results for the management of newly admitted and day assessment patients.[5]

Other

It is important to realise that proteinuria is not seen in all cases of pre-eclampsia and is not mandatory for the clinical diagnosis.[5] Hypertension and other clinical characteristics that may be used for the clinical diagnosis, in the absence of proteinuria, are the new onset of the following:[4,5]

■ liver function abnormalities;
■ elevated serum creatinine;
■ platelet count <100 000 with evidence of haemolysis;
■ neurologic signs, such as headache or visual disturbances;
■ epigastric pain;
■ fetal growth restriction.

Oedema

Oedema is too common a finding in pregnancy and has been withdrawn by consensus reports from the diagnosis of pre-eclampsia.[4,5] However, closer surveillance of patients may be prudent when a sudden increase of oedema occurs.

Plasma urate

Fractional clearance of urate decreases with pre-eclampsia resulting in elevated serum urate. Hyperuricaemia is commonly found during the laboratory evaluation of an elevated blood pressure in pregnancy, and the level correlates weakly with the severity of disease.[9,10] Clinicians commonly use an elevated serum uric acid to confirm a suspected case of pre-eclampsia; however, recent evidence suggests that it is not key for planning intervention.[10]

Mild versus severe pre-eclampsia

There has long been interest in classifying the severity of pre-eclampsia both for prognosis and management. However, pre-eclampsia can be an unpredictable and progressive disease, and diligent maternal and fetal surveillance is required in all cases. Nevertheless, categorizing 'mild' from 'severe' pre-eclampsia may assist clinicians in patient management strategies, such as hospital admission, use of magnesium sulphate for seizure prophylaxis, and an indication for expediting delivery.

Severe pre-eclampsia is defined as:[1]

■ systolic blood pressure ⩾160 mmHg or diastolic blood pressure ⩾110 mmHg on two occasions;
■ proteinuria >5 g/24 h or dipstick 3–4+ on two occasions 4 h apart;
■ oliguria less than 500 mL in 24 h;

- persistent cerebral disturbances;
- pulmonary oedema;
- epigastric pain;
- impaired liver function;
- thrombocytopenia ($<100\,000$ cells/mm^3);
- fetal growth restriction.

HELLP (haemolysis, elevated liver enzymes and low platelets) syndrome

The HELLP syndrome occurs in 2–12 per cent of patients with pre-eclampsia,[11] and is characterised with the following:

- haemolysis;
- abnormal peripheral blood smear;
- elevated liver enzymes;
- raised serum bilirubin levels;
- raised alanine transaminase levels $>72\,IU/L$;
- raised lactic dehydrogenase levels $>600\,IU/L$;
- thrombocytopenia ($<100\,000$/mm^3).

See Jaundice and liver disease in pregnancy.

Gestational hypertension

Gestational hypertension is defined as follows:[4,5]

- hypertension arising in pregnancy after 20 weeks' gestation;
- no proteinuria;
- no other clinical characteristics suggestive of pre-eclampsia;
- hypertension that resolves within 3 months of delivery.

Perinatal and maternal complications are generally low with gestational hypertension. However, gestational hypertension diagnosed prior to 30 weeks progresses to pre-eclampsia in approximately 40 per cent of cases. This incidence falls to 10 per cent when gestational hypertension is found after the 37th week.[12] Thus, diligent surveillance of both mother and fetus is required when non-proteinuric hypertension is discovered in pregnancy regardless of the gestation.

Chronic hypertension

Chronic hypertension is defined as follows:[4,5,13]

- hypertension that is present prior to pregnancy;
- diagnosed prior to 20 weeks' gestation;

- hypertension diagnosed for the first time during pregnancy that does not return to normal 3 months postpartum.

Essential hypertension is defined as hypertension without an apparent cause. Secondary hypertension is hypertension associated with disorders such as aortic coarctation, and renal, renovascular or endocrine disease.[5] In cases where patients present for prenatal care after 20 weeks, it may be difficult to distinguish gestational hypertension, or pre-eclampsia, from chronic hypertension. Obtaining pre-pregnancy records from the patient's previous practitioners (emergency room or general practitioner visits) may be helpful. In addition, one can differentiate pre-eclampsia from chronic hypertension by the development of proteinuria and/or the clinical characteristics listed above. One may have to monitor the patient's blood pressure through the postpartum period to determine the hypertensive classification.

Chronic hypertension and superimposed pre-eclampsia

The development of superimposed pre-eclampsia occurs in approximately 20–25 per cent of women with chronic hypertension.[14,15] Both perinatal and maternal risks rise significantly with this transition, and heightened surveillance is strongly recommended. The diagnosis of superimposed pre-eclampsia can be quite difficult even for the most skilled clinicians, especially in those women with pre-existing proteinuria. It is thus important in early pregnancy to obtain baseline liver and renal function evaluations as well as quantification of proteinuria either via a 24-h urine or protein/creatinine ratio.

Findings after 20 weeks' gestation that are suggestive of superimposed pre-eclampsia include the following:[4]

- new onset of proteinuria (no proteinuria in early pregnancy);
- sudden increase in proteinuria (as compared to baseline elevated levels in early pregnancy);
- sudden increase in blood pressure that had previously been well controlled;
- new evidence of thrombocytopenia ($<100\,000$ cells/mm);
- elevated transaminases to abnormal levels.

■ Initial evaluation

Clinical history

Elevated blood pressures are commonly discovered during routine antenatal visits. However, there may be antecedent symptoms, such as a sudden increase in swelling involving non-dependent regions, e.g. the face, eyelids and hands. Rapid onset of carpal tunnel syndrome and sudden weight gain (>2.5–3 kg/week) should alert the clinician to search for other signs and symptoms of pre-eclampsia. Headaches and indigestion are common in pregnancy, but those that are resistant to common therapies demand closer inspection. A history of visual disturbances is generally unreliable as an indicator of pre-eclampsia. The sensitivity of detecting the disease is greater when the prevalence is higher, thus a search for risk factors is prudent in the initial evaluation. Risk factors include family history, nulliparity, cohabitation prior to pregnancy of <3 months (common in teenage pregnancies), donor sperm insemination, oocyte donation, embryo donation, obesity, multiple gestation, previous history of pre-eclampsia or poor pregnancy outcome, and coexisting medical conditions, such as chronic hypertension, renal disease, diabetes mellitus and thrombophilias.[16,17]

Physical examination

Several measurements of the blood pressure should be undertaken following local protocols in order to confirm the elevation. Facial swelling may discriminate pre-eclampsia from the normal lower-extremity oedema commonly seen in the third trimester. A thorough physical examination is required to assist in differentiating mild from severe disease. This examination should include the following:

- a fundoscopic examination to look for chronic and acute changes;
- a cardiopulmonary examination to exclude tachycardia, raised jugular–venous pulsations and evidence of pulmonary oedema;
- an abdominal examination to evaluate hepatic tenderness;
- symphysiofundal height measurement for evidence of fetal growth restriction;

- determination of hyperreflexia, indicating cerebral irritation due to oedema.

For those patients where delivery may be considered, vaginal examination to assess cervical favourability is reasonable.

Laboratory tests

Other than proteinuria, where its presence generally differentiates gestational hypertension and pre-eclampsia, there are no laboratory tests that are diagnostic for pre-eclampsia. However, laboratory evaluations are useful to assist in the diagnosis as well as assessing progression and severity of the condition. The tests include the following:[4]

- haemoglobin, haematocrit and blood smear;
- platelet count;
- quantification of proteinuria;
- creatinine;
- serum uric acid;
- serum transaminase and lactic dehydrogenase levels.

Fetal assessment

An ultrasound scan should be considered in all patients with the diagnosis of pre-eclampsia, to evaluate for fetal growth restriction. Further fetal evaluation and surveillance may include fetal cardiotograph, Doppler velocimetry or biophysical profile. The frequency of fetal surveillance is dependent on the severity of the disease.

■ Differential diagnosis

There are other disease processes that may mimic or even coincide with pre-eclampsia. Although the presentation can be similar, there may be subtle differences for each disease that will assist the clinician in instituting a specific treatment strategy.

Thrombotic thrombocytopenic purpura (TTP)/haemolytic–uraemic syndrome (HUS)

These two disease processes present with microangiopathic haemolytic anaemia (MHA) and severe thrombocytopenia, thus the confusion in relation to HELLP syndrome.

Thrombotic thrombocytopenic purpura is commonly described as a pentad of findings: MHA, thrombocytopenia, neurological symptoms (headache, confusion and seizures), fever and renal dysfunction. However, the pentad presents in only 40 per cent of cases. The majority will usually present with MHA, thrombocytopenia and neurological findings.[18] Presentation in the mid-trimester should lead the clinician to suspect TTP.

Haemolytic–uraemic syndrome (HUS) commonly presents postpartum with the characteristic acute renal disease, thrombocytopenia and MHA.[19] HUS is rare in adults but must be considered when the HELLP syndrome does not resolve in the first few days postpartum. Since these conditions can lead to rapid maternal deterioration, accurate diagnosis and early treatment is essential. Plasma exchange has been advocated as the first-line treatment in pregnancy.[20]

Acute fatty liver of pregnancy

Patients present, generally in the third trimester, with non-specific symptoms such as nausea, vomiting, headache, malaise or abdominal pain. Some patients may describe symptoms suggestive of a viral illness. Physical and laboratory findings may include jaundice, hypertension, hypoglycaemia, hyperbilirubinaemia, coagulopathy, elevated creatinine and elevated transaminases. Compared to the HELLP syndrome, proteinuria is less commonly present.[20] Transaminases are elevated to the levels seen in the HELLP syndrome, but not commonly to those levels seen in acute viral hepatitis. Liver biopsy can be diagnostic, but is infrequently required for the diagnosis. See Jaundice and liver disease in pregnancy.

Systemic lupus erythematosus

Systemic lupus erythematosus (SLE) is more common in women of reproductive age.[21] This may present for the first time in pregnancy. SLE may manifest itself with renal, haematological and/or neurological alterations. Hypertension is common in association with renal dysfunction, making the differentiation from pre-eclampsia difficult in early gestations. Evidence of dermatologic (malar or discoid rash) and arthritic complaints in conjunction

with the other clinical findings, as well as an atypical presentation for pre-eclampsia will commonly suggest this alternative diagnosis. A high titre of antinuclear antibodies and positive autoantibodies to double-stranded DNA will allow the clinician to suspect the diagnosis further. The diagnosis of SLE is based on clinical and laboratory criteria.[22]

Acute renal disease

An atypical presentation of acute renal insufficiency and hypertension should lead the clinician to include acute renal disease in the differential diagnosis of hypertension in pregnancy. The differential diagnosis of acute renal failure should be divided in to three categories: prerenal, intrinsic, or postrenal renal failure. Prerenal renal failure may be secondary to hypovolaemia, such as from haemorrhage or increased vascular resistance from non-steroidal anti-inflammatory drugs. Intrinsic renal disease may be from acute tubular necrosis or glomerulonephritis. Postrenal renal disease may be from bilateral urinary obstruction from the gravid uterus (especially in multiple pregnancy).

The clinician should review the clinical history of risk factors or exposures, consider a renal ultrasound for evidence of obstruction, determine the fractional excretion of sodium from urinary electrolytes, and review the urinary sediment for evidence of hyaline (prerenal), renal tubular (acute tubular necrosis) or red-cell casts (glomerulonephritis).

■ Management

The management of pre-eclampsia presents a common conflict to the clinician: what is good for the mother may not be good for the fetus and vice versa. Delivery is always better for the mother, but may not be so for the fetus. The safety of the mother should always be paramount, and balancing the risks to the mother with the risks to the fetus will test the clinical skills of the patient's care giver. The duty of care is to the mother; in the UK, the fetus *in utero* has no legal rights. Although the 'cure' for pre-eclampsia is ultimately delivery, reducing both maternal and fetal risk complications may include corticosteroids for fetal lung maturity, reducing the risk of intracerebral haemorrhage with antihypertensives, and magnesium sulphate to prevent convulsions. Proceeding with delivery or expectant management will depend on the gestational age, fetal condition, obstetric condition and severity of maternal condition.[17] There are common algorithms that have been developed to assist in the management of these patients.[17,23]

An initial patient presentation demands a formulated management plan and an exit strategy (possible delivery). In general, delivery should be considered for delivery at >37–38 weeks' gestation for mild disease and >34 weeks for severe disease.[17] Expectant management for severe preeclampsia requires clinicians experienced with this form of intensive surveillance.

■ References

1. ACOG practice bulletin. Diagnosis and management of preeclampsia and eclampsia. Number 33, January 2002. *Obstet Gynecol* 2002; **99:** 159–67.

2. Capeless EL, Clapp JF. Cardiovascular changes in early phase of pregnancy. *Am J Obstet Gynecol* 1989; **161:** 1449–53.

3. Wilson M, Morganti AA, Zervoudakis I, *et al*. Blood pressure, the renin–aldosterone system and sex steroids throughout normal pregnancy. *Am J Med* 1980; **68:** 97–104.

4. Report of the National High Blood Pressure Education Program Working Group on High Blood Pressure in Pregnancy. *Am J Obstet Gynecol* 2000; **183:** S1–S22.

5. Brown MA, Hague WM, Higgins J, *et al*. The detection, investigation and management of hypertension in pregnancy: full consensus statement. *Aust NZ J Obstet Gynaecol* 2000; **40:** 139–55.

6. Meyer NL, Mercer BM, Friedman SA, Sibai BM. Urinary dipstick protein: a poor predictor of absent or severe proteinuria. *Am J Obstet Gynecol* 1994; **170:** 137–41.

7. Neithardt AB, Dooley SL, Borensztajn J. Prediction of 24-hour protein excretion in pregnancy with a single voided urine protein-to-creatinine ratio. *Am J Obstet Gynecol* 2002; **186:** 883–6.

8. Rodriguez-Thompson D, Lieberman ES. Use of a random urinary protein-to-creatinine ratio for the diagnosis of significant proteinuria during pregnancy. *Am J Obstet Gynecol* 2001; **185:** 808–11.

9. Lam C, Lim KH, Kang DH, Karumanchi SA. Uric acid and preeclampsia. *Semin Nephrol* 2005; **25:** 56–60.

10. Thangaratinam S, Ismail KM, Sharp S, Coomarasamy A, Khan KS. Accuracy of serum uric acid in predicting complications of pre-eclampsia: a systematic review. *BJOG* 2006; **113:** 369–78.

11. Sibai BM. The HELLP syndrome (hemolysis, elevated liver enzymes, and low platelets): much ado about nothing? *Am J Obstet Gynecol* 1990; **162:** 311–16.

12. Saudan P, Brown MA, Buddle ML, Jones M. Does gestational hypertension become pre-eclampsia? *Br J Obstet Gynaecol* 1998; **105:** 1177–84.

13. ACOG Practice Bulletin. Chronic hypertension in pregnancy. ACOG Committee on Practice Bulletins. *Obstet Gynecol* 2001; **98(Suppl):** 177–85.

14. Caritis S, Sibai B, Hauth J, *et al*. Low-dose aspirin to prevent preeclampsia in women at high risk. National Institute of Child Health and Human Development Network of Maternal–Fetal Medicine Units. *N Engl J Med* 1998; **338:** 701–5.

15. McCowan LM, Buist RG, North RA, Gamble G. Perinatal morbidity in chronic hypertension. *Br J Obstet Gynaecol* 1996; **103:** 123–9.

16. Duckitt K, Harrington D. Risk factors for pre-eclampsia at antenatal booking: systematic review of controlled studies. *BMJ* 2005; **330:** 565.

17. Sibai B, Dekker G, Kupferminc M. Preeclampsia. *Lancet* 2005; **365:** 785–99.

18. Ridolfi RL, Bell WR. Thrombotic thrombocytopenic purpura. Report of 25 cases and review of the literature. *Medicine (Baltimore)* 1981; **60:** 413–28.

19. Weiner CP. Thrombotic microangiopathy in pregnancy and the postpartum period. *Semin Hematol* 1987; **24**: 119–29.
20. Egerman RS, Sibai BM. Imitators of preeclampsia and eclampsia. *Clin Obstet Gynecol* 1999; **42**: 551–62.
21. Silman AJ, Hochberg MC. *Epidemiology of the rheumatic diseases.* New York: Oxford University Press, 2001.
22. Tan EM, Cohen AS, Fries JF, *et al.* The 1982 revised criteria for the classification of systemic lupus erythematosus. *Arthritis Rheum* 1982; **25**: 1271–7.
23. Sibai BM. Diagnosis and management of gestational hypertension and preeclampsia. *Obstet Gynecol* 2003; **102**: 181–92.

BREAST LUMPS IN PREGNANCY

Peter Frecker

Nowadays women are asked to be 'breast aware' so that they present early with breast cancer, that is to say, as soon as they perceive any change in their breast (Box 1).

During pregnancy, changes to the breast can be marked and some women may seek advice for what to the examining physician are considered normal physiological developments. These changes include:

- breast lobules becoming more prominent;
- enlarged Montgomery's tubercle;
- thickening of an area of the breast;
- accessory breast tissue in the axilla is a common anatomical anomaly, which will enlarge naturally during pregnancy. It may cause a little discomfort and be perceived as a serious problem.

Pregnant women may become more conscious of their breasts and present with lesions that have been there for a long time, including lipomas, sebaceous cysts, neurofibromas or haemangiomas. Lymph nodes adjacent to the axillary tail of the breast can fluctuate in size and it must not be forgotten that one is occasionally

Box 1 Differential diagnosis of breast lumps in pregnancy

- Physiological
- Prominent breast lobule
- Montgomery's tubercle
- Accessory breast tail
- Incidental
- Lipoma
- Sebaceous cyst
- Neurofibroma
- Haemangioma
- Lymph nodes
- Fibroadenoma
- Cyst
- Conditions related to pregnancy
- Lactating nodule
- Galactocoele
- Abscess
- Malignancy
- Carcinoma

situated within that part of the breast; the so-called intramammary node. Many of these concerns can be allayed by experienced midwives.

■ Lactating nodule

This is also known as adenosis of pregnancy and the difference between this and the very common fibrocystic disease of the breast, which is unrelated to pregnancy, is blurred. The breast undergoes huge proliferation in pregnancy and many women may note one particular area to be more thickened than the rest, an asymmetrical swelling or an actual well-defined lump such that imaging and biopsy may be contemplated. In this last case the ultrasonographer may recognise it as a solid lump, but of similar echogenicity to the surrounding breast tissue, and the pathologist will describe it as normal breast tissue of pregnancy. Hopefully, as with other benign breast lumps seen in pregnancy, resort to excision biopsy can be avoided.

Although fibrocystic disease of the breast does not occur in pregnancy, the condition is included for completeness. It has been labelled 'benign breast change syndrome', the symptoms of which include cyclical pain and thickening of the breast, typically in the upper outer quadrant. It should be emphasised that this is a very common problem and that the diagnosis begins with 'benign' and no 'disease' is mentioned. The pathologists looking at pieces of such breasts histologically will call it fibrocystic disease due to its cyclical proliferative features plus the sclerotic features that are perceived to be the basis of the mild inflammation. However, this term is very similar to that of fibroadenoma, which is also common and quite different; hence it is falling out of use.

Fibroadenoma

Fibroadenomas are common benign breast lumps seen in teenagers, women in their twenties and there is another rise in incidence for women in their forties. Typically they appear mobile within the breast, are of a rubbery consistency on palpation, with a slightly irregular or bosselated surface and frequently are multiple. Excision is avoided as long as imaging and biopsy support the benign diagnosis. The natural history of these lumps is that they enlarge over a period of months and then remain unchanged, even for years, but eventually shrink and possibly appear as a calcified spot on mammograms in later life. In pregnancy they may appear as a new diagnosis, enlarge to cause concern, or infarct. This last complication may demand a surgical excision, which is liable to wound complication.

Cyst and galactocoele

A simple breast cyst can be large compared to the multiple tiny cysts of fibrocystic disease. It may present as a lump of sudden onset. They are often found to be multiple when the breast is scanned and are most common in women in their thirties and forties, being an age group of pregnancy more these days than for our ancestors. We assume that the explanation for not seeing this in pregnancy nearly as frequently as for the non-pregnant population is because the simple cyst is essentially a degenerative change in the breast in direct contrast to what is happening as a consequence of pregnancy. Galactocoeles are more common in pregnancy and present as the same spherical shape with a smooth surface as the simple cyst. The diagnosis, for both, is confirmed by needle puncture and aspiration.

Abscess

This problem is more common for the lactating woman than the pregnant one. They do not usually present a diagnostic problem because of the general systemic upset, localised pain, tenderness and redness of the overlying skin, and usually with the sign of fluctuance. The main difficulty is to determine whether it is an abscess or (the not much less painful) mastitis. If an abscess is mistaken for mastitis and nothing is done other than to prescribe antibiotics, then the abscess may be partially treated in any case, become better defined, and one is left with a clear decision to aspirate or drain it at operation.

Carcinoma (Fig. 1)

This is a disastrous diagnosis for any young woman but in pregnancy it is doubly difficult. If the appropriate scan is requested or biopsy made, in good time, then the evidence is that the prognosis is no worse than that for a similar lesion occurring in a woman of similar age who is not pregnant. The problem is that the irregular hard lump is seen as being something to do with the pregnancy, or mastitis, and the diagnosis can be missed. It should therefore be considered mandatory to take a careful account as to what has happened to the breast and then to examine both breasts and both axillae thoroughly. In this way, failure or delay in diagnosis may be avoided. Referral to a breast specialist should be triggered by the following findings:

- slight asymmetry of the breasts;
- a subtle dimpling of the skin;

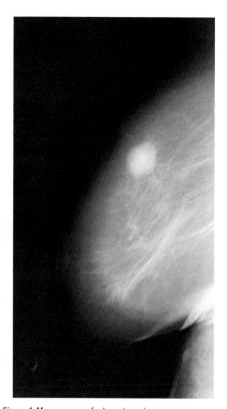

Figure 1 Mammogram of a breast carcinoma.

- apparent inflammation but without the commensurate tenderness;
- nipple retraction;
- an ill-defined lump.

■ Useful website

www.breastcancercare.org.uk

BREAST TENDERNESS IN PREGNANCY AND THE PUERPERIUM

Peter Frecker

Breast pain, of mild degree, is a very common symptom during pregnancy and in the puerperium. As a consequence, the clinician of first contact can usually be confident to reassure the woman as to its benign cause and strategies for coping with it. The breast surgeon, therefore, sees many women with the benign breast change syndrome (BBC) but few with breast pain due to the changes of pregnancy and lactation. BBC is, by definition, not seen in pregnancy, but we recognise that the cycle of proliferative and degenerative changes with a mild inflammation has some parallels with what happens in pregnancy, where it is all proliferative, although pathologically can develop hyperplasia, adenosis and neo-duct formation.

Some heavy-breasted woman may need advice as to the type of support (bra) to wear given that the pain, whatever the cause, is exacerbated by poor support of the breast. Others may need to be told about engorgement of the breast and how to breast feed the baby.

■ Sepsis

Mastitis is manifested by redness, swelling and oedema of the breast, together with fever and tachycardia in severe cases. This is treated with antibiotics. The woman should be encouraged to continue breast feeding the baby, perhaps expressing and discarding the milk from the infected side. If an abscess develops, the pain is more intense and exquisite tenderness may develop over the infected area (Fig. 1). This can be managed by either serial aspiration, with antibiotics, or surgical drainage under a general anaesthetic. It can be

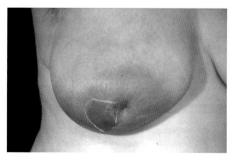

Figure 1 Breast abscess. Reproduced with kind permission from Richard Sainsbury.

difficult for the mother to continue to feed the baby through such an episode.

An ultrasound scan of the breast may be helpful to distinguish between mastitis and abscess. A needle can be inserted, speculatively, to see whether or not there is pus present. The mother, who may have other young children, requires help and continued attention from health professionals during this difficult time.

Diabetic women can pose extra complications; for example, it may be that they harbour an unusual organism that leads to necrosis of the skin over a part of the breast. Diabetic granulomatous mastopathy is a rare non-specific inflammatory condition, characterised by pain and lumps, and mimicking carcinoma. Diagnosis is made histologically usually by a core biopsy that can be performed in an outpatient clinic.

■ Carcinoma

Breast cancer normally presents as a painless lump. However, the breast in pregnancy and during lactation is difficult to assess clinically, and there may be breast pain and tenderness in addition to a carcinoma or actually caused by the malignancy; for example, in a case of inflammatory carcinoma. The assessment of the breast with the usual means of imaging is also difficult and, if suspicion remains, investigations must be pursued. (See Box 2 in Breast/nipple discharge in pregnancy.)

BREAST/NIPPLE DISCHARGE IN PREGNANCY

Peter Frecker

■ Physiological

The function of the breast is to produce milk and preparation for lactation occurs during the pregnancy, consequently discharge is to be expected. The breast specialist sees many young women with a trivial nipple discharge who are not pregnant and, in the absence of a definitive diagnosis (e.g. hyperprolactinaemia), would

class this symptom as a variant of normal. This discharge is from several ducts, typically bilateral, and clear or slightly coloured. The differential diagnosis is summarised in Box 1.

Box 1 Causes of breast/nipple discharge in pregnancy

- ■ Intrinsic to pregnancy (physiological)
- ■ Skin disorders – eczema
- ■ Benign breast problems
  - ● duct ectasia
  - ● intraductal papilloma
- ■ Malignancy
  - ● Paget's disease of the nipple (carcinoma presenting at the nipple)
  - ● ductal carcinoma *in-situ* (this may occur concurrently with an invasive malignancy of the breast)

■ Duct ectasia

There is no particular association with pregnancy but this condition occurs in approximately 1 in 15 women, at some time in their lives, and is usually of no more than a nuisance value. However, acute severe sepsis about the nipple/areola complex can occur and becomes a chronic problem in some women.

Ectasia is a term used to describe dilatation or distension of a hollow organ. The primary problem is a non-specific inflammatory condition labelled as periductal mastitis, which can be complicated by secondary bacterial infection and enlargement or ectasia of ducts. The condition is seen typically in women in their 30s and 40s, and there is an association with smoking. The discharge is from multiple ducts, usually bilateral, and can be of various colours and, on occasions, tinged with blood.

Some of the women with this problem may have nipple inversion as a consequence, or a possible cause, of the problem. This inversion may interfere with the woman's ability to breast feed. Rarely, a fistula will develop, or occur following a procedure to drain an abscess, between a duct and an opening on the areola, or beyond. The patient may complain of staining on the bra only, but close inspection will reveal the opening of the mammillary fistula eccentric to the nipple.

■ Blood

A persistent blood-stained discharge, unilaterally, raises the possibility of ductal carcinoma *in situ* (DCIS) or actual invasive carcinoma. It is important to ascertain the exact nature of the discharge. It can be almost black in duct ectasia, whilst in DCIS it is usually bright red and persistent.

A phenomenon that is seen rarely, and for which there is no good explanation amongst primiparous women, is copious discharge of blood, bilaterally, towards the end of pregnancy and in the puerperium. Investigation is required but very often no serious pathology is found.

A further cause of a blood-stained nipple discharge, unilaterally, is the intraductal papilloma (Fig. 1). This is a benign polypoid lesion, which may be visualised on the wall of a duct, close to the nipple, on a scan.

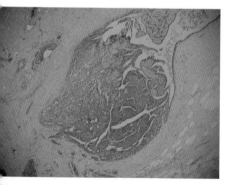

Figure 1 Histological picture showing an intraductal papilloma.

The woman presenting with discharge of blood needs to be examined with these diagnoses in mind. If a mass is found on examination, then this should be investigated in the usual way (Box 2). If there is no associated mass, then some form of

Box 2 Breast/nipple discharge: establishing a diagnosis

- History
- Clinical examination
- Cytology of the discharge
- Ultrasound scan and/or mammogram
- If there is a mass lesion:
  - fine-needle aspiration for cytology
  - core biopsy
  - excision biopsy

imaging is required. Ultrasound scanning can be diagnostic and mammograms, with protection of the fetus as necessary, can be undertaken. If these investigations are normal, then any diagnostic biopsies, for final confirmation of a benign pathology, can usually be delayed until after parturition. Applying some of the discharge to slides for cytology may provide further reassurance in the interim.

Clearly nipple discharge of blood requires referral to a breast specialist. Rarely, both intraductal papilloma and DCIS can present with persistent clear discharge.

■ Paget's disease

This is carcinoma presenting at the nipple (Fig. 2). The usual presentation is of an unhealed ulcer, but in some cases the complaint may be of a slight discharge, with or without blood, not having noticed the erosive lesion. Close examination leads the clinician on to imaging and nipple biopsy. The main differential diagnosis is eczema, the distinguishing features being that the much more common benign problem is usually bilateral and affects the periareolar area rather than the nipple itself. It is usually associated with itching and the florid inflammation. The patient with eczema may also present complaining of nipple discharge because they have noticed the staining on the bra, due to serum 'leaking' from the rash, and has not made the link between that and the irritation.

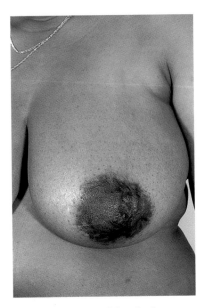

Figure 2 Paget's disease of the nipple.

BREATHLESSNESS IN PREGNANCY: CARDIAC CAUSES

Velmurugan C Kuppuswamy and Sandy Gupta

■ Introduction

Breathlessness is a common complaint in pregnancy, and may be a phenomenon related to the physiological changes associated with pregnancy. However, shortness of breath in association with any of the following conditions should arouse suspicions of an underlying cardiac pathology:

- orthopnoea – breathlessness when lying flat;
- paroxysmal nocturnal dyspnoea – sudden onset of breathlessness at night;
- dysarrhythmia – erratic heart rhythm.

After suicide, cardiac disease is the most common indirect cause of maternal mortality in the UK.[1] Cardiac myopathies and congenital heart disease constitute two of the main life-threatening

conditions for the mother and her baby (Fig. 1). New-onset heart disease, such as rheumatic heart disease, in pregnancy in the UK is very uncommon; but may be a problem in some ethnic populations. In addition, there are other simple non-cardiac causes for shortness of breath in pregnant women, such as iron-deficiency anaemia, and exacerbation of underlying respiratory conditions needs to be ruled out before embarking on the more serious cardiac causes. This chapter aims to discuss the cardiac causes of dyspnoea, which can be basically divided into cardiomyopathies and congenital abnormalities.

■ Cardiomyopathies

Cardiomyopathy in pregnancy mainly comprises three types: peripartum; dilated and hypertrophic. While dilated and hypertrophic cardiomyopathies may affect anyone and present at any time during pregnancy, peripartum cardiomyopathy occurs mostly in young women of Afro–Caribbean origin during the last trimester of pregnancy or in the first 6 weeks postpartum.

Peripartum cardiomyopathy

It is a rare condition, occurring in 1 in 3000–15 000 pregnancies. The pathogenesis is poorly understood, but some form of myocarditis, possibly viral, has been postulated.[2] Maternal mortality can be as high as 20 per cent; however, fetal outcome is good.[3]

The management is similar to that of any form of cardiomyopathy with impaired systolic ventricular function. The major challenge is the assessment of recurrent risk in future pregnancies. The patient should have regular surveillance with an echocardiogram for assessment of left ventricular function, which may predict the risk of recurrence and outcome in future pregnancies. However, there is a substantial risk of recurrence of symptomatic heart failure and permanent impairment of left ventricular function in any subsequent pregnancy.[4]

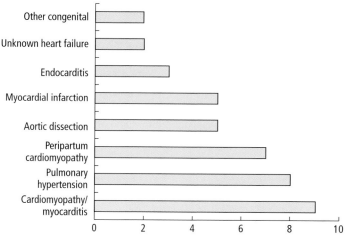

Figure 1 Cardiac causes of maternal deaths in the UK: confidential enquiry into maternal deaths 1997–1999 (total maternal deaths, $n = 409$; cardiac, $n = 41$).

Dilated cardiomyopathy

This condition is poorly tolerated in pregnancy. The risk of maternal death is 7 per cent if the patient is in New York Heart Association (NYHA) functional classification >II. In addition to maternal death, there is elevated risk of heart failure, which has to be distinguished from the shortness of breath of pregnancy by careful clinical assessment. Heart failure should be managed as in the non-pregnant patient, but angiotensin-converting enzyme inhibitors are associated with renal agenesis in the fetus and should be avoided until after delivery.

Hypertrophic cardiomyopathy (HOCM)

Women with hypertrophic cardiomyopathy usually tolerate pregnancy well, as the left ventricle seems to adapt in a physiological way.[5] This is especially advantageous in this condition where the left ventricular cavity dimensions tend to be small. Women with a murmur and an increased gradient across the left ventricular outflow tract may present for the first time in pregnancy.[6]

Maternal death is uncommon[1] and there is no evidence to suggest the risk of sudden death is increased by pregnancy.[2] However, considerable distress may be caused by the diagnosis and by the genetic implications. The diagnostic echocardiogram, electrocardiogram (ECG), exercise testing and ambulatory ECG monitoring and genetic counselling are carried out as in the non-pregnant patient.

Women with severe diastolic dysfunction can cause concern with pulmonary congestion or even sudden pulmonary oedema. Beta-blockers should be continued and a small dose of diuretic may help, but rest in conjunction with the beta-blocker to prevent tachycardia is recommended.

Atrial fibrillation in women with HOCM is frequently managed with low-molecular-weight heparin and beta-blockade. Cardioversion may be considered, if rate control fails, after excluding thrombus in the left atrial appendage with a transoesophageal echocardiogram.

Finally, the genetic risk needs to be discussed, including the phenomenon of anticipation, which determines an earlier onset and more severe form in succeeding generations in some families.

Normal vaginal delivery with good analgesia and a low threshold for forceps assistance is the safest mode of delivery for the mother with any form of cardiomyopathy, since it is associated with reduced blood loss and less rapid haemodynamic changes than Caesarean section.[7]

■ Congenital heart disease

Congenital heart disease is the most common birth defect in the world – about 1 per cent of newborns around the world have congenital heart disease. In the UK, approximately 250 000 adults have congenital heart disease equally divided between the sexes. Some have simple defects, such as small atrial or ventricular septal defects that may remain clinically silent until diagnosed on routine examination, whereas others have complex abnormalities that require surgical intervention for survival.

Fifty years ago, 90 per cent of this population would not have lived up to adulthood. Advances in cardiology and cardiac surgery have led to more than 85 per cent of these infants surviving into childbearing age and the number is growing by approximately 1600 new cases every year.

Table 1 Pregnancy-related risks for women with congenital heart disease by specific lesion (Modified and reproduced with permission from *Pregnancy and congenital heart disease*, 18 February 2006)[8]

Lesion	Exclude before pregnancy	Potential hazards	Recommended treatment during pregnancy and peripartum
Low-risk lesions			
Ventricular septal defects[7]	Pulmonary arterial hypertension	Arrhythmias	Antibiotic prophylaxis for unoperated or residual defect
		Endocarditis (unoperated or residual defect)	
Atrial septal defects (unoperated)[7]	Pulmonary arterial hypertension	Arrhythmias	Thromboprophylaxis, if bed rest is required
	Ventricular dysfunction	Thromboembolic events	Consider low-dose aspirin during pregnancy
Coarctation (repaired)[9]	Recoarctation	Pre-eclampsia (coarctation is the only congenital heart lesion known as an independent predictor of pre-eclampsia)	Beta-blockers, if necessary, to control systemic blood pressure
	Aneurysm formation at site of repair (MRI)	Aortic dissection	Consider elective Caesarean section before term in case of aortic aneurysm formation or uncontrollable systemic hypertension
	Associated lesion, such as bicuspid aortic valve (with or without aortic stenosis or aortic regurgitation), ascending aortopathy	Congestive heart failure	Antibiotic prophylaxis
	Systemic hypertension Ventricular dysfunction	Endarteritis	
Tetralogy of Fallot[10]	Severe right ventricular outflow tract obstruction	Arrhythmias	Consider preterm delivery in the rare case of right ventricular failure
	Severe pulmonary regurgitation	Right ventricular failure	Antibiotic prophylaxis
	Right ventricular dysfunction	Endocarditis	
	DiGeorge syndrome		

Table 1 Continued

Lesion	Exclude before pregnancy	Potential hazards	Recommended treatment during pregnancy and peripartum
Moderate-risk lesions			
Mitral stenosis[13]	Severe stenosis	Atrial fibrillation	Beta-blockers
	Pulmonary venous hypertension	Thromboembolic events	Low-dose aspirin
		Pulmonary oedema	Consider bed rest during third trimester with additional thromboprophylaxis
			Antibiotic prophylaxis
Aortic stenosis[14]	Severe stenosis (peak pressure gradient on Doppler ultrasonography >80 mmHg, ST segment depression, symptoms)	Arrhythmias	Bed rest during third trimester with thromboprophylaxis
	Left ventricular dysfunction	Angina	Consider balloon aortic valvotomy (for severe symptomatic valvar stenosis) or preterm Caesarean section if cardiac decompensation ensues (bypass surgery carries 20% risk of fetal death)
		Endocarditis	Antibiotic prophylaxis
		Left ventricular failure	
		Endocarditis	
Fontan-type circulation[12]	Ventricular dysfunction	Heart failure	Consider anticoagulation with low-molecular-weight heparin and aspirin throughout pregnancy
	Arrhythmias	Arrhythmias	Maintain sufficient filling pressures and avoid dehydration during delivery
	Heart failure (NYHA >II)	Thromboembolic complications	Antibiotic prophylaxis
		Endocarditis	
High-risk lesions			
Marfan syndrome[17]	Aortic root dilatation >4 cm	Type A dissection of aorta	Beta-blockers in all patients
			Elective Caesarean section when aortic root >45 mm (≈35 weeks' gestation)
Eisenmenger syndrome; other pulmonary arterial hypertension[18]	Ventricular dysfunction	30–50% risk of death related to pregnancy	Therapeutic termination should be offered
	Arrhythmias	Arrhythmias	If pregnancy continues, close cardiovascular monitoring, early bed rest and pulmonary vasodilator therapy with supplemental oxygen should be considered
		Heart failure	Close monitoring necessary for 10 days postpartum
		Endocarditis for Eisenmenger syndrome	

MRI, magnetic resonance imaging; NYHA, New York Heart Association.

Furthermore, these women are at heightened risk of maternal and fetal complications should they conceive. The medical profession should, therefore, be aware of the clinical presentations, diagnosis and management of these conditions.

The congenital cardiac lesions in pregnancy can be broadly classified based on the related risks for the pregnant women into low-, moderate- and high-risk lesions (Box 1). The ensuing discussion will focus on the clinical manifestation and diagnosis of individual congenital cardiac lesions. The management of pregnancy and labour depends on the risk category of the patient (Table 1).

Box 1 Classification of congenital heart disease in pregnancy based on risk involved

Low-risk lesions
- Ventricular septal defect
- Atrial septal defects (unoperated)
- Coarctation repaired
- Tetralogy of Fallot repaired

Moderate-risk lesions
- Mitral stenosis
- Aortic stenosis
- Fontan-type circulation

High-risk lesions
- Marfan syndrome
- Eisenmenger syndrome

Low-risk conditions
Ventricular septal defect
A small ventricular septal defect (VSD) with normal right-sided pressures confers no added risk in pregnancy. However, antibiotic prophylaxis is required against infective endocarditis. Paradoxical embolism is not common in VSD with a large pressure gradient across the defect. Large defects causing pulmonary vascular disease are discussed under pulmonary hypertension and Eisenmenger syndrome/complex.

Unoperated atrial septal defect
Unrepaired atrial septal defects (ASDs) are well tolerated in the presence of a normal pulmonary vascular resistance. The pre-existing tendency to atrial arrhythmia may increase with the increasing cardiac output in pregnancy. The combination of a potential right to left shunt and the hypercoagulable state of pregnancy increases the risk of paradoxical embolism, especially with increases in intrathoracic pressure during labour. This also applies to known patent foramen ovale. There is a role for thromboembolic prophylaxis but not antibiotics in ASD; however, the benefits have to be weighed against the risks.

Repaired coarctation of the aorta
In current-day practice almost all patients born with coarctation of aorta have the condition corrected by early childhood. Pregnancy poses little risk in repaired coarctation as long as there is no aneurysm at the site of repair.[9] This should be confirmed with magnetic resonance imaging or computed tomography before conception.

Repaired tetralogy of Fallot
Tetralogy of Fallot is the most common cyanotic congenital heart disease and was among the first complex congenital defects to be successfully repaired surgically. Most patients with tetralogy of Fallot reaching adulthood have had their anomaly repaired, and are currently asymptomatic and leading a near-normal life. Pregnancy is well tolerated in this group of women;[10] however, severe pulmonary insufficiency may ensue and may cause decompensation during pregnancy. This emphasises the need to assess women with congenital heart disease, even after a 'successful' repair, on a regular basis to ensure that any cardiac lesions that may limit cardiac reserve sufficiently to complicate pregnancy can be corrected before conception.[11]

Moderate-risk conditions
Fontan-type circulation
The various forms of Fontan operation (Fig. 2) create two separate circulations in series in the

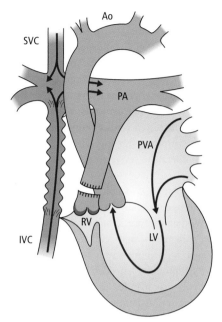

Figure 2 The total cavopulmonary connection variant of the Fontan operation for a single functional ventricle. The superior vena cava (SVC) and inferior vena cava (IVC; via a conduit) are connected directly to the right pulmonary artery and the main pulmonary artery ligated. The ventricle supports the systemic circulation and there is no mixing. A rudimentary second ventricle can be seen. Ao, aorta; LV, left ventricle; PA, pulmonary artery; PVA, pulmonary venous atrium; RV, right ventricle; SVA, systemic venous atrium.

presence of a functionally univentricular heart. These patients are therefore not cyanosed, but experience a long-term low-output state and are at risk of ventricular failure and atrial arrhythmia. They are generally anticoagulated with warfarin, which should be converted to full-dose, low-molecular-weight heparin for the duration of pregnancy. Maternal outcome depends on functional capacity and ventricular function, which is more likely to be adequate if the single ventricle is morphologically left.[12] If these are satisfactory and the woman accepts the 30 per cent rate of first trimester fetal loss, twice that of the general population, then there is no reason to advise against pregnancy as has occurred in the past.

Mitral stenosis

The commonest chronic rheumatic valvular lesion in pregnancy in the UK is mitral stenosis, particularly in the ethnic population from Indian subcontinent, China, Eastern European and East African countries. Since rheumatic mitral stenosis can remain silent up until the third decade, symptoms may often first appear during pregnancy. Congenital fusion of the commissures, or 'parachute mitral valve', and left atrial myxoma are other causes of mitral stenosis during pregnancy.

Haemodynamic abnormalities in a pregnant woman with mitral stenosis include elevated left atrial, pulmonary venous and arterial pressures, which is a function of valve area and flow across the valve.[13] The maternal complications include pulmonary oedema, pulmonary hypertension and right ventricular failure. Tachycardia that may be precipitated by exercise, fever or emotional stress may decrease the diastolic left ventricular filling time and further elevate left atrial pressure, reducing the cardiac output. The end result is biventricular failure. The elevated pressure may also predispose pregnant women to develop atrial arrhythmias, which, with the loss of atrial contractility associated with rapid ventricular response, may have unfavourable effects further leading to pulmonary oedema.

Clinical presentation Pregnant women with mitral stenosis present clinically with symptoms of both left and right ventricular failure, depending on the severity and duration of the valvular disease. Symptoms of left-sided heart failure are more common and include orthopnoea, paroxysmal nocturnal dyspnoea and exertional dyspnoea. Unless the patient has long-standing valve disease, symptoms of right ventricular failure are less common and include peripheral oedema and ascites, which in pregnancy can be difficult to recognise.

Careful examination looking specifically for an opening snap and a diastolic rumbling murmur with presystolic accentuation, which are characteristic auscultatory findings in mitral stenosis, may be rewarding. The presence of elevated jugular venous pressure, hepatomegaly, a loud pulmonary component of the second heart sound and right ventricular heave on examination also supports a diagnosis of mitral stenosis. Most pregnant women with mitral stenosis may present with atrial fibrillation plus or minus cardiac failure.

Assessment and diagnosis Transthoracic echocardiography is the diagnostic modality of choice for evaluation of mitral stenosis in pregnant women. It may confirm the diagnosis and help determine the severity of the stenosis. In addition, the echocardiogram allows assessment of pulmonary pressures, right ventricular function, mitral regurgitation, other valves and the configuration of the subvalvular apparatus, which is important in determining the success of percutaneous mitral balloon valvuloplasty. Invasive diagnostic testing, such as right heart catheterisation, is seldom warranted.

Aortic stenosis

Symptomatic aortic valve disease is less common than mitral valve disease in pregnant women. In the UK, congenital aortic stenosis secondary to membrane on the bicuspid aortic valve appears to be the predominant cause.[14] In contrast, rheumatic heart disease is the most common cause in developing countries and the ethnic population in the UK. During pregnancy, women with bicuspid aortic valves are at risk for aortic dissection related to the hormonal effects on connective tissue.

The pressure gradient across the aortic valve is responsible for the haemodynamic changes in aortic stenosis. The increase in left ventricular systolic pressure needed to maintain sufficient pressure in arterial circulation leads to increased stress on the ventricular wall. To compensate for this, left ventricular hypertrophy develops, which can result in diastolic dysfunction, fibrosis, diminished coronary flow reserve and late systolic failure.

An increase in stroke volume and a fall in peripheral resistance are largely responsible for the increase in the gradient across the aortic valve. The clinical consequences of the increased aortic gradient depend on the degree of pre-existing left ventricular hypertrophy and left ventricular systolic function. When compensatory changes in the left ventricle are inadequate to meet the demands imposed by the need for increased cardiac output late in pregnancy, symptoms develop. This usually occurs with moderate to severe aortic stenosis.

Clinical findings Clinical presentation and symptoms depend on the degree of aortic stenosis. Women with aortic valve areas $>1.0\,cm^2$ tolerate pregnancy well and are asymptomatic. Women with more severe aortic stenosis may have symptoms of left-sided heart failure, which primarily may manifest as exertional dyspnoea. Blackout or near-fainting presyncope is rare and pulmonary oedema (fluid in the lungs) is even more unusual.

As symptoms of aortic stenosis may resemble those of normal pregnancy, clinicians may be misled. Physical findings vary with the severity of the disease. The left ventricular impulse is sustained and displaced laterally. A systolic ejection murmur is heard along the right sternal border and radiates toward the carotid arteries and a systolic ejection click may be heard. A fourth heart sound may be present, suggesting abnormal diastolic function. The presence of slow rising pulse and narrow pulse pressure (difference between systolic and diastolic blood pressure) suggests haemodynamically significant aortic stenosis.

Assessment and diagnosis Diagnosis can be confirmed with echocardiography. The aortic gradient and valve area can be calculated by Doppler flow studies. In addition, echocardiography can detect left ventricular hypertrophy. Estimation of ejection fraction and left ventricular dimensions may be useful to predict outcome during pregnancy, labour and delivery. Women with an ejection fraction less than 55 per cent are at high risk for development of heart failure during pregnancy. Cardiac catheterization is indicated, if the clinical picture is consistent with severe aortic stenosis, if non-invasive data are inconclusive and if percutaneous balloon valvuloplasty is required. Fetal echocardiography is indicated if the mother has congenital aortic stenosis, since the risk that the fetus has similar anomalies is about 15 per cent.

High-risk lesions

Marfan syndrome

Marfan syndrome in pregnant women with normal aortic root carries a dissection risk of about 1 per cent. While the risk of dissection is tenfold with a aortic root diameter >4 cm, the main maternal risk in Marfan syndrome is type A aortic dissection, repair of which carries a 22 per cent maternal mortality.[15] Patients with poor family history, cardiac involvement and aortic root >4 cm diameter or a rapidly dilating aorta are at high risk of dissection and should be advised against pregnancy.[16,17] Those who elect to proceed with pregnancy should be treated with beta-blockers and undergo elective Caesarean section. Patients should also be aware of the 50 per cent recurrence risk.

Aortic dissection can occur without pre-existing disease in pregnancy, probably because of the hormonal changes and increased cardiovascular stress of pregnancy. Bicuspid aortic valve with dilated aortic root may also be a risk factor for aortic dissection in pregnancy, with similar histological findings to that of Marfan syndrome.

Eisenmenger syndrome

Pulmonary hypertension of any cause carries a high risk of maternal death. The risk of death for a patient with Eisenmenger syndrome is 40–50 per cent.[18] Women should be advised against pregnancy. Laparoscopic sterilisation may be considered but not without significant risk. The progesterone subdermal implant at least as effective as sterilisation without any added cardiovascular risk. In the event of pregnancy, therapeutic termination should be offered. Women who elect to continue should be referred to the specialist centre.

■ Care in pregnancy

Antenatal care

The level of antenatal care and monitoring should be determined prior to conception or as soon as pregnancy is confirmed. The main management recommendations for individual cardiac lesions are summarised in Table 1.

General obstetricians based in a district general hospital in the UK on average only ever see a few patients with moderate to severe congenital heart disease; therefore, these patients should be referred to a specialist centre for counselling. Moderate- to high-risk patients should ideally be managed in a tertiary multidisciplinary set-up with 24-h access to a cardiologist, anaesthetist, obstetrician and a neonatologist. Low-risk patients may continue with their antenatal care locally, taking into consideration the specialist recommendations (Table 1).

The antenatal care and delivery should be carefully planned. The patient should be involved in the decision-making process and understand the 'minimal risk approach'. Some patients may benefit from hospitalisation during the third trimester of pregnancy for bed rest, closer cardiovascular monitoring and for oxygen therapy (in patients with cyanotic heart disease). Patients admitted for bed rest should receive appropriate thromboprophylaxis with low-molecular-weight heparin.

Patients with Eisenmenger syndrome (or other forms of pulmonary arterial hypertension), Marfan syndrome with aortic root diameter >4 cm or severe left-side obstructive lesions should be advised of the high maternal morbidity and mortality associated with pregnancy. In the case of unplanned pregnancy, early termination should be considered. If the patient chooses to proceed with pregnancy, however, the need for care in a tertiary multidisciplinary unit cannot be overemphasised.

Anticoagulation in pregnancy and labour

Women with congenital heart disease are at heightened risk of thromboembolic events secondary to chronic or recurrent arrhythmia, sluggish blood flow or metallic heart-valve prostheses. The risk of thromboembolism is elevated sixfold during pregnancy and 11-fold in the puerperium;[19] therefore, achieving adequate anticoagulation is important. However, this is not without risk, and is associated with substantial maternal and fetal complications. Warfarin, an effective oral anticoagulant, crosses the placenta and thus carries major risks for the fetus. In contrast, heparin does not cross the placenta and is, therefore, safe.[20] However, it is reported to be less effective for thromboprophylaxis, particularly in women with metallic valve prosthesis. Therefore, any advice on anticoagulant treatment during pregnancy must weigh the risks and benefits for both mother and fetus, and decisions regarding treatment should be made jointly by the couples.[21]

■ References

1. Lewis G, Drife JO. Why mothers die 2000–2002. *The sixth report of confidential enquiries into maternal deaths in the United Kingdom.* London: RCOG Press, 2004.

2. Person GD, Veille JC, Rahimtoola S, *et al.* Peripartum cardiomyopathy. National Heart, Lung and Blood Institute and Office of rare diseases. (National Institute of Health) workshop recommendations and review. *JAMA* 2000; **283**: 1183–8.

3. O'Connell JB, Costanzo-Nordin MR, Subramanian R, *et al.* Peripartum cardiomyopathy: clinical, hemodynamic, histologic and prognostic characteristics. *J Am Coll Cardiol* 1986; **8**: 52–6.

4. Elkyam U, Tummala PP, Rao K, *et al.* Maternal and fetal outcomes of subsequent pregnancies in women with peripartum cardiomyopathy. *N Engl J Med* 2001; **355**: 1567–71.

5. Thaman R, Varnava A, Hamid MS, *et al.* Pregnancy related complications in women with hypertrophic cardiomyopathy. *Heart* 2003; **89**: 752–6.

6. Autore C, Conte MR, Piccininno M, *et al.* Risk associated with pregnancy in

7. Oakley C, ed. *Heart disease in pregnancy.* London: BMJ Publishing Group, 1997. [A thorough review of the management of heart disease in pregnancy.]

8. Uebing A, Steer PJ, Yentis SM. Pregnancy and congenital heart disease. *BMJ* 2006; **332**: 401–6.

9. Beauchesne LM, Connolly HM, Ammash NM, *et al.* Coarctation of the aorta: outcome of pregnancy. *J Am Coll Cardiol* 2001; **38**: 1728–33. [Retrospective analysis of 118 pregnancies in women with coarctation.]

10. Veldtman GR, Connolly HM, Grogan M, *et al.* Outcomes of pregnancy in women with tetralogy of Fallot. *J Am Coll Cardiol* 2004; **44**: 174–80.

11. Meijer JM, Pieper PG, Drenthen W, *et al.* Pregnancy, fertility, and recurrence risk in corrected tetralogy of Fallot. *Heart* 2005; **91**: 801–5.

12. Canobbio MM, Mair DD, van der Velde M, *et al.* Pregnancy outcomes after the Fontan repair. *J Am Coll Cardiol* 1996; **28**: 763–7. [Retrospective analysis of 33 pregnancies in women post-Fontan procedure.]

13. Bryg RJ, Gordon PR, Kudesia VS, *et al.* Effect of pregnancy on pressure gradient in mitral stenosis. *Am J Cardiol* 1989; **63**: 384–6.

14. Lao TT, Sermer M, MaGee L, *et al.* Congenital aortic stenosis and pregnancy – a reappraisal. *Am J Obstet Gynecol* 1993; **169**: 540–5.

15. Weiss BM, von Segesser LK, Alon E, *et al.* Outcome of cardiovascular surgery and pregnancy: a systematic review of the period 1984–1996. *Am J Obstet Gynecol* 1998; **179**: 1643–53.

16. Lind J, Wallenburg HC. The Marfan syndrome and pregnancy: a retrospective study in a Dutch population. *Eur J Obstet Gynecol Reprod Biol* 2001; **98**: 28–35.

17. Elkyam U, Ostrzega E, Shotan A, *et al.* Cardiovascular problems in pregnant

hypertrophic cardiomyopathy. *J Am Coll Cardiol* 2002; **40**: 1864–9.

women with the Marfan syndrome. *Ann Intern Med* 1995; **123:** 117–22.

18. Yentis SM, Steer PJ, Plaat F. Eisenmenger's syndrome in pregnancy: maternal and fetal mortality in the 1990s. *Br J Obstet Gynaecol* 1998; **105:** 921–2.

19. Hanania G. Management of anticoagulants during pregnancy. *Heart* 2001; **86:** 125–6.

20. Sanson BJ, Lensing AWA, Prins MH, *et al.* Safety of low-molecular-weight heparin in pregnancy: a systematic review. *Thromb Haemost* 1999; **81:** 668–72.

BREATHLESSNESS IN PREGNANCY: RESPIRATORY CAUSES

Simon Quantrill

■ Introduction

Breathlessness in pregnancy is usually due to physiological changes and less commonly to other conditions. The incidence of these conditions in pregnancy is difficult to estimate owing to a lack of relevant studies. Breathlessness, which is the sensation of difficulty in breathing, should be distinguished from tachypnoea, which is an increased respiratory rate. Respiratory rate is crucial to assessing the severity of illness and is often poorly noted by clinicians. Cyanosis is unreliable as a marker of hypoxia, particularly in pregnancy, where there is likely to be a degree of anaemia.

■ Causes of breathlessness

Table 1 lists those causes of breathlessness in pregnancy most likely to be encountered or which are well-recognised as specific complications of pregnancy, but are rare, such as amniotic fluid embolism. When assessing the breathless pregnant patient, the approach should be similar to that undertaken in the non-pregnant patient, as most potential causes are the same. It is helpful to divide these causes into physiological, upper airways, respiratory, chest wall, cardiac (see Breathlessness in pregnancy: cardiac causes) and metabolic.

Physiological

Physiological breathlessness usually starts in the first or second trimester and increases in incidence as gestation progresses. It occurs in 60–70 per cent of pregnant women and is thus the norm. The main diagnostic problem is in distinguishing between a physiological cause and a more serious condition, such as those listed in Table 1. Physiological breathlessness of pregnancy is usually relatively mild, rarely severe, and actually improves or at least does not worsen as term approaches. Breathlessness at rest is uncommon, and activities of daily living and exercise tolerance are not usually affected.

Many studies have been conducted into changes of lung function during pregnancy, with conflicting results. These changes occur as a result of homeostasis owing to the increasing need for oxygenation of the growing fetus. The most significant and well-documented alteration is of increased minute ventilation by 20–40 per cent (tidal volume × respiratory rate) owing to a higher tidal volume. Respiratory rate is not significantly altered or only very slightly increased so most of this higher tidal volume can be ascribed to greater inspiratory effort. This in turn is what leads to the sensation of breathlessness through activation of chest wall proprioceptors and may explain why patients sometimes complain of 'difficulty getting air in'.

Chest X-ray and lung function tests are essential for excluding other causes of breathlessness but there is no specific diagnostic test for physiological dyspnoea of pregnancy. The diagnosis is, therefore, made on clinical grounds together with a normal chest X-ray and lung function tests.

Dysfunctional breathing is common in young women and hence would be expected to occur commonly in pregnancy. Patients typically complain of breathlessness, which appears to be out of proportion to the clinical findings and

Table 1 Non-cardiac causes of breathlessness in pregnancy

Site	Conditions
Physiological	Physiological breathlessness of pregnancy Dysfunctional breathing Vocal cord dysfunction
Upper airways	Nasal obstruction

Respiratory	*Obstructive airways disease:* asthma, cystic fibrosis, bronchiectasis, COPD, obliterative bronchiolitis
	Parenchymal and interstitial lung disease: pneumonia, aspiration pneumonitis, ALI/ARDS, extensive
	    tuberculosis, pulmonary metastases, sarcoidosis, drug-induced, lymphangioleiomyomatosis,
	    lymphangitis carcinomatosa, extrinsic allergic alveolitis, fibrosing alveolitis, COPD
	Vascular: pulmonary embolism, amniotic fluid embolism, pulmonary hypertension (primary and secondary)
	Pleural: pleural effusion, empyema, pneumothorax

Chest wall	Obesity Kyphoscoliosis Ankylosing spondylitis Neuromuscular disease, e.g. multiple sclerosis, polio
Metabolic	Anaemia Thyrotoxicosis Acute or chronic renal failure Metabolic acidosis/diabetic ketoacidosis Systemic sepsis

ALI, acute lung injury; ARDS, adult respiratory distress syndrome; COP, cryptogenic organising pneumonia; COPD, chronic obstructive pulmonary disease.

their ability to perform activities of daily living. It occurs at rest and while talking as well as during exercise. Frequently there are unusual descriptions of dyspnoea including 'difficulty in taking a full breath' or 'a feeling of blockage in the chest'. Physical examination, as for physiological breathlessness of pregnancy, is normal apart from a possible increased respiratory rate.

The term 'dysfunctional breathing' covers a number of phenotypes (clinical manifestations) of which hyperventilation is one of the best known. Although these conditions are clearly not life-threatening, they may cause considerable distress to sufferers, who may also have underlying psychological problems or psychiatric illness.

Vocal cord dysfunction could also be grouped under dysfunctional breathing and leads to similar descriptions of breathlessness. However, this condition frequently manifests as attacks of breathlessness and may simulate asthma, with which it often coexists. Around 10 per cent of all acute asthma admissions may in fact be due to vocal cord dysfunction. It can be diagnosed by clinical history, simple spirometry, which shows a narrowed inspiratory flow–volume loop, and laryngoscopy, which demonstrates adduction of the vocal cords on inspiration and sometimes expiration. Examination may reveal frank stridor or inspiratory wheeze on auscultation of the chest, transmitted from the vocal cords, but is usually normal between attacks.

Upper airways

Nasal obstruction (see Blocked nose in pregnancy) due to rhinitis may occur in up to 30 per cent of pregnant women, as a result of mucosal oedema, hyperaemia, capillary congestion and mucus hypersecretion, which are caused by increased oestrogen levels. This occurs mostly in the third trimester and may lead to a sensation of breathlessness, particularly if severe.

Respiratory
Obstructive airways disease
Asthma is by far the most common obstructive airways disease likely to be encountered in pregnancy, occurring in 0.4–7 per cent of women,

but will usually have been diagnosed previously. It is characterised by intermittent breathlessness and wheeze, worse on exertion, which responds rapidly to inhaled beta-agonists. Examination reveals widespread expiratory wheeze when uncontrolled or during exacerbations. Diagnosis can be confirmed by peak flow monitoring over a 2-week period typically revealing overall reduced peak flows and significant variability. There is frequently diurnal variation with symptoms worsening at night or in the early morning. Uncontrolled asthma is defined by any of the following features: persistent troublesome symptoms, nocturnal symptoms, frequent use of inhaled beta-agonists, exacerbations and limitation of physical activity.

There is some evidence that asthmatic symptoms worsen in one-third of patients, improve in one-third and are unchanged in the remaining third during pregnancy. However, it is also known that more than one-third of women reduce the use of their inhaled corticosteroids during pregnancy, which leads to an increased need to use the emergency department for this condition. Non-steroidal anti-inflammatory drug (NSAID) usage may trigger or worsen asthma.

Cystic fibrosis and *bronchiectasis* will usually have been diagnosed prior to pregnancy and are characterised by frequent chest infections and increased cough with viscous discoloured sputum. Breathlessness occurs if the disease is moderate or severe. Haemoptysis and chest pain may occur during exacerbations and there is a greater frequency of pneumothorax, especially in cystic fibrosis. Malabsorption with steatorrhoea is common with cystic fibrosis and sinusitis is common to both conditions.

Auscultation usually reveals inspiratory crackles over the affected areas. The diagnosis can be confirmed by chest X-ray, but high-resolution computerised tomography (HRCT) scanning may be necessary for some cases of cystic fibrosis and is the investigation of choice for suspected bronchiectasis. This investigation may be necessary in pregnancy, but may be deferred, if the immediate clinical management is unlikely to be significantly altered by the result.

Chronic obstructive pulmonary disease (COPD) can only develop with a smoking history of a minimum of 20 pack-years (number of cigarettes smoked per day multiplied by number of years smoked, divided by 20, the latter figure being the number in a packet), and so is most likely to occur in pregnant women who are older than 35 years of age. The main symptom is breathlessness on exertion with reduced exercise tolerance. It may be accompanied by a cough with morning sputum production (chronic bronchitis). Examination may reveal reduced breath sounds generally or wheeze during exacerbations. Although confined to older women, this condition is very common, accounting for more admissions to hospital than any other respiratory disease. It often goes undetected as lung function (FEV1; see Lung function section below) can decline significantly before symptoms develop. Spirometry is, therefore, the cornerstone of diagnosis, whilst chest X-ray may be normal or reveal only hyperexpanded lungs.

Obliterative bronchiolitis is a relatively uncommon condition that is difficult to diagnose. Clinical and radiological features may be indistinguishable from asthma, with small airways obstruction, and there may be a history of childhood respiratory illness.

Parenchymal and interstitial lung disease

Pneumonia does not occur more frequently in pregnancy and usually presents as an acute illness with a short history of breathlessness, cough and fever. There may be sputum production, pleuritic chest pain and a preceding history of sore throat, cold or influenza-like symptoms. Occasionally, e.g. with mycoplasma pneumonia, the illness may be of several weeks' duration. Examination may reveal increased respiratory rate, auscultatory crackles or bronchial breathing. Diagnosis is confirmed by chest X-ray, which shows consolidation (Fig. 1). *Pneumocystis* pneumonia, which most often complicates human immunodeficiency virus (HIV) disease usually presents with a several week history of dry cough and worsening breathlessness. Chest X-ray in this condition usually reveals bilateral interstitial infiltrates, although it may be normal. Bronchoscopy is often necessary to obtain specimens for cytological analysis.

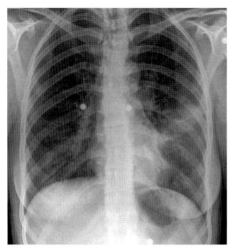

Figure 1 Pneumonia of the lingula lobe.

Aspiration pneumonitis is more common during pregnancy due to the propensity for gastro-oesophageal reflux, and can occur during labour or during induction of general anaesthesia. The result may be a clinical condition indistinguishable from pneumonia resulting in respiratory failure owing to acute lung injury or adult respiratory distress syndrome (ARDS).

Acute lung injury or *ARDS* occurs in 0.2–0.3 per cent of pregnancies and may be caused by pneumonia, aspiration pneumonitis, eclampsia or amniotic fluid embolism in pregnancy, with which the patient will have presented initially. The diagnosis is suggested by a deteriorating clinical condition and worsening of chest X-ray consolidation throughout both lung fields.

Tuberculosis (TB) may lead to breathlessness when there is extensive bilateral involvement of lung parenchyma. There may be a history of cough, sputum, weight loss, haemoptysis and night sweats, frequently with underlying risk factors, such as ethnicity or family history. Sputum should be examined for acid-fast bacilli and a chest X-ray performed, which will show extensive consolidation (if the patient presented with breathlessness), often with cavitation. If there is

no sputum production, then bronchoscopy is necessary to collect bronchial washings.

Pulmonary metastases, e.g. from choriocarcinoma, are rare and easily diagnosed by chest X-ray, which shows one or more nodules of varying size. Symptoms usually occur when metastases are extensive, and include breathlessness, cough and haemoptysis, but chest auscultation will often be normal. Choriocarcinoma may also cause pleural effusions when pleural metastases are present.

Sarcoidosis is common in young women, especially of Afro–Caribbean origin in which it is often more severe. It may cause breathlessness, if there are pulmonary infiltrates, or, rarely, extensive mediastinal lymphadenopathy compressing the main bronchi. In such cases there may also be cough, weight loss and other organ involvement, such as skin or eyes. Auscultation of the chest may be normal or reveal inspiratory crackles or wheeze. There may be palpable lymphadenopathy and skin lesions. The diagnosis can be confirmed by chest X-ray alone in conjunction with the clinical picture. Serum angiotensin-converting enzyme is usually raised and a biopsy may be necessary, e.g. of bronchial mucosa by bronchoscopy.

Drug-induced interstitial lung disease may be caused, for example, by nitrofurantoin or amiodarone. Nitrofurantoin, which is used for long-term treatment of recurrent urinary tract infections, can cause acute and chronic forms of interstitial lung disease with severe life-threatening hypoxia. Amiodarone, which is used in the treatment of cardiac arrhythmias, can cause an acute pneumonitis (incidence 0.1–0.5 per cent with a dose of 200 mg daily) and subsequent pulmonary fibrosis (incidence 0.1 per cent). It is more common with increasing dose and duration of therapy. These conditions usually present with breathlessness and dry cough. Auscultation of the chest may reveal fine bibasal inspiratory crackles.

Lymphangioleiomyomatosis is a rare condition, but it occurs exclusively in young women of reproductive age and should, therefore, be considered in the differential diagnosis of breathlessness in pregnancy. Clinical manifestations include interstitial lung disease, recurrent pneumothoraces, which may be bilateral, and an association with tuberous sclerosis, which is often apparent. Chest auscultation may be normal or reveal fine inspiratory crackles. There is some evidence that lymphangioleiomyomatosis worsens during pregnancy. Diagnosis may be suspected clinically and with chest X-ray, but HRCT scanning is needed for confirmation.

Lymphangitis carcinomatosa occurs in advanced metastatic breast cancer, and can cause severe breathlessness and dry cough. As with drug-induced interstitial lung disease, there may be profound hypoxia.

Extrinsic allergic alveolitis is relatively uncommon and associated with an identifiable trigger antigen, such as inhalation of thermophilic *Actinomycetes* spores in mouldy hay (farmer's lung). Progressive breathlessness, wheeze and cough occur with pulmonary infiltrates on chest X-ray, often in the upper lobes.

'*Fibrosing alveolitis*' usually occurs later in life, but may be associated with autoimmune diseases, which occur more frequently in young women, such as rheumatoid disease, scleroderma and systemic lupus erythematosus, and should, therefore, be considered in the differential diagnosis of breathlessness in pregnancy. It is now classified into a number of conditions of which usual interstitial pneumonia and non-specific interstitial pneumonia are the most common. Progressive breathlessness and cough are typical, with bilateral, fine, mid–late inspiratory crackles on auscultation. Finger clubbing may be present, but is often absent in earlier and milder disease. Chest X-ray usually shows peripheral bibasal interstitial shadowing, but HRCT scanning is necessary to define the type of disease and likely response to treatment. Lung function testing, as with the other interstitial lung diseases, reveals a reduced transfer factor (diffusion capacity).

Cryptogenic organising pneumonia may also be associated with the above autoimmune diseases, and may present more acutely with breathlessness, cough and hypoxia. The parenchymal shadowing is often more patchy than in fibrosing alveolitis. The chronic nature of some of the above conditions may not necessarily be compatible with pregnancy, although some may have a relatively acute onset.

Vascular

Pulmonary embolus remains an important cause of breathlessness that needs to be excluded. The risk of *pulmonary embolism* (PE) in pregnancy is higher with increasing age, body mass index, Caesarean section, family history of thromboembolism, thrombophilia, previous thromboembolism and pre-eclampsia. Pregnancy itself is also a major risk factor for venous thromboembolism and PE remains one of the most common causes of maternal death in the UK. PE may present with breathlessness and chest pain, but also may be asymptomatic: 40 per cent of patients with a proximal deep vein thrombosis and no chest symptoms will have a positive ventilation/perfusion (V/Q) scan. There may be tachycardia and hypotension in more severe cases, and usually a degree of hypoxia. Chest examination will usually be normal except for an increased respiratory rate. Chest X-ray is important in excluding other possible causes of breathlessness, and diagnosis is confirmed by V/Q scanning. Computerised tomographic pulmonary angiography (CTPA) may be needed for diagnosis when the V/Q scan is inconclusive.

Amniotic fluid embolism is rare, occurring in 0.01–0.001 per cent of pregnancies, and presents with sudden onset of breathlessness during labour or within 30 minutes of delivery. There is cardiovascular shock as well as disseminated intravascular coagulation and the mortality is 60–90 per cent, making it a leading cause of maternal death.

Primary pulmonary hypertension is a rare condition occurring most commonly in young women and presenting with breathlessness on exertion. There may be ankle oedema and other signs of right-sided heart failure, such as a raised jugular venous pressure, but the onset and progression are insidious and the diagnosis is frequently missed early in the course of the disease.

Secondary pulmonary hypertension is a consequence of chronic lung disease or pulmonary embolism, and will present with similar symptoms and signs. There may be significant hypoxia with both types of pulmonary hypertension.

Pleural

Pleural effusion secondary to pneumonia or TB, for example, may cause breathlessness, particularly if moderate or large in size (Fig. 2). Rare causes of pleural effusion in pregnancy include lymphangioleiomyomatosis (chylothorax), choriocarcinoma, breast carcinoma and other malignancies, and ruptured diaphragm during labour. Chest examination reveals dullness to percussion, and absent or reduced breath sounds over the effusion. Small effusions may be asymptomatic. It is debatable whether labour itself predisposes to the development of pleural effusions. Studies of chest X-rays postpartum revealed an increased number of effusions but, when ultrasonography was used, no increased incidence was observed.

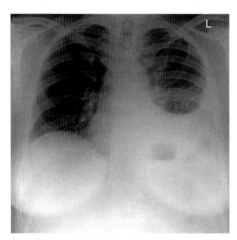

Figure 2 Pleural effusion left side.

Empyema and *pneumothorax* are discussed elsewhere with reference to non-cardiac causes of chest pain (see Chest pain in pregnancy: non-cardiac causes).

Chest wall

Obesity (body mass index >30) frequently leads to breathlessness and reduced exercise tolerance. Examination may otherwise be normal. *Kyphoscoliosis, ankylosing spondylitis* and *neuromuscular disorders* may cause respiratory

failure because of abnormal lung mechanics or diaphragmatic paralysis. Any patient with one of these conditions complaining of breathlessness should have arterial blood gases checked for evidence of hypoxia and hypercapnia.

Splinting of the diaphragm may occur in ovarian hyperstimulation syndrome (OHSS) and also with gross polyhydramnios. Appropriate management will depend on the severity of the OHSS and the stage of the pregnancy, see Amniotic fluid abnormalities.

Metabolic

Anaemia is common in pregnancy, but will usually lead to reduced exercise tolerance and tiredness rather than breathlessness as such. The conjunctivae and nail beds should be examined and a note made of general pallor; however, these signs are unreliable and the blood haemoglobin level should always be checked.

Thyrotoxicosis may occasionally present with breathlessness. Typical features include weight loss, sweating, diarrhoea, irritability, tremor, tachycardia and eye signs. There may be a goitre on examination of the neck. Diagnosis is confirmed by thyroid function testing.

Acute and chronic renal failure, metabolic acidosis and *systemic sepsis* can cause breathlessness, but the diagnosis should be apparent from the clinical picture.

Usually the diagnosis of breathlessness in pregnancy can be made from the history and physical examination, but a chest X-ray is essential to exclude the more important conditions listed above. Many chronic diseases affect fertility and consequently occur uncommonly *de novo* in pregnancy. A focused history should thus be obtained.

■ History

History of presenting complaint

- Onset of symptoms in relation to timing of the pregnancy.
- Duration, chronicity, nature and severity of breathlessness.
- Exercise tolerance, especially in relation to activities of daily living, e.g. climbing stairs.

- Presence or absence of cough, sputum or haemoptysis.
- Relief with inhalers.
- Palpitations.
- Chest pain.
- Weight loss, fevers, anorexia, malaise.
- Leg pain.
- Nasal and sinus problems.
- Sore throat, arthralgia and myalgia.

Past medical history

This includes the following:

- asthma, hay fever, eczema;
- TB, previous BCG (bacille Calmette–Guérin), cystic fibrosis, bronchiectasis, other lung disease;
- sarcoidosis, kyphoscoliosis, neuromuscular disease, heart disease, recurrent urinary tract infections;
- malignancy (e.g. breast cancer), immunosuppression (e.g. HIV positive);
- psychiatric illness;
- previous history of PE or thrombophilia.

Drug history

- Amiodarone, nitrofurantion, NSAIDs and inhalers.

Psychological history

- Symptoms of anxiety or depression.

Family history

- Clotting disorders, asthma, atopy, TB, lung cancer and sarcoidosis.

Social history

- Ability to continue leading normal life, especially going to work, climbing stairs, doing housework, carrying shopping.
- Living in or travel to area of high TB prevalence, and contact with TB.

■ Physical examination

- *General appearance*: confusion, sweating, tremor, pyrexia, cyanosis, pallor, obesity, clubbing, lymphadenopathy, BCG scar, goitre, exophthalmos, lid lag. These may reflect the severity of the disease or point to potential aetiologies.
- *Cardiovascular*: arrhythmia, low or high blood pressure, raised jugular venous pressure (JVP), parasternal heave, gallop rhythm, murmur, pericardial rub.

- *Respiratory*: rate, effort, accessory muscle usage, kyphoscoliosis, tracheal shift, dullness to percussion, wheeze, bronchial breathing, reduced or absent breath sounds, crackles.
- *Breast*: lumps, although mammography, if indicated, may be better than examination.
- *Neurological:* muscle wasting, fasciculation, upper or lower limb weakness, sensory loss, cerebellar signs.

■ Investigations

Radiology

Concern is often raised by the patient, partner or other medical or non-medical staff, regarding the risk of ionising radiation to the growing fetus. Doses of ionising radiation for various radiological investigations are shown in Table 2.

Table 2 Radiation dose from various radiological modalities

Radiological modality	Estimated fetal radiation dose (rads)
Chest X-ray	0.00007
Perfusion scan	0.175
Ventilation/perfusion (*V/Q*) scan	0.215
CTPA	<0.100
HRCT thorax	0.100
Conventional CT thorax	0.265

CT, computerised tomography; CTPA, computerised tomographic pulmonary angiogram; HRCT, high-resolution computerised tomography.

The accepted cumulative dose of radiation to which the fetus can be exposed during pregnancy is estimated to be 5 rads. This is the equivalent of 71 000 chest X-rays, 50 CTPAs or 30 *V/Q* scans, figures worth bearing in mind when considering and discussing the need for these investigations with the pregnant patient. However, it is not known what the fetal risk of developing cancer is later in life for any given radiation dose. The American College of Radiology state that radiological procedures should only be performed in pregnancy if the result is necessary for the care of the patient. When considering any potential adverse effects to the fetus, the risks of not performing important radiological investigations must be taken into account and conveyed to the patient. It can be seen that, for most of the common tests, exposure to radiation is minimal. The tests themselves are essential to arriving at a clear diagnosis that enables a proper management plan to be instituted.

In the first instance, a chest X-ray is crucial to diagnosing or excluding important respiratory conditions such as pneumonia, pleural effusion, pneumothorax, tuberculosis and sarcoidosis (Figs 1 and 2). Without this simple investigation, it is impossible to manage the patient correctly or make any sensible assumptions about the cause of breathlessness. Similarly, *V/Q* scanning is essential to the diagnosis of PE. CTPA is useful in the diagnosis of PE when *V/Q* scanning shows only an intermediate probability of PE, and the clinical suspicion is intermediate or high. HRCT is used in the diagnosis of bronchiectasis and interstitial lung disease, but could be avoided until the postpartum period if the result is unlikely to change the immediate clinical management of the condition.

Although the radiation dose from thoracic CT scanning may be acceptable to the fetus, of greater consideration might be the potential excess risk of breast cancer to the pregnant woman herself: A dose of 1 rad may increase the lifetime risk of breast cancer by as much as 14 per cent in exposed women younger than 35 years old. CTPA delivers 2–3.5 rad to each breast.

Lung function

The most important lung function tests, forced expiratory volume (amount blown out) in one second (FEV1) and FEV1/forced vital capacity (FEV1/FVC) ratio are unchanged in pregnancy (FVC is the total volume of air the subject is able to blow out in one manoeuvre). Normal spirometry (FEV1, FVC and FEV1/FVC ratio) performed with a simple hand-held spirometer (Fig. 3) should exclude any obstructive lung disease (asthma, cystic fibrosis, bronchiectasis, COPD) of sufficient severity to cause breathlessness, although it may also be normal in well-controlled asthma. Spirometry indicative of obstructive lung disease is typified by a low

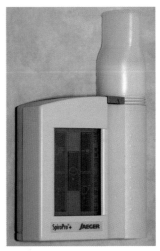

Figure 3 Hand-held spirometer.

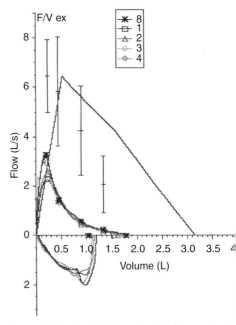

Figure 4 Spirometry (flow/volume loop) showing results of several attempts, indicating good reliability. ex, expected.

FEV1/FVC ratio (<70 per cent), low FEV1 (<80 per cent) and a characteristic 'scooped out' flow–volume curve, caused by obstruction to the small airways (Fig. 4).

Spirometry should only be performed and interpreted by trained personnel, and one should be wary of misleading computer printout diagnoses! Attention should also be paid to the inspiratory flow–volume loop, which may be significantly narrowed in cases of vocal cord dysfunction. Peak flow recordings are essential for the diagnosis of asthma and most useful if measured over a period of at least 2 weeks.

More extensive lung function tests, such as diffusion capacity (transfer factor) and static lung volumes, which are useful in diagnosing and monitoring interstitial lung disease, need to be performed in a respiratory laboratory. Walking oximetry involves asking a patient to walk for 6 minutes with a hand-held oximeter attached to the finger. It is a useful test in the diagnosis of unexplained breathlessness for two reasons: (1) it demonstrates how far a patient can walk in that time and with how many stops; and (2) it shows whether there is any oxygen desaturation during the test. In this way, an objective measure can be determined of how far the patient can walk, and whether or not there is any significant respiratory disorder.

Blood tests

In the investigation of the pregnant patient with excessive breathlessness, blood should be taken for haemoglobin, white cell count, urea and electrolytes, D-dimers and thyroid function tests. Negative D-dimers effectively exclude a diagnosis of PE and should obviate the need for V/Q scanning, but D-dimers increase progressively until term and are, therefore, of most use in early pregnancy. Positive D-dimers are relatively non-specific and may be raised with infections, for example.

Arterial blood gases should be taken in any patient needing further investigation or suspected of having a PE or pneumonia in particular, as significant hypoxia (low PaO_2) usually occurs in these conditions.

■ When should the breathless pregnant patient be referred to a respiratory specialist?

The following is a list of suggested criteria for referral to a respiratory specialist, when considering the breathless pregnant patient:

■ unduly troublesome breathlessness;
■ worsening breathlessness;
■ acute breathlessness;
■ when a CT of the thorax is indicated;
■ when detailed lung function testing, such as diffusion capacity, static lung volumes or walking oximetry, is needed;
■ uncertainty about performing or interpreting spirometry;
■ abnormal chest X-ray or lung function result;
■ uncertainty regarding diagnosis.

■ Summary

Breathlessness in pregnancy is usually physiological in nature, but can generally be distinguished from more serious causes by taking a careful history, performing a physical examination and a chest X-ray. Simple lung function testing should be performed where necessary, and is essential for diagnosing or excluding important respiratory conditions.

■ Further reading

Brewis RAL, Corrin B, Geddes DM, Gibson GJ, eds. *Respiratory Medicine*, 2nd edn. London: WB Saunders, 1995.

Mallick S, Petkova D. Investigating suspected pulmonary embolism during pregnancy. *Respir Med* 2006; **100:** 1682–7.

Pereira A, Krieger BP. Pulmonary complications of pregnancy. *Clin Chest Med* 2004; **25:** 299–310.

Pulmonary disease in pregnancy. *Clin Chest Med* 1992; **13**(4): December.

www.brit-thoracic.org.uk [Guidelines for the diagnosis and management of asthma, COPD, pulmonary embolism, TB, pneumonia, interstitial lung disease, pleural disease and pneumothorax.]

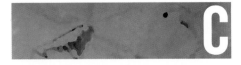

CERVICAL CYTOLOGY, ABNORMAL

Karina Reynolds and Nicola Fattizzi

The cervical smear is an important test that screens for premalignant disease of the cervix. Cervical cells are collected from the cervical transformation zone. Prior to puberty, the squamocolumnar junction is located within the endocervical canal. As a result of the hormonal changes at puberty, there is eversion of the columnar epithelium towards the vagina. At the same time there is a change in the vaginal pH, which becomes more acidic (pH 4–5). This stimulates 'metaplasia' whereby the columnar epithelium changes to squamous epithelium. This area, essentially where columnar cells have transformed to squamous cells, is called the transformation zone. It is in this area that most premalignant changes occur; therefore, it is essential that the squamocolumnar junction is sampled when taking a smear (Fig. 1).

Until recently, smears have been taken with a spatula and spread on to a glass slide. The current National Institute for Health and Clinical Excellence (NICE) guidelines suggest that liquid-based cytology (LBC) should be the method of processing the cells; this should result in a reduction of inadequate smear rates. Current National Health Service Cervical Screening Programme (NHSCSP) guidelines recommend starting screening at the age of 25 years and undertaking smears every 3 years until the age of 50 years, and then every 5 years until the age of 65. This reflects the rarity of cervical cancer below the age of 25 years.

Dyskaryosis is a cytological term essentially meaning abnormal (dys) nuclei (karyosis). On microscopy there is a change in the nuclear–cytoplasmic ratio with an increase in the size of the nucleus compared with the cytoplasm. Increased mitoses and lobulation may also be seen (Figs 2 and 3).

■ Colposcopy referral recommendations

Abnormalities in cervical cytology include the following.

Inadequate smear

The smear is considered to be inadequate in several circumstances where definitive diagnosis is not possible owing to inadequate interpretation in the laboratory. The smear may be poorly prepared at the point of collection (too thick, poorly fixed or air-dried), may be obscured by blood or inflammatory cells, or may not contain the right type or amount of cells (i.e. a slide that contains too few cells or consists entirely of endocervical cells). The rate of inadequate smears should be reduced with the introduction of LBC.

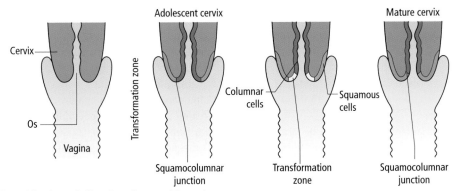

Figure 1 Development of transformation zone of the cervix.

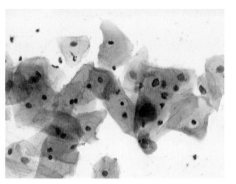

Figure 2 Normal cervical cytology.

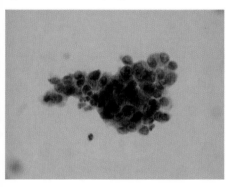

Figure 3 Severe dyskaryosis, change in the nuclear–cytoplasmic ratio.

Borderline smear

Two main conditions can be encountered when a diagnosis of borderline nuclear abnormality is made. The first is the least important clinically, consisting of those cases in which human papillomavirus (HPV) change and actual mild dyskaryosis are difficult to differentiate. The second condition includes all situations where it is difficult to differentiate benign, reactive or reparative changes from significant degrees of dyskaryosis, or even invasive cancer on occasions.

Premalignant disease

Premalignant disease of the cervix is a subclinical condition and so women with cervical dyskaryosis are asymptomatic. Symptoms and signs are suggestive of invasive disease or coexisting conditions. Those symptoms requiring investigation include vaginal discharge, and intermenstrual, postcoital and postmenopausal bleeding.

Dyskaryosis and HPV change are often present in the same smear, but the presence of HPV should not of itself modify recommendations for management. These should be based on the severity of the dyskaryosis. According to the NHSCSP guidelines, women with mild dyskaryosis should be seen and assessed in colposcopy, but not necessarily treated; patients with either moderate or severe smears should be referred for colposcopy after one test. The degree of dyskaryosis (mild, moderate and severe) often correlates with the changes that are found at histology (CIN I, CIN II and CIN III; see later). However, this is not always the case.

Cervical intraepithelial neoplasia (CIN) is a histological diagnosis characterized by nuclear abnormalities (large abnormal nuclei and reduced cell cytoplasm) as well as cellular disorganization (loss of cell stratification and maturation throughout the thickness of the cervical epithelium) and increased mitotic activity. The extent of the above features identifies the degree of CIN (Figs 4 and 5). If the mitoses and

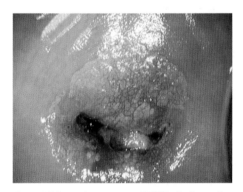

Figure 4 Colposcopic appearance of CIN III after the application of acetic acid.

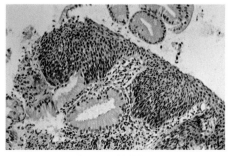

Figure 5 Histological picture of CIN III.

immature cells are present only in the lower one-third of the epithelium, the lesion is designated as CIN I, whereas involvement of the middle and upper thirds is diagnosed as CIN II and CIN III, respectively.

Prospective studies show that the spontaneous regression rate of biopsy-proven CIN I ranges from 60 per cent to 85 per cent, with regression typically occurring within a 2-year follow-up period. This information has led to the recommendation that patients diagnosed with CIN I do not necessarily require treatment. If CIN I is not treated, cytological and colposcopic follow-up should be performed until spontaneous regression has occurred or treatment is required. If the lesions progress during follow-up or persist at 2 years, treatment should be carried out. Unlike CIN I, CIN II and CIN III require treatment.

Colposcopy is a diagnostic tool, the definitive diagnosis being made on histology of the colposcopically directed biopsy.

There are two main types of treatment as follows.

- *Excisional treatments* – generally preferred: knife cone biopsy, laser cone biopsy, large loop excision of the transformation zone (LLETZ or loop). Hysterectomy is occasionally required. With an excisional approach, the transformation zone is completely removed and available for full histological assessment after treatment. In a 'see-and-treat' approach, the histological diagnosis will not be available prior to treatment.
- *Destructive treatments*: including cryocautery, laser ablation and electrodiathermy cold coagulation. A histological diagnosis is mandatory prior to treatment.

Glandular neoplasia

High-grade cervical glandular intraepithelial neoplasia (CGIN) is a premalignant disease of the cervix but is rarer than CIN. The incidence of glandular neoplasia on cytology is in the order of 0.05 per cent of routine smears. This is a challenging disease given that cytological screening is unsatisfactory and colposcopic features usually require expert interpretation. The

diagnosis is often made by chance whilst treating CIN, as these conditions often coexist. Fortunately, most cases of CGIN occur within 1 cm of the squamocolumnar junction but recurrence rates are high (14 per cent), even when the treatment margins are free of disease, as the condition is often multifocal.

Treatment ranges from conservative (in selected cases who wish to retain fertility) to hysterectomy. Conservative options include conization. On follow-up, it is recommended that regular endocervical cytology in addition to conventional cytology and colposcopy should be performed.

It is important to emphasise that this type of cervical cytological abnormality can be related to disease higher in the genital tract, and this needs to be considered depending on symptoms and colposcopic findings (Fig. 6).

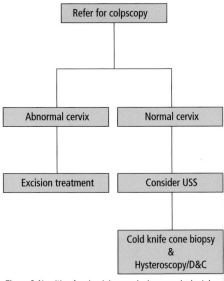

Figure 6 Algorithm for glandular neoplasia on cervical cytology.

Malignant disease

The smear test is a screening test for premalignant disease and not a diagnostic test for cervical cancer. Cervical cytology from a cervix with an invasive lesion often contains inflammatory cells only.

Useful websites

Guidelines for the NHS Cervical Screening Programme: www.bsccp.org.uk/docs/public/pdf/nhscsp20.pdf
The British Society for Colposcopy and Cervical Pathology: www.bsccp.org.uk

CERVICAL SWELLING (CERVIX UTERI)

Karina Reynolds and Nicola Fattizzi

The cervix uteri is the lower part of the uterus (womb) and is comprised mainly of fibrous tissue (Fig. 1). It is lined by squamous epithelium on the ectocervix and columnar epithelium on the endocervix. The position of the squamo-columnar junction varies depending on the age of the woman. Likewise the size of the cervix increases at the time of puberty, during the reproductive age and pregnancy, before reducing in size after the time of the menopause.

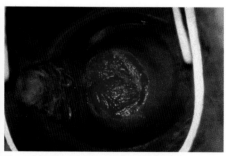

Figure 1 Normal cervix showing a cervical ectropion.

Cervical swellings can be divided into categories as listed below.

Physiological, e.g. nabothian follicles

Nabothian cysts represent a common cause of cervical swelling (Fig. 2). These retention cysts occur very frequently and are the end result of spontaneous 'healing' of cervical eversion by squamous metaplasia, which covers over and obstructs endocervical glands. These cysts can

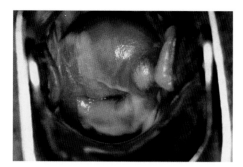

Figure 2 Nabothian follicle on the cervix.

become large and polypoid. Clinically they may mimic a carcinoma by making the cervix look abnormal. When numerous and large, they result in cervical hypertrophy. They represent a clinical diagnosis and no action is necessary.

Reactive

In non-infectious cervicitis, a swollen, erythematous and friable cervix with an associated purulent endocervical discharge may develop. This may be secondary to insults, such as chemical irritation, copper-containing intrauterine contraceptive devices (IUCDs), inappropriate tampon use, pessaries, surgical instrumentation and therapeutic intervention.

Cervical stenosis can occur for many different reasons, causing either a haematometra or a pyometra and, subsequently, the cervix may appear swollen and oedematous. In older women, cervical stenosis may be due to atrophy but, in younger women, cervical scarring may result from trauma (lacerations during labour or at the time of abortion) or surgery (cone biopsy, cryotherapy, cervical cauterization or radiation therapy for cervical cancer).

Note that the diagnosis of haematometra or pyometra in an older woman should always suggest the possibility of an associated malignancy.

The diagnosis may be inferred from the patient's history and biopsy if necessary.

Infective (bacterial, viral and fungal)

Both acute and chronic cervical infections (acute and chronic cervicitis) can frequently result in some degree of cervical swelling. The organisms most commonly responsible for active inflammation in the cervix include *Candida albicans*, *Trichomonas vaginalis*, *Neisseria gonorrhoeae* and Herpes simplex virus. An acute inflamed cervix is swollen and red, often with a mucopurulent plug exuding from the external os; with Herpes it can also become necrotic. Diagnosis is confirmed by taking appropriate swabs from the vagina and endocervical canal.

Cervical warts (Fig. 3) are an uncommon finding and are usually due to human papillomavirus (HPV) types 6 and 11. They may reflect exposure to the oncogenic types of HPV (16 and 18) and should be biopsied as there may be coexisting cervical intraepithelial neoplasia at their base.

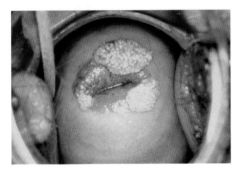

Figure 3 Cervical wart/condyloma.

Specific forms of chronic cervicitis that may result in some degree of cervical swelling include tuberculous cervicitis and cervical involvement in schistosomiasis. Cervical tuberculosis is rare in the UK but may spread from upper genital tract disease, which in turn originates from pulmonary tuberculosis. The clinical presentation is either as a predominantly hypertrophic or ulcerative lesion, which may be mistaken for carcinoma. The cervix may also be involved with similar features, mainly when tuberculosis presents with a non-caseating granulomatous lesion, in syphilis, granuloma inguinale and lymphogranuloma venereum.

Diagnosis in these cases may be made on biopsy and a high index of suspicion. The differential diagnosis may be made only by means of Ziehl–Neelsen-stained sections, culture or animal inoculation of cervical tissue.

■ Haemorrhagic

Endometriotic cysts can occur on the cervix either in isolation or as part of the picture of endometriosis (see Pelvic pain and Mentrual periods, heavy and/or irregular). Diagnosis will be made by biopsy.

■ Neoplastic

Benign

Endocervical polyps (Fig. 4) represent a very common swelling on the uterine cervix. They are most often focal and observed in multigravida during the fourth to sixth decades of life. Their size can range from a few millimetres to some centimetres; rarely, a cervical polyp can become so large that it protrudes beyond the introitus and is mistaken for a carcinoma. A polyp is defined essentially as a lump on the end of a stalk without any commitment as to the nature of the lump. In reality several different cervical lesions can mimic a cervical polyp and

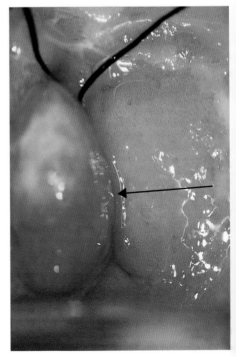

Figure 4 Cervical polyp (arrow) with IUCD strings visible.

can only be classified histologically, as the macroscopic appearances may be similar.

The different types include the following.

- *Mesodermal stromal polyp*, also known as pseudosarcoma botryoides, is a benign, exophytic mass almost always observed in the vagina and cervix of pregnant patients. It can be confused with the malignant sarcoma botryoides.
- *Decidual pseudopolyp* – during gestation, decidual change can occur on the ectocervix, with the finding of a raised plaque or pseudopolyp and, as a consequence, can be mistaken for invasive carcinoma. It can occur in the endocervix, resulting in the formation of a polypoid protrusion from the ectocervical external os.
- *Cervical leiomyoma* (fibroid) – cervical myomas are usually single and can cause enlargement and distortion of the cervix, with stretching and narrowing of the canal. The differential diagnosis includes a leiomyoma arising in the fibromuscular tissue of the cervix and a pedunculated leiomyoma, which arises submucosally in the corpus of the uterus and has elongated sufficiently to protrude through the cervical os.
- *Papillary adenofibroma* – a benign cervical neoplasm typically observed in perimenopausal and postmenopausal women, so-called because of its resemblance to adenofibroma of the ovary.
- *Adenomyoma*.
- *Fibroadenoma*.
- *Granulation tissue* is very friable and usually occurs following some form of surgery.

All these lesions may present with discharge, contact bleeding (postcoital and intermenstrual) or pressure symptoms, depending on size. However, the vast majority are asymptomatic and are usually incidental findings at the time of routine cervical cytology. The final diagnosis is histological after removal.

Malignant
Primary
As a result of the introduction of the National Health Service Cervical Screening Programme, the incidence of -primary invasive cancer of the cervix has reduced, such that a general practitioner will see one case of cervical cancer every

7–9 years. It occurs at least ten times less commonly than breast cancer in the UK.

The majority of cervical cancers are squamous in type. They are usually exophytic cauliflower-type growths or typical epitheliomatous ulcers with accompanying necrosis and haemorrhage (Figs 5 and 6). Small or early lesions may be clinically indistinguishable from cervicitis or ectopy. As the carcinoma grows, it may virtually replace the cervix resulting in a

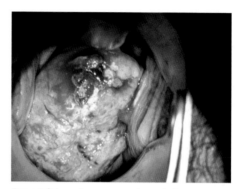

Figure 5 Colpscopic appearance of a cervical cancer.

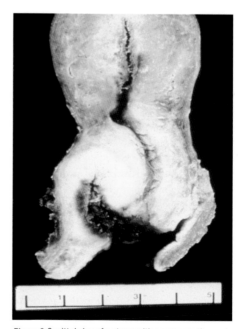

Figure 6 Sagittal view of a uterus with a cancer on the cervix.

bulky, irregular, friable growth and may become distorted if the adjacent vaginal fornices become involved. These features are responsible for the common presenting symptoms of inter-menstrual and postcoital bleeding as well as increased vaginal discharge. Pain is a late feature of this disease. In the event of an endophytic-type squamous cell carcinoma or an adeno-carcinoma, the tumour growth tends to occur within the endocervical canal, frequently invad-ing deeply into the cervical stroma to produce an enlarged, hard, barrel-shaped cervix. In many of these patients, the macroscopic cervical appearances can be normal.

Other rarer malignant tumours that can cause a cervical swelling include lymphoma and leukaemia of the cervix, which are neoplasms of the haematopoietic system whose manifestation in the cervix is usually a reflection of widespread disease. Most patients present with a cervical mass, but they may also complain of vaginal bleeding and discharge. The cervix is typically diffusely enlarged and barrel-shaped. Less commonly the tumour may appear as a polypoid endocervical mass protruding through the cervical os. Some-times a lymphoma-like lesion (pseudolym-phoma), a marked inflammatory extensive lesion of the cervix, can be confused with lymphopro-liferative diseases and can be differentiated only by histology. Different types of sarcoma (adenosarcoma, embryonal rhabdomyosarcoma, carcinosarcoma and leiomyosarcoma) are very rarely encountered as causes of cervical swelling.

Another rare neoplasm of the uterine cervix with a poor prognosis is malignant melanoma. It may initially be misdiagnosed (mainly in the achromic forms) and discovered at an advanced stage when immunohistochemistry is useful – a definitive diagnosis can only be made on immunohistochemical methods and exclusion of other primary sites of melanoma.

Secondary

Secondary tumours do occur in the cervix but are usually from other parts of the genital tract. It is uncommon to find an isolated secondary from another anatomical site in the body.

CHEST PAIN IN PREGNANCY: CARDIAC CAUSES

Velmurgan C Kuppuswamy and Sandy Gupta

Chest pain is the commonest presenting com-plaint in accident and emergency, but fortunately

---

Box 1 Differential diagnosis of chest pain in pregnancy

Cardiac causes

Ischaemic
- Acute coronary syndrome
- Coronary atherosclerosis
  - coronary spasm
  - coronary dissection
  - coronary thrombosis
- Coronary arteritis

Non-ischaemic
- Aortic dissection
- Pericarditis
- Mitral valve prolapse

Non-cardiac causes

Pulmonary
- Pulmonary embolism/infarction
- Pneumothorax
- Pneumonia with pleural involvement

Gastrointestinal
- Oesophageal spasm
- Oesophageal reflux
- Oesophageal rupture
- Peptic ulcer disease

Neuromusculoskeletal
- Thoracic outlet syndrome
- Lesions of cervical/thoracic spine
- Costochondritis/Tietze's syndrome
- Herpes zoster
- Chest wall pain
- Pleurisy

Psychogenic
- Anxiety
- Depression
- Cardiac psychosis

it is not common in pregnancy. The differential diagnosis for chest pain in pregnant women is the same as non-pregnant women and includes cardiovascular, pulmonary, gastrointestinal, neuromusculoskeletal and pschygeneic aetiologies (Box 1). Cardiopulmonary causes, although less common, carry high mortality in pregnancy and therefore need to be excluded as a priority in patients presenting with chest pain. This section will primarily focus on the life-threatening causes of chest pain in pregnancy.

Coronary heart disease

Acute myocardial infarction (MI) the commonest form of acute coronary syndrome in pregnancy is rare in pregnant women, occurring in 1:10 000 pregnancies.[1] The incidence of MI in pregnancy may be increasing, reflecting the trend towards older maternal age. The mortality from MI in pregnancy may be as high as 37–50 per cent and the risk of death is greatest if the infarct occurs late in pregnancy, in women under 35 years old, or if delivery is within 2 weeks of the infarction.[2]

Cardiac troponin I is unaffected by normal pregnancy, labour and delivery; therefore, it is the investigation of choice in the diagnosis of acute coronary syndrome.[3] Thrombolysis is contraindicated for 10 days post-Caesarean section and in late pregnancy in case of premature labour, in view of the heightened risk of haemorrhage. Primary angioplasty may be the best option but there is a lack of evidence to guide management; therefore, the risk of maternal death must be weighed against the risks of radiation, antiplatelet drugs and intracoronary thrombolysis.[4,5]

Women with established coronary heart disease (CHD) should be assessed and treated before conception. Coronary spasm, in-situ coronary thrombosis and coronary dissection occur more frequently than atherosclerotic CHD.

Spontaneous coronary dissection

Sudden severe chest pain in a previously fit pregnant woman may be caused by dissection of the coronary artery. Therefore, thrombolytics

should not be given, but immediate coronary angiography performed with a view to primary angioplasty with stenting may improve survival. Dissection can occur in one or more coronary arteries, and the indication for intervention depends on the site and apparent size of the evolving infarct.

Coronary arteritis and *in-situ* thrombosis

Old Kawasaki disease leading to coronary arteritis with aneurysm formation and thrombosis may present with angina or infarction in pregnancy, and may need coronary artery bypass surgery. Coronary arteritis may be associated with ongoing autoimmune vascular disease and present with infarction in pregnancy or the puerperium. Coronary angiography may be essential for recognition of the mechanism and anatomy of the infarct to tailor appropriate management. Coronary arteritis commonly occurs in the peripartum period and should be differentiated from postpartum cardiomyopathy in the presence of heart failure.

Non-ischaemic causes

Mitral valve prolapse (MVP) is the most common congenital heart lesion and the diagnosis is frequently made in young women of childbearing age.[6] Mitral valve prolapse usually presents with atypical chest pain and mid-systolic murmur associated with a mid-systolic click. The management of this disorder during pregnancy has not been well studied. Women with an otherwise normal heart tolerate pregnancy well and develop no further cardiac complications. Furthermore, the incidence of antepartum and intrapartum complications or signs of fetal distress is no greater than in pregnant women without known cardiac disorder.[7] Antibiotic prophylaxis and regular surveillance with echocardiogram in patients with moderate to severe mitral regurgitation is imperative.[8]

Aortic dissection

Acute aortic dissection is a sudden event in which a tear in the intimal wall of the aorta

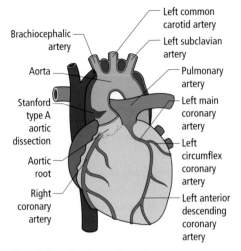

Figure 1 Dissection of ascending aorta.

Table 1 Aortic dissection versus early labour

Symptoms and signs	Aortic dissection	Early labour
Nausea	Present	Present
Anxiety	Present	Present
Restlessness	Present	Present
Epigastric discomfort	Present	Present
Excessive sweating	Present	Present
Arm discrepancy in blood pressure	Present	Absent
Discrepancy in radial pulse	Present	Absent
New-onset diastolic murmur	Present	Absent
Burning sensation in the chest	Present	Absent

allows blood to escape from the true lumen of the vessel, rapidly separating the inner layer from the outer layer of the tunica media (Fig. 1). Patients with Marfan's syndrome have elevated risk of dissection secondary to an abnormal number of microfibres in the tissue of the aorta, which may lead to progressive weakness of the tunica media.[9–11] The parietal pericardium is attached to the ascending aorta just proximal to the origin of the innominate artery. Rupture of any part of the ascending aorta leads to extravasation into the pericardial sac. Rapid death results from the subsequent haemopericardium. Dissections of the transverse arch of the aorta are more complex because the brachiocephalic, left common carotid and left subclavian arteries may be compromised.

Clinical manifestations

Aortic dissection is rare in pregnancy and may be initially overlooked because its manifestations are similar to those for early labour. Pregnant women often experience epigastric discomfort that they may interpret as burning in the chest. Although it is not a symptom of early labour, burning in the chest can be an early symptom of aortic dissection. Blood pressures that differ from one arm to the other or radial pulses that differ in intensity from one arm to the other, the new onset of a diastolic

aortic murmur, and increased severity of chest pain are important characteristics that can be used to distinguish early aortic dissection from early labour. Table 1 summarises the clinical features that distinguish signs of aortic dissection from that of early labour.

Diagnosis and treatment

Acute aortic dissection may be apparent on a chest radiograph as a widened mediastinum, particularly in the upper part of the mediastinum and toward the left side of the thorax. Cardiomegaly and pericardial effusions are also common radiographic findings in patients with ascending aortic dissection. An echocardiogram should be obtained primarily to evaluate left ventricular function, aortic valve competence and size of the aortic root. However, neither a chest radiograph nor an echocardiogram is sufficient for a definitive diagnosis of aortic dissection to be made. Computed tomography, if available, is the emergency diagnostic procedure of choice for aortic dissection.

After definitive diagnosis, repair with a composite graft is the procedure of choice. Preservation of the aortic valve or its replacement with a homograft avoids the need for long-term anticoagulants.[12] Normothermic bypass, progesterone per vaginam and continuous fetal heart monitoring reduce the risk to the fetus.[13]

Acute dissection with origin beyond the left subclavian artery and not involving the proximal aorta should be managed medically. This does no

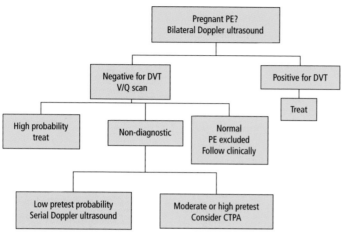

Figure 2 Algorithm for diagnosis and management of pulmonary embolism in pregnancy. CTPA, computerised tomographic pulmonary angiogram; DVT, deep vein thrombosis; PE, pulmonary embolism; V/Q, ventilation/perfusion.

usually need surgery and can be followed by serial magnetic resonance imaging scans. Progressive dilatation to 5 cm or more, recurrent pain or signs consistent with fresh dissection, such as the development of organ or limb ischemia, are all indications for repair. The baby, if viable, should be delivered by Caesarean section before going on to bypass. The anaesthetic management of Caesarean section followed by repair of aortic dissection should minimise fetal exposure to depressant drugs while ensuring a well-controlled haemodynamic environment for the mother.[13] Pregnant women with Marfan's syndrome should be considered at high risk. A successful outcome hinges on rapid diagnosis and prompt referral to the specialist centres.

Pulmonary embolism

Pregnancy is an important risk factor for venous thrombosis and venous thromboembolism is a leading direct cause of preventable death in pregnancy. Diagnosis of venous thromboembolism is complicated in that the symptoms of dyspnoea and lower extremity oedema are relatively common complaints of pregnant patients. Physicians should maintain an appropriately high index of suspicion and request prompt diagnostic imaging in an appropriate sequence (Fig. 2). Diagnosis of deep venous thrombosis with Doppler ultrasonography of the lower extremity poses no health risk to the fetus but other radiographic studies pose a low radiation risk to the fetus. Clinicians should aggressively pursue objective evidence of venous thromboembolism,[14] as anticoagulant therapy poses a greater health risk to mother and fetus than the radiation dose required for diagnosing pulmonary embolism. Once the diagnosis is made, anticoagulation with intravenous unfractionated heparin or subcutaneous low-molecular-weight heparin should be used antepartum followed by warfarin therapy after delivery.[15]

Conclusion

Other causes of chest pain, such as musculoskeletal and gastrointestinal, which are benign but more common in pregnancy, should be excluded. Most women with heart disease have successful pregnancies, but nowadays most cardiologists and obstetricians see only small numbers. Women with known or suspected heart disease, unexplained chest pain or other symptoms of pregnancy, or women who are planning a pregnancy should be referred to a specialist centre. A multidisciplinary approach with experienced cardiologists working as a team with obstetricians, anaesthetists, clinical geneticists and neonatologists constitutes the optimal care for pregnant women with known, suspected or new-onset heart disease.

◼ References

1. Royal College of Obstetricians and Gynaecologists. *Why mothers die 1997–1999, the confidential enquiries into maternal deaths in the United Kingdom.* London: Royal College of Obstetricians Gynaecologist, 2001. [An analysis of all UK maternal deaths published every 3 years. Each cardiac death, and the adequacy of management, is examined in detail.]

2. Webber MD, Halligan RE, Schumacher JA. Acute infarction, intracoronary thrombolysis, and primary PTCA in pregnancy. *Cathet Cardiovasc Diag* 1997; **42:** 28–43.

3. Shade GH, Ross G, Bever FN, *et al.* Troponin I in the diagnosis of acute myocardial infarction in pregnancy, labour and post partum. *Am J Obstet Gynecol* 2002; **187:** 19–20.

4. Chaithiraphan V, Gowda RM, Khan IA, *et al.* Peripartum acute myocardial infarction: management perspective. *Am J Therapeut* 2003; **10:** 75–7.

5. Sebastian C, Scherlag M, Kugelmass A, *et al.* Primary stent implantation for acute myocardial infarction during pregnancy: use of abciximab, ticlopidine and aspirin. *Cat het Cardiovasc Diagn* 1998; **45:** 275–9.

6. Elkayam U. Pregnancy and cardiovascular disease. In: Braunwald E, ed. *Heart Disease. A Textbook of Cardiovascular Medicine,* 7th edn. Philadelphia: WB Saunders, 2001: 1972–3.

7. Oakley C, ed. *Heart Disease in Pregnancy.* London: BMJ Publishing Group, 1997. [A thorough review of the management of heart disease in pregnancy.]

8. Bonow RO, Carabello B, de Leon AC Jr, *et al.* Guidelines for the management of patients with valvular heart disease: Executive summary. A report of the American College of Cardiology/American Heart Association Task Force on Practice Guidelines (Committee on Management of Patients with Valvular Heart Disease). *Circulation* 1998; **98:** 1949–84.

9. Baughman KL. The heart and pregnancy. In: Topol EJ, ed. *Textbook of Cardio-vascular Medicine,* 2nd edn. Philadelphia: Lipincott Williams & Wilkins, 2002: 733–51.

10. Elkyam U, Ostrzega E, Shotan A, *et al.* Cardiovascular problems in pregnant women with the Marfan syndrome. *Ann Intern Med* 1995; **123:** 117–22.

11. Lalchandani S, Wingfield M. Pregnancy in women with Marfan's syndrome. *Eur J Obstet Gynecol Reprod Biol* 2003; **110:** 125–30.

12. Gopal K, Huson IM, Ludmir J, *et al.* Homograft aortic root replacement during pregnancy. *Ann Thorac Surg* 2002; **74:** 243–5.

13. Weiss BM, von Segesser LK, Alon E, *et al.* Outcome of cardiovascular surgery and pregnancy: a systematic review of the period 1984–1996. *Am J Obstet Gynecol* 1998; **179:** 1643–53.

14. Anon. Outcome of pulmonary vascular disease in pregnancy: a systematic overview from 1978 though 1996. *J Am Coll Cardiol* 1998; **31:** 1650.

15. Laurent P, Dussarat GV, Bonal J, *et al.* Low molecular weight heparins: a guide to their optimum use in pregnancy. *Drugs* 2002; **62:** 463–77.

CHEST PAIN IN PREGNANCY: NON-CARDIAC CAUSES

Simon Quantrill

◼ Introduction

This chapter should be read in conjunction with the one on cardiac causes of chest pain. It may be difficult to distinguish between the two, especially as cardiac chest pain frequently presents 'atypically'. Non-cardiac causes of chest pain are summarised in Table 1. There are few data on the relative frequency with which these conditions

Table 1 Non-cardiac causes of chest pain in pregnancy

More likely	Less likely
Unexplained, 'non-specific'	
Chest wall	
Intercostal myalgia/neuralgia	Tietze's syndrome
Muscular strain	Intercostal myositis
Costochondritis	Osteoarthritis of cervical or thoracic spine; thoracic disc lesion
Trauma ±rib fracture	Vertebral or sternal fracture ±osteoporosis or osteomalacia
Mastalgia	
Shingles	
Chest wall abscess (e.g. staphylococcal, TB)	
Cocaine abuse	
Pleura	
Pneumonia	
Infection not visible on chest X-ray (e.g. viral pleuritis, including 'Bornholm disease')	
Pleural effusion due to pneumonia or tuberculosis (TB)	Pleural effusion due to rheumatoid disease, lymphangioleiomyomatosis, malignancy (e.g. choriocarcinoma, breast cancer)
	Empyema
	Haemothorax
Pneumothorax	Pneumomediastinum
Pulmonary embolus	
Sickle chest syndrome	Connective tissue disease (e.g. systemic lupus erythematosus)
Mediastinum	
Oesophageal reflux	
Oesophageal spasm	
	Mediastinitis (e.g. spontaneous or due to oesophageal rupture)
	Aortic aneurysm
	Mediastinal tumour (e.g. lymphoma)
Extrathoracic	
Peptic ulceration	Kidney: pyelonephritis, stones
	Gallbladder disease (e.g. acute cholecystitis)
	Liver disease (e.g. hepatitis)
	Acute and chronic pancreatitis

cause chest pain in pregnancy, except for pulmonary embolus (PE), which remains a major cause of maternal mortality. None of the listed conditions are more likely to occur during pregnancy (except for PE) and so the approach to diagnosis should be the same irrespective of the woman being pregnant. Globally, sickle cell disease may prove to be the most significant cause of non-cardiac chest pain, although non-specific, unexplained and costochondritis are the most common. If the chest pain is pleuritic, then it may suggest an underlying chest wall or respiratory disorder, although this is not invariable.

■ Causes of non-cardiac chest pain

'Non-specific' is a label that is very often used when no other diagnosis can be made. It can also be associated with a history of underlying anxiety or depression.

It is essential to understand the anatomy and physiology of the thorax, especially its innervation, in order to diagnose the cause of chest pain. Thus, diseases that affect only the lung parenchyma, such as interstitial lung disorders, will not give rise to chest pain, as the lungs themselves have no pain fibres in their afferent nerve supply. For chest pain from an intrathoracic cause, there must be parietal pleural involvement. Pneumonia causes chest pain if the infection extends to the pleura: often there will be an associated pleural effusion, although this may be small and difficult to spot. Pain is caused by inflammation of the parietal pleura and not by the fluid itself; accumulation of such pleural fluid will usually give rise to breathlessness (see Breathlessness in pregnancy: respiratory causes) but not pain.

Chest wall

Diagnoses such as '*intercostal myalgia*', '*muscular strain*' and '*costochondritis*' are invariably made on clinical grounds alone after excluding other more serious conditions. There are no laboratory or radiological tests that will confirm these conditions, and the diagnosis must therefore be based on history and examination together with a normal chest X-ray in particular. There are no data to indicate the frequency of these diagnoses in pregnancy. Costochondritis is very common in the general population and results in pain and tenderness, mainly over the upper anterior chest wall. Tietze's syndrome is an uncommon form of costochondritis characterised by chest pain due to inflammatory swelling of the costochondral junctions.

Shingles, the rash caused by the Varicella zoster virus, which reactivates in the dorsal ganglia after prior chickenpox infection, may result in severe chest wall pain. This may persist after the initial rash has subsided when it is called postherpetic neuralgia, and may occur in approximately 20 per cent of cases for unknown reasons, although psychosocial factors may be important. Usually the rash of shingles is obvious, being dermatomal, but pain may precede the development of the rash as well as persist afterwards.

Pleura

Viral pleuritis is a common disorder, but diagnosis is usually based on exclusion of other causes together with a history of coryza or influenza-like symptoms, such as fever, sore throat, generalised arthralgia/myalgia, malaise and cough. Examination may reveal a high

temperature and occasionally a pleural rub, usually best heard in the lower lateral zone of the thorax. 'Bornholm disease' refers to viral pleuritis with sudden onset of pleuritic chest pain and high temperature, caused usually by Coxsackie B virus. The pain is often severe with chest wall tenderness on palpation and there may be associated pericarditis/myocarditis. Other causative organisms include Coxsackie A and echovirus. Virological diagnosis is based on throat swabs, faecal tests and paired sera samples taken at least 10 days apart. In routine clinical practice it is hard to identify the causative virus and may take up to 2 weeks to obtain results. By that time the patient is likely to have recovered. The diagnosis is therefore usually a clinical one.

Pneumonia is characterised by symptoms of breathlessness, productive cough with sputum plus fever. The chest X-ray will show areas of consolidation. Symptoms may vary considerably, but the chest X-ray is by definition abnormal (see Fig. 1 in Breathlessness in pregnancy: respiratory causes). Findings on physical examination commonly include a high temperature and crackles on auscultation. Bronchial breathing occurs when the consolidation is dense and more extensive.

Pulmonary embolus can cause lateral chest pain due to pulmonary infarction at the edge of the lung (often resulting in a wedge-shaped area of necrosis), which then spreads to the pleura, resulting in pain. Central chest pain due to pulmonary embolus may have the same aetiology, but can also be caused by angina following a large embolus, which puts strain on the right ventricle. The most common symptom of pulmonary embolus is breathlessness, with haemoptysis occurring in only about 9 per cent of cases. Clinical examination will reveal signs concomitant with the size of the embolus, but which usually include an increased respiratory rate and tachycardia, cyanosis, hypotension and loud second heart sound (P2) occurring with major emboli. There may be a swollen leg with the typical appearance of a deep vein thrombosis (DVT), left-sided in 85 per cent of cases.

Diagnosis is made radiologically by ventilation/ perfusion (V/Q) scanning, and PE or DVT can be excluded if D-dimers are negative (see Bleeding disorders in pregnancy, including thrombocytopenia).

The *acute chest syndrome of sickle cell disease* may cause severe chest pain, which is typically lateral, but often not pleuritic in nature. Its incidence in pregnancy is unknown. These patients will be known to have sickle cell disease and are often admitted with a crisis whose predominant features will include pain, especially in the limbs. An underlying cause for the chest pain includes pulmonary embolism – due to thrombus, fat or bone marrow – and infection, but is found in only 38 per cent of patients. Respiratory infection is commonly due to *Chlamydia pneumoniae*, *Mycoplasma pneumoniae* and respiratory syncytial virus, but many other organisms may be responsible. These are usually identified from blood samples sent for serology, although the results may be available too late to alter management. Acute respiratory failure may occur in 13 per cent of cases. Fat embolism can be diagnosed by sputum containing fat macrophages or samples obtained from bronchoscopy, although this may only be possible in patients who are intubated.

Tuberculous pleuritis may cause chest pain when tuberculosis (TB) affects the pleura causing a pleural effusion (Fig. 1). Typical symptoms also include fever, weight loss and night sweats, which are usually drenching and nocturnal. Weight loss may be difficult to determine in pregnancy, but failure to gain weight appropriately as gestation progresses may be significant. Breathlessness will depend on the size of the effusion. When TB is restricted to the pleural cavity, it is considered closed and non-transmissible. However, when cough, sputum or haemoptysis are present, then the diagnosis of open transmissible TB is likely, as it will signify concomitant pulmonary involvement. Physical examination will reveal dullness to percussion, and reduced or absent breath sounds over the effusion. The diagnosis of pleural TB is usually made by pleural biopsy as simple aspiration of the effusion will rarely be smear positive

(acid-fast bacilli seen on direct microscopy of fluid) and often culture negative. Pleural biopsy, however, gives a diagnostic yield of at least 60 per cent on histology, rising to 90 per cent if the biopsy is cultured.

Pneumothorax usually presents with the sudden onset of pleuritic chest pain and breathlessness. The pain often subsides quite rapidly, as it is probably due to the sudden shearing off from the chest wall of the parietal pleura. Although primary spontaneous pneumothorax can occur in anyone, it is 9–22 times more common in smokers and usually occurs in those with a tall, thin body habitus. The incidence of primary spontaneous pneumothorax is 1.2/100 000 in females, although it is seven times more common in men than women; therefore, its incidence in pregnancy is likely to be low.

There is no reason to suppose that pneumothorax should be any more common in pregnancy with the exception of during labour, when repeated strenuous Valsalva manoeuvres could theoretically increase the risk of subpleural bleb (small bulla-like structure) rupture, which is the main cause of spontaneous pneumothorax. The clinical diagnosis may be difficult, as physical examination reveals a hyper-resonant percussion note and significantly reduced breath sounds on the affected side only when the pneumothorax is of a sufficiently large size. Tracheal deviation in practice is often difficult to determine and only occurs with very large 'tension' pneumothoraces. Chest X-ray is essential to the diagnosis and should be reviewed by a skilled practitioner, as small pneumothoraces are easily missed.

Pneumomediastinum has also been described in pregnancy and may present with chest pain and breathlessness. This condition is even less common than pneumothorax, although the two may coexist due to a similar underlying cause. Pneumomediastinum may be due to oesophageal rupture and has been reported in association with hyperemesis gravidarum. Subcutaneous surgical emphysema that causes a 'crunching' sensation under the fingertips, may be found on palpation of the upper thorax and neck, and a crunching sound heard on auscultation of the chest.

Empyema may present with pleuritic or non-specific chest pain and occurs most frequently as a complication of pneumonia, developing from a simple parapneumonic effusion. It is more likely to occur when there is underlying immunosuppression. Although pneumonia is well described in pregnancy, there are no series or even case reports focused specifically on thoracic empyema in pregnancy. Typically the history is of several weeks' general malaise, with tiredness, fevers, chest pain and breathlessness, sometimes with a preceding chest infection or documented pneumonia. Weight loss may occur, but again in pregnancy may be difficult to determine. Physical examination reveals similar findings to a pleural effusion with a dull percussion note, and reduced or absent breath sounds over the affected area. An empyema can be loculated in which case the signs are less typical. Chest X-ray may show an identical picture to that of a pleural effusion, but also demonstrate a pleural collection not typical of a straightforward effusion, owing to loculation. Ultrasound of the chest is a useful tool for demonstrating loculated fluid, estimating the amount of fluid present and guiding drainage. Simple needle aspiration is essential for diagnosis and may reveal pus, but the fluid does not need to be frankly purulent to be classified as empyema and an analysis of fluid pH may be necessary: a pH of <7.2 is usually taken as an indication that complete drainage is needed.

Connective tissue disease, such as *rheumatoid arthritis (RA), systemic lupus erythematosus (SLE)* or *Sjögren's disease* may cause pleural effusions accompanied by chest pain; however, the presentation is often with breathlessness and no pain. The connective tissue disorder will usually be pre-existing and therefore easily identified as a possible or likely cause of the effusion. Occasionally, one of these conditions may present for the first time with pleuritis and this could occur in pregnancy, especially as they are generally more common in young women. A history of arthralgia, rashes and dry eyes may be volunteered. The pleural fluid aspirate and a blood sample should be analysed for the relevant autoantibodies (rheumatoid factor, antinuclear factor, Ro and La antibodies) following a diagnostic tap.

Thoracic *malignancy* occurs rarely in pregnancy and if involving the pleura would tend to cause breathlessness more often than chest pain. Pleural effusion may occur but is due to involvement of the visceral pleura, which is not innervated, and/or blockage of lymphatics. *Breast cancer* frequently spreads to bone and pleura, and is the most common malignancy of young women. Bronchial carcinoma usually occurs in later life at an age beyond that of most pregnancies and has rarely been reported. Chest pain due to any thoracic malignancy will be most likely caused by rib metastases, in which case it will be persistent and often severe, interrupting sleep.

Mediastinum

Oesophageal reflux is extremely common in pregnancy and can result in chest pain, usually manifest as 'heartburn', a burning sensation in the centre of the chest worse after meals. Up to two-thirds of pregnant women may have reflux, caused by relaxation of the gastro-oesophageal sphincter owing to high progesterone levels. Smoking and alcohol are aggravating factors. However, the expression of heartburn may be different in individual women who may complain of chest pain indistinguishable from other causes. Usually the diagnosis can be made on clinical grounds alone (see Heartburn in pregnancy).

Extrathoracic

Peptic ulcer disease is less common in pregnant women, but the resultant upper abdominal pain may manifest as lower chest pain instead. Endoscopy may be necessary if symptoms fail to clear with drug treatment or complications such as gastrointestinal bleeding are apparent (see Epigastric pain in pregnancy).

Other abdominal diseases, such as *cholecystitis, gallstones, kidney stones, pyelonephritis* or *acute pancreatitis*, for example, may occasionally present with lower chest pain, which leads to diagnostic difficulty. One of these disorders might be suspected if there are other typical features in the history, such as pain occurring shortly after eating meals (especially with a high fat content) for gallstones; fever and/or rigors with cholecystitis and pyelonephritis; frequency, dysuria and haematuria with pyelonephritis and sometimes kidney stones; spasmodic pain with gallstones and kidney stones; or the presence of possible triggers for acute pancreatitis such as alcohol or known gallstones.

The following provides an approach to the history and examination in the pregnant patient with chest pain (refer also to cardiac causes of chest pain).

■ History – key features to be elucidated

History of the presenting complaint

- Duration, onset, severity, nature and radiation of chest pain.
- Relation of pain to meals.
- Aggravating or relieving factors.
- Breathlessness.
- Cough, sputum, haemoptysis.
- Fever, weight loss.
- Arthralgia, myalgia, sore throat.
- Trauma, e.g. fall.
- Leg pain.

Psychological

- Symptoms of anxiety or depression.

Past medical history

- TB or contact history.
- Previous history of thrombosis or embolism, e.g. DVT in previous pregnancy.
- Sickle cell disease.
- Underlying immunosuppression, e.g. HIV disease.
- Connective tissue disease, e.g. SLE, RA, Sjögren's syndrome.
- Asthma.
- Chickenpox.
- Shingles.

Medication

- Prednisolone.
- Previous use of oral contraceptive pill.

Family history

- Clotting disorders.
- TB.

Social history

- Smoking, ethnicity, travel history, contact with TB.

■ Physical examination – key findings to look for

- *General examination*: fever, sweating, cyanosis, lymphadenopathy, jaundice, anaemia, inflamed throat, evidence of connective tissue disease.
- *Cardiovascular system*: tachycardia, hypotension, raised jugular venous pressure (JVP), parasternal heave, loud second heart sound (P2), gallop rhythm, pericardial rub.
- *Respiratory system*: increased respiratory rate, chest wall tenderness, chest wall masses, tracheal deviation, dullness to percussion, crackles, bronchial breathing, reduced or absent breath sounds on auscultation.
- *Breast*: lumps.
- *Abdomen*: right upper quadrant, epigastric or loin tenderness; enlarged liver.

■ Investigations

Chest radiography delivers negligible radiation and is crucial to diagnosing or excluding important conditions such as pneumonia and pleural effusion. Similarly, pulmonary embolism cannot be reliably diagnosed without a *V/Q* scan. The consequences of misdiagnosis are potentially far worse than the negligible risk of harm to the fetus from these tests. Ultrasonography is usually the first investigation of choice for possible abdominal pathology.

■ Summary

Non-cardiac causes of chest pain are broadly the same in pregnancy as in the non-pregnant state. The most common causes will be non-specific and often no definite aetiology will be found. More serious causes should be apparent from the history, examination and simple investigations.

■ Further reading

Brewis RAL, Corrin B, Geddes DM, Gibson GJ, eds. *Respiratory Medicine*, 2nd edn. London: WB Saunders, 1995.

Pulmonary disease in pregnancy. *Clin Chest Med* 1992; **13**(4): December.

Warrell DA, Cox TM, Firth JD, Benz EJ, eds. *Oxford Textbook of Medicine*, 4th edn. Oxford: Oxford University Press, 2004.

www.brit-thoracic.org.uk: Guidelines for the diagnosis and management of pneumonia, TB, pulmonary embolism, pleural disease, pneumothorax.

COLLAPSE IN PREGNANCY

Greg Davis

Pregnant women are normally young and healthy and, apart from simple fainting, collapse is very uncommon, with cardiac arrest estimated to occur only once in 30 000 pregnancies.

In pregnancy, collapse usually indicates a life-threatening emergency. Typically the sequence of events is that the woman becomes agitated, possibly short of breath, then confused before losing consciousness and collapsing. It is imperative that resuscitation should commence immediately even though the diagnosis may not be clear initially. Immediate assessment will determine if the woman is conscious, breathing and whether there is significant blood loss. Resuscitation should follow the standard Advanced Life Support protocols and the diagnosis may only become clear as the resuscitation proceeds.

A flow chart for the diagnosis of the woman collapsing in pregnancy is shown in Fig. 1.

The causes of collapse are shown in Box 1 and these will be covered in this sequence in the chapter.

■ Syncope

Blood pressure normally falls in the second trimester of pregnancy owing to reduced peripheral resistance. Venous pooling occurs in the lower limbs and more muscle activity is necessary than in the non-pregnant state to ensure adequate venous return. Consequently, pregnant women are more prone to fainting by anything that exacerbates these normal physiological changes. Standing still for prolonged periods, e.g. on public transport, standing up quickly and lying supine in late pregnancy are more likely to cause

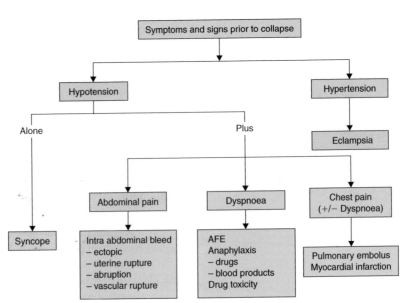

Figure 1 Flow chart for the diagnosis of the woman collapsing in pregnancy. AFE, amniotic fluid embolism.

Box 1 Causes of collapse in pregnancy

- Syncope
- Haemorrhage due to:
  - blood loss – ruptured ectopic pregnancy, placental abruption, uterine rupture
  - coagulopathy – sepsis, abruption, amniotic fluid embolism
- Embolism – pulmonary, amniotic fluid, air, fat
- Intracranial bleeding
- Eclampsia
- Myocardial infarction
- Anaphylaxis
- Drug toxicity
- Transfusion reaction

fainting than in the non-pregnant woman. Hot weather increases peripheral vasodilatation and also makes fainting more likely.

The diagnosis is usually suggested by the history (either from the recovering woman or observers) and the situation in which it has occurred, e.g. when standing on a crowded stuffy train. Loss of consciousness is not sudden and is preceded by a feeling of light-headedness or dizziness, a cold sweat and nausea. Observers will note pallor, sweating and a rapid weak pulse. If the woman does not sit or lie down, these signs and symptoms will be quickly followed by a complete loss of consciousness and resulting collapse. There may be injury due to falling and, less commonly, seizures due to cerebral anoxia if the woman is kept in an upright or semi-recumbent position. The woman will usually regain consciousness quickly when she is placed in the recovery position and give a history of symptoms confirming the diagnosis on recovering. If seizures have occurred, a careful history and examination will be necessary to exclude a more serious cause. Sometimes the diagnosis may only be made after further investigation to rule out an intracranial or metabolic cause for the seizure(s).

■ Haemorrhage

Haemorrhage due to any cause may lead to collapse in pregnancy. Pregnant women have a significant increase in blood volume (up to 40 per cent by the end of pregnancy) but may lose up to 35 per cent of their blood volume without showing signs of hypovolaemia. The degree of blood loss may be completely or partially concealed and, when decompensation occurs, it is often more rapid than in the non-pregnant. Fetal distress may be the first sign of hypovolaemia as the mother's blood flow is diverted from her pelvic organs (normally 30 per cent of cardiac output in late pregnancy) to maintain blood pressure and cerebral perfusion. The symptoms of hypovolaemia (shock) are shortness of breath, agitation, thirst and the woman complaining of feeling cold and shivering. Signs to be observed are fetal distress, pallor, a cold clammy skin, a rapid weak pulse, low blood pressure and progressive loss of consciousness as blood pressure falls.

Blood loss

Ectopic pregnancy

Ectopic pregnancy usually presents between 6 and 10 weeks of pregnancy, and it has been estimated that 50 per cent of cases will have been seen by a doctor and the diagnosis missed prior to hospital presentation. One in 80–90 pregnancies is ectopically situated and this increases to one in 20 if the woman has had fertility treatment. Other risk factors for ectopic pregnancy are: previous ectopic pregnancy; use of progesterone-only contraception; tubal damage, including previous sterilisation; and a history of a fertility problem.

Any woman of reproductive age admitted to hospital with loss of consciousness should be assumed to be (1) pregnant and (2) have a ruptured ectopic pregnancy until proved otherwise. There may be a history of severe abdominal pain and then a progressive loss of consciousness. There will be signs of shock. Her abdomen may be distended and, depending on the level of consciousness, very tender with signs of peritonism (guarding and rebound tenderness).

The latter are not invariable, however, and distension and tenderness may be difficult to assess if the woman is unconscious and/or large.

A large intra-abdominal bleed causing shock is usually a straightforward diagnosis and immediate surgery is required. In women of this age group without a history of trauma, ruptured ectopic pregnancy is the most likely diagnosis and is confirmed by a positive pregnancy test on blood (or urine) taken during resuscitation. Blood should be taken for full blood count, cross-match and quantitative human chorionic gonadotrophin (HCG). If resuscitation is effective and the woman's condition is stabilised sufficiently prior to surgery to allow further investigation, ultrasound scanning will reveal an empty uterus and the presence of intra-abdominal bleeding. The detection of a pelvic mass on ultrasound scanning is not necessary to confirm the diagnosis.

Abruption

In the second half of pregnancy, placental abruption is the most likely cause of blood loss sufficient to cause collapse. The bleeding behind the placenta does not, of itself, usually cause hypovolaemia and collapse. However, the extravasation of blood into the myometrium can lead to a severe coagulopathy and disseminated intravascular coagulation with subsequent diffuse bleeding and resulting haemorrhagic shock. The uterus is usually tender, firm and the fundus may be rising. With electronic fetal heart rate monitoring the fetal heart rate is either clearly abnormal or absent. While resuscitation is taking place, blood should be taken for full blood count, group and cross-match, and coagulation tests. The woman must be closely observed once haemodynamically stable and delivery of the baby is under way or completed, as coagulopathy may not be obvious at first and only develop subsequently.

Uterine rupture

Spontaneous uterine rupture is rare during pregnancy, but more likely if the woman has a history of myomectomy or classical Caesarean section. Rupture is more likely to occur in labour and the risk is thought to be increased by induction with prostaglandins in women with a previous Caesarean delivery and in obstructed labour, particularly in multiparous women. Most uterine ruptures are not associated with collapse and present with pain and fetal distress. 'Catastrophic' uterine rupture usually presents in labour with the sudden onset of severe, generalised abdominal pain, fetal distress and shock, and may proceed rapidly to collapse and death. A history of uterine surgery and the degree of abdominal pain suggest uterine rupture or a major intra-abdominal bleed; resuscitation and immediate surgery are required to save the mother's life. The fetus is usually dead unless the rupture occurs in hospital and delivery is accomplished very quickly.

Trauma

Abdominal trauma in pregnancy, whether due to automobile accidents, falls or domestic violence may lead to abruption, uterine rupture and/or significant intra-abdominal bleeding resulting in collapse. Other causes of intra-abdominal bleeding are rare in pregnancy, but the rupture of congenital or pregnancy-related vascular aneurysms, e.g. splenic or adrenal arteries, is thought to be more common in pregnancy, owing to increased blood flow, changes in the vessel walls and vasodilatation. The presentation will be similar to that of spontaneous uterine rupture (see earlier) but with a history of trauma. It is important to remember that this history may not be forthcoming if the trauma is a result of domestic violence.

Coagulopathy

Serious blood loss causing collapse is often exacerbated by coagulopathy in pregnancy. The coagulopathy may be part of the disease process, e.g. severe pre-eclampsia, abruption, amniotic fluid embolism, or due to the consumption of coagulation factors as a result of massive blood loss. Coagulation factors should be measured in severe pre-eclampsia but are unlikely to be abnormal if the platelet count is normal. Coagulopathy should be anticipated where collapse has occurred from abruption, amniotic fluid embolism or massive haemorrhage of any cause.

■ Embolism

Pulmonary embolism

Venous thromboembolism occurs in one in 1000–2000 pregnancies and is a leading cause of maternal death in developed countries. While a lower limb deep venous thrombosis (DVT) is the likely precursor for pulmonary embolism (PE), this is often undiagnosed and the initial presentation may be sudden cardiopulmonary arrest. Risk factors for DVT are prolonged bed rest, maternal age >35 years, parity of three or greater, a personal or family history of DVT, varicose veins, smoking or a known hypercoagulable state, such as antiphospholipid syndrome. If the DVT is untreated, 20 per cent of women will develop PE. A total of 15 per cent of pregnant women who develop a PE will die, with two-thirds dying within 30 minutes of the embolic event. This emphasises the point that making the diagnosis of PE takes second place to resuscitation.

Pulmonary embolism should be suspected when there is sudden cardiac and/or pulmonary compromise in the absence of other precipitating factors such as blood loss. Collapse may be preceded by chest pain and shortness of breath. During resuscitation, oxygen saturation should be assessed, although it will be low, so this is not helpful diagnostically. When stable, the woman should have a chest X-ray to exclude intrathoracic pathology, such as pneumothorax, and will need a low-dose ventilation/perfusion (V/Q) scan to confirm the diagnosis of PE. Because of the profound disturbance of maternal physiology in this situation, the V/Q scan is very likely to be diagnostic. If suspicion of PE is high, then treatment should be commenced whilst waiting for the results of investigations (see Chest pain in pregnancy, non-cardiac and Leg pain in pregnancy).

Amniotic fluid embolism

Amniotic fluid embolism (AFE) is a rare phenomenon occurring in one in 8000–80 000 pregnancies and its incidence increases with maternal age. It usually occurs during labour after rupture of the membranes; however, it has been reported after amniocentesis and first trimester curettage. Classically it is thought to be associated with hypertonic uterine activity and abruption, but these factors are not invariable. The pathophysiology is not clear, but there is respiratory and cardiovascular collapse, which may be profound and fatal within 30–60 minutes. If the woman lives longer than this, a coagulo-pathy invariably develops rapidly and contributes to the haemorrhagic shock. There are similarities in the presentation to anaphylactic shock and AFE has been termed the anaphylactoid syndrome of pregnancy.

The presentation is similar to PE with shortness of breath and rapid collapse. Chest pain is not a feature of AFE; however, if the woman is unconscious, there may be no history to help with this distinction. Provided the woman survives the initial collapse following embolism, the progressive coagulopathy confirms the diagnosis of AFE and distinguishes it from PE. The diagnosis is clinical and the purpose of investigations is to guide treatment. Blood should be taken for a full blood count, coagulation studies and cross-match. If AFE has occurred, these blood tests will need repeating frequently to assess the need for the replacement of blood products. The taking of blood and provision of blood products should be coordinated by a haematologist because of the rapidly changing situation. The detection of fetal squames in central venous blood confirms the diagnosis, but is of little clinical benefit and pursuit of the diagnosis must not interfere with the woman's resuscitation.

■ Intracranial bleeding

Although rare in pregnant women, intracranial bleeding of any cause may lead to loss of consciousness and collapse. This may occur as a result of trauma or spontaneously as seen in subarachnoid haemorrhage. If traumatic in origin, the cause will usually be obvious and should be suspected in any pregnant woman presenting with significant head injury. Although there may be a preceding history of headache (see Headache in pregnancy), spontaneous acute intracranial bleeding due to subarachnoid haemorrhage, rupture of a berry or saccular aneurysm or arteriovenous malformation (Fig. 2) may present with a sudden loss of consciousness and collapse. In most cases, blood pressure will be normal or elevated, and signs of raised intracranial pressure will be detected with papilloedema and cranial nerve abnormalities. The abrupt history, these signs and the absence of bleeding all indicate an intracranial cause that will normally need immediate neurosurgical review and probable intervention.

■ Eclampsia

Eclampsia occurs in one in 2000 pregnancies (in the developed world) and about one-third of eclamptic fits occur antenatally. There may be a history of preceding severe pre-eclampsia with hypertension, proteinuria, and abnormal renal, liver or other haematological dysfunction. These women may present with symptoms and signs of imminent eclampsia: severe headache, persistent visual disturbances, epigastric pain and/or hyper-reflexia. In making the diagnosis, it should be remembered that these symptoms are also indications for convulsion prophylaxis with magnesium sulphate. If pregnant women with these symptoms do fit, it is likely that the seizures are due to a hypertensive encephalopathy. However, in 20 per cent of cases, the fit is the initial presentation with normal or only mildly elevated blood pressure. In these women, cerebral vasoconstriction leading to ischaemia and cerebral oedema due to cell death is the most likely cause of the fitting (Fig. 3). Cerebrovascular accidents complicating pre-eclampsia and eclampsia are now an important cause of maternal death in developed countries.

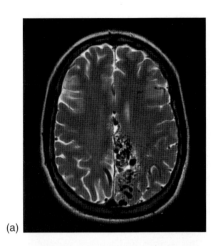

(a)

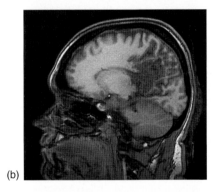

(b)

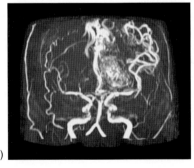

(c)

Figure 2 Scans showing a large arteriovenous malformation (AVM) in a pregnant woman who was found collapsed at home. She subsequently had a number of witnessed generalised tonic/clonic seizures. Mother and baby did well and mother had no further seizures after delivery. (a) Axial T2-weighted MRI showing AVM (cluster of dark blood vessels). (b) Sagittal T1-weighted MRI showing AVM (area of low signal posteriorly). (c) Intracranial MR angiogram showing aberrant vasculature.

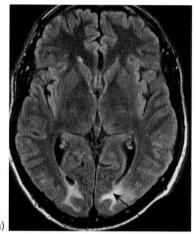 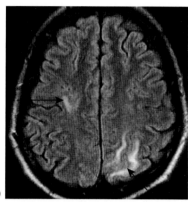

(a)   (b)

Figure 3 This 34-year-old woman presented with severe pre-eclampsia at 34 weeks' gestation and was found collapsed in a hospital bathroom. She appeared to be postictal and it was assumed she had suffered an eclamptic seizure. Owing to the uncertainty, a magnetic resonance imaging scan was performed. (a) This axial FLAIR image demonstrates increased signal (marked by arrows), owing to cerebral oedema of the subcortical white matter in the occipital lobes. The increased signal would be even more marked if the changes were a result of infarction. (b) The sporadic nature of the changes seen with pre-eclamptic encephalopathy is shown in this FLAIR image further cephalad, which again shows changes in the left posterior parietal lobe (small arrow), but less marked signal increase in the right posterior frontal white matter (large arrow). FLAIR, fluid-attenuated inversion recovery.

The fit may be witnessed in which case the woman usually complains of feeling 'unwell', collapses and loses consciousness. The fit is typically generalised tonic/clonic and short lived, and there may be urinary incontinence or injury to the mouth and/or tongue. Supportive care should be undertaken during the fit and magnesium sulphate administered to terminate the fit and provide subsequent prophylaxis to prevent recurrence.

If the fit is not witnessed, then diagnosis may be more difficult. A history of pre-eclampsia is suggestive. If conscious, the woman will be confused and her vital signs normal. In particular, blood pressure will be normal or elevated, in sharp contrast to most other causes of maternal collapse. As a result of the fit, there may be external trauma, damage to mouth and/or tongue or evidence of incontinence.

◼ Myocardial infarction

Although most pregnant women are young and healthy, increasingly, older and less medically fit women are having babies. Women with ischaemic heart disease are at risk of myocardial infarction, although it remains a very rare cause of cardiac arrest in pregnancy. The diagnosis should be suspected when significant chest pain precedes the collapse. There may or may not be a history of cardiac disease. As above, the diagnosis must be made as resuscitation continues. The woman should have an electrocardiogram and cardiac enzymes tests performed when she is stable.

◼ Anaphylaxis

Anaphylaxis is a severe, rapid-onset, allergic reaction, which may result in death. It is a multisystem disorder that usually involves shortness of breath, anxiety, flushing or itching, and may progress to collapse due to hypoxia (upper airway oedema, bronchospasm) and/or shock (vasodilatation, fluid shift, myocardial depression). In pregnant women, it is most often seen after the administration of penicillin for Group B streptococcus prophylaxis in labour or after a dose of a non-steroidal anti-inflammatory drug. It has also been observed in women sensitive to latex if inadvertently used during the labour, e.g. use of a urinary catheter containing latex.

The diagnosis is usually clear because of the close association between the woman taking the drug and the subsequent reaction; however, the skin changes are often transient and may be missed. If so, the sudden onset of airway obstruction in the absence of a history of airways disease makes other causes unlikely. There are no investigations that are helpful in making the diagnosis, which is confirmed by the response to appropriate treatment with adrenaline and intravenous fluids.

■ Drug toxicity

Local anaesthetics

Although not strictly a 'toxic' effect, the commonest cause of collapse in pregnant women is probably temporary respiratory paralysis as a result of an epidural block for analgesia ascending too high and paralysing the woman's diaphragm and accessory respiratory muscles. This can happen after a 'top-up', but is more likely after the initial dose of local anaesthetic. There is usually very effective analgesia and motor paralysis initially, and then the woman complains of feeling short of breath or finding it difficult to breathe. She becomes more anxious and dyspnoeic, before quite rapidly progressing to respiratory arrest. The close correlation between the administration of local anaesthetic and the progressive respiratory distress confirms the diagnosis.

A more truly toxic effect occurs with intravascular injection of a local anaesthetic agent, again typically with the insertion or topping up of an epidural block, although it has also been described with the insertion of pudendal nerve blocks. Pregnant women appear to be more susceptible, probably because of increased vascularity in the vessels around the epidural space, and the increased pressures in the subarachnoid and epidural spaces that occur with contractions. Generally, the longer acting agents, e.g. bupivacaine, are more toxic than shorter-acting agents like lignocaine. Signs and symptoms usually occur within minutes of the injection of local anaesthetic. Women may complain of a funny taste, and become confused and short of breath. Respiratory paralysis follows and cardiac arrest may occur as a result of anoxia and/or myocardial depression. Seizures may also occur owing to anoxia. Because both occur after injection of local anaesthetic, it can be difficult to differentiate between a high block and intravascular injection. The latter usually has the characteristic metallic taste and quicker onset.

Treatment is essentially the same, namely cardiorespiratory support as required until the effect wears off, so a lack of certainty in the final diagnosis is not critical. Once again, acute management of the clinical problem, respiratory arrest owing to muscle paralysis, is more important and the exact diagnosis can usually be made after the woman has recovered.

Magnesium toxicity

Magnesium sulphate is effective as an anticonvulsant owing to its action as a blocker of neuromuscular junctions. With its widespread use for convulsion prophylaxis in obstetrics, overdose has become more common, particularly as it is often given in emergency situations where clinical errors are more likely to occur. With increasing levels of magnesium there is progressive loss of reflexes, flushing and shortness of breath, leading to respiratory arrest unless the rise in magnesium levels is halted. At higher levels still there are alterations in cardiac conduction and, ultimately, cardiac arrest.

■ Transfusion reaction

Transfusion reactions are common but do not usually cause collapse; however, they are an allergic response to foreign biological material and anaphylaxis can develop. Symptoms usually occur soon after the transfusion begins and the cause is, therefore, obvious. The symptoms are similar to anaphylaxis with skin changes that may be transient, raised body temperature, generalised urticaria and airway obstruction.

■ Conclusion

Collapse in pregnancy is rare, and therefore frightening and often unfamiliar to the clinicians present, i.e. midwifery and obstetric staff. The diagnosis of the underlying cause of the collapse may not be immediately obvious. As has been emphasised in this section, resuscitation must begin even if the diagnosis is unclear. The differential diagnosis is not extensive but, in this clinical situation, rational thought often deserts us. Prompt introduction of appropriate resuscitation may make the difference between the woman living or dying, and give the time necessary to make a diagnosis. It is also the reason for including collapse in the emergency practice drills of all maternity staff.

COLLAPSE IN THE PUERPERIUM

Greg Davis

Most of the causes of collapse in the puerperium are also seen in pregnancy and this chapter should be read together with Collapse in pregnancy. However, collapse in the puerperium is more common, principally due to postpartum haemorrhage. This will therefore be the main focus of this section, with shorter discussion of the other causes described in Collapse in pregnancy, which are relevant to the puerperium. Once again it is important to emphasise that resuscitation must be proceeding while the diagnosis is being made.

A flow chart for the diagnosis of the woman collapsing in the puerperium is shown in Fig. 1.

Immediate puerperal collapse, symptoms and signs

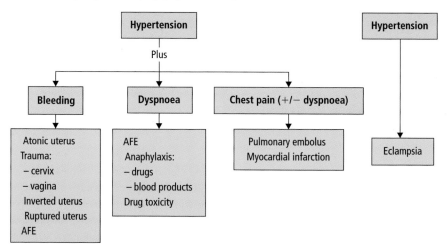

Delayed puerperal collapse, symptoms and signs

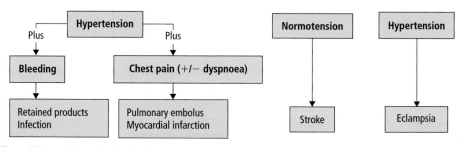

Figure 1 Diagnostic flow chart for the collapsed woman in the puerperium. AFE, amniotic fluid embolism.

Although an arbitrary classification, for the purposes of this discussion:

- *immediate collapse* is seen in the first 24 hours after delivery and usually within the first few hours;
- *delayed collapse* occurs after 24 hours and within 6 weeks of delivery.

It is rare for collapse more than 6 weeks following delivery to be due to a pregnancy-related cause.

The causes of collapse are shown in Box 1 and these will be covered in this sequence in the chapter.

Box 1 Causes of collapse in the puerperium

Immediate collapse
- Haemorrhage due to:
  - blood loss – atonic uterus, genital tract trauma, placenta praevia, uterine rupture
  - coagulopathy – severe pre-eclampsia, abruption, amniotic fluid embolism, sepsis
- Embolism – pulmonary, amniotic fluid, air, fat
- Eclampsia
- Myocardial infarction
- Anaphylaxis
- Drug toxicity
- Transfusion reaction

Delayed collapse
- Haemorrhage
- Eclampsia
- Infection/sepsis
- Pulmonary embolus
- Myocardial infarction

■ Haemorrhage

In contrast to antepartum haemorrhage, the bleeding associated with postpartum haemorrhage is usually obvious, although it may initially be obscured by blankets covering the newly delivered woman. The symptoms and signs of hypovolaemia (shock) may develop rapidly with progressive loss of consciousness as blood pressure falls. A systematic examination to determine the cause of the bleeding should be undertaken while resuscitation is proceeding (Fig. 2). In most cases of collapse resulting from severe haemorrhage, there will be a combination of factors contributing to the blood loss. For example blood loss from significant vaginal trauma with a poorly contracted uterus may lead to a coagulopathy owing to consumption of clotting factors. Other staff will need to be involved in the resuscitation and will also contribute to establishing the diagnosis. While inserting large-bore cannulae, blood should be taken for blood count and cross-match.

In summary, the causes of postpartum haemorrhage can be simply classified as the four 'T's:

- *trauma* (vaginal, cervical);
- *tone* or lack of it (uterine atony);
- *tissue* (retained products of conception or blood clot);
- *thrombin* or lack of it (coagulopathy).

Blood loss
Atonic uterus
Uterine atony (lack of contractility) is common and should be anticipated if the labour has been prolonged, required oxytocin augmentation or forceps, or vacuum assistance has occurred. Bleeding will continue from the placental bed site while the uterus remains atonic, and this must be corrected with oxytocics and abdominal massage of the uterus. The degree of uterine contraction should be assessed by palpation frequently to determine the effects of the measures taken. If the uterus fails to respond, rupture of the uterus should be considered, although it is uncommon.

Genital tract trauma
If the uterine fundus is well contracted on palpation, bleeding must be coming from the lower segment of the uterus, cervix or vagina. Bleeding from the cervix or lower uterine

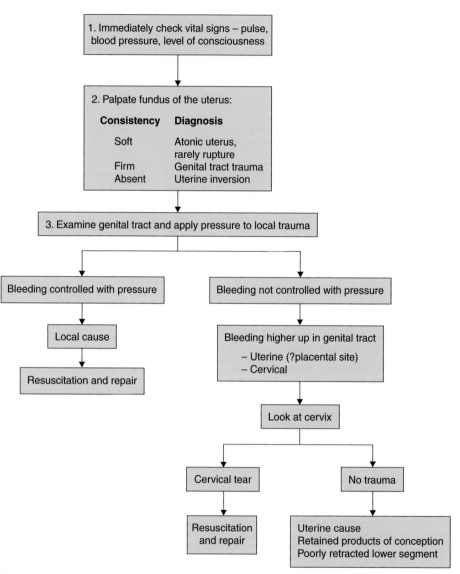

Figure 2 Assessment of a woman with postpartum haemorrhage.

segment should be excluded by using a pack to apply firm pressure to vaginal trauma. Pressure will usually control the bleeding from vaginal trauma. If significant bleeding continues despite the application of pressure, the cervix must be examined for lacerations. In a collapsed woman, this is usually done under anaesthesia together with exploration of the uterine cavity looking for retained products of conception.

Uterine cause
If vaginal and cervical trauma are excluded by examination, then the bleeding is due to either retained placenta/products of conception/blood clot or a poorly retracted lower segment. Gentle exploration of the uterine cavity digitally or using a large blunt curette will allow the removal of any remaining tissue. Great care must be taken in these circumstances because of the ease

with which the uterus can be perforated. Rarely, a uterine rupture may be detected in this manner. If no tissue is detected, it is likely that the lower segment is not retracting and this usually occurs when the placenta has been implanted in the lower segment.

Coagulopathy

In most instances of postpartum haemorrhage sufficient to cause maternal collapse, there will be an accompanying coagulopathy of some degree. This will also contribute to the overall blood loss. It is most frequently a consumptive coagulopathy due to excessive blood loss and a resulting depletion of clotting factors, but there are also well-recognised coagulopathic conditions peculiar to pregnancy. Repeated blood testing will be necessary to monitor the effect of blood factor replacement during resuscitation. Input from a haematologist will be required to assist with expediting the testing, interpretation of the results and procurement of replacement factors. In general, coagulopathy due to consumption is more readily corrected than that due to a coagulopathic condition of pregnancy.

Severe pre-eclampsia

Coagulopathy is a feature of severe pre-eclampsia and is usually preceded by a progressive fall in the platelet count. It is not usually of sufficient severity to cause collapse alone, but may be a contributing factor as described previously.

Abruption

Although placental abruption is discussed in the previous chapter as a cause of collapse in pregnancy, collapse after placental abruption is more likely to occur in the puerperium. To a variable extent the blood loss may be tamponaded behind the placenta prior to delivery. Significant abruption is usually closely followed by delivery of the baby, either because of rapid labour or urgent Caesarean section. However, a severe coagulopathy may ensue and disseminated intravascular

coagulation lead to diffuse bleeding and resulting haemorrhagic shock. The diagnosis has usually been made from the history of pain, bleeding, fetal distress and the onset of labour. The uterine fundus is tender, firm and may be larger than expected. While resuscitation is taking place, blood should be taken for full blood count, group and cross-match, and coagulation tests.

Amniotic fluid embolism

Amniotic fluid embolism (AFE) is described in more detail in Collapse in pregnancy and below. Rapidly escalating, profound coagulopathy is invariable in AFE provided the mother survives the initiating event.

Sepsis

Maternal sepsis and, in particular, sepsis due to chorioamnionitis is a potent cause of coagulopathy.

■ Embolism

Pulmonary embolism

Collapse from pulmonary embolism is more likely to occur in the postpartum period than antenatally. Puerperal factors that increase the risk of pulmonary embolism are dehydration in labour, Caesarean section and immobility following delivery. It should be remembered that the widespread use of prophylaxis against thrombosis for Caesarean section has led to a significant fall in maternal deaths from this cause.

The presentation in the puerperium is no different to that seen at other times. There may be chest pain and shortness of breath followed by cardiac and/or pulmonary compromise in the absence of precipitating factors such as blood loss. Pulmonary embolism is not usually seen immediately after delivery but is more likely in first two to three days of the puerperium (see Chest pain in pregnancy: non-cardiac causes).

Amniotic fluid embolism

Although rare, amniotic fluid embolism is most likely to present at the time of, or immediately after delivery. As with pulmonary embolism, there is shortness of breath and rapid collapse, usually without chest pain. The proximity to delivery makes AFE a more likely diagnosis than pulmonary embolism and this will be confirmed by the rapidly developing coagulation disorder, which is a feature of AFE but not pulmonary embolism (see Collapse in pregnancy).

Eclampsia

Eclampsia is more likely to occur postpartum than prior to delivery but is rare more than 5 days following birth. In postpartum eclampsia, the woman will usually be hypertensive, although this may have only developed during labour or after delivery of the baby. The woman will usually complain of feeling unwell and may have symptoms of imminent eclampsia (see Collapse in pregnancy). She will often be agitated and her reflexes will be abnormally brisk with more than two beats of clonus present. If the fit is witnessed, she will be observed to lose consciousness and then have a generalised tonic/clonic convulsion. There may be damage to the mouth and/or tongue, or evidence of incontinence.

The woman should be kept from harm while magnesium sulphate is administered to stop the seizure and prevent recurrence. Eclamptic fits are not typically prolonged, but are likely to recur without treatment for the fit and raised blood pressure. After the seizure, blood should be collected for complete blood count, urea, electrolytes and creatinine, coagulation and liver function tests, if not done recently. The urine should be checked for the presence of significant proteinuria unless it is already known to be present.

The diagnosis is often clear because the woman will be hypertensive and there will be evidence of pre-eclampsia with proteinuria and/or haematological abnormalities. If the fit is not witnessed, a history of pre-eclampsia is usually suggestive, although the blood pressure may be normal or slightly elevated. If there are no features of pre-eclampsia or the fitting is prolonged and/or focal in nature, further investigation will be needed. This will usually require a computerised tomography (CT) scan and, often, magnetic resonance imaging to exclude arteriovenous malformations, mass lesions or other intracranial causes. Metabolic causes, such as hypoglycaemia, will be excluded by the laboratory investigations. Drug withdrawal can also be a cause of fitting and may need a high level of vigilance.

Myocardial infarction

Collapse in the puerperium due to myocardial infarction is even less common than during pregnancy as the load on the heart diminishes rapidly after birth. However, it may occur if there are additional demands on an already diseased heart, e.g. fluid overload during labour, severe hypertension following the administration of ergometrine, and should be suspected when significant chest pain precedes the collapse. There may or may not be a history of cardiac disease, and electrocardiography and cardiac enzymes will be diagnostic.

Anaphylaxis

Anaphylaxis may occur in the puerperium as in pregnancy, again usually as a result of the use of antibiotics for the treatment of infection. As described in 'Collapse in pregnancy', the diagnosis is usually clear because of the close association between the administration of the drug and the reaction occurring.

Drug toxicity

Respiratory paralysis and collapse due to a high epidural or spinal block, intravenous injection of local anaesthetic or overdose with magnesium sulphate are equally likely to occur in the immediate postpartum period. Again, the close correlation between administration of the drug and the onset of respiratory distress confirms the diagnosis.

Transfusion reaction

As transfusion is more common in the postnatal period, transfusion reactions are more likely, although they do not usually lead to collapse. However, should collapse occur, the onset of symptoms at the time of transfusion will make the diagnosis clear.

■ Delayed puerperal collapse

Although postpartum haemorrhage can occur more than 24 hours following birth, it is unlikely to cause collapse and other causes are more likely. Delayed haemorrhage is often associated with sepsis due to retained products of conception, and collapse may occur due to the combination of blood loss and septic shock. Prior to the widespread use of antibiotics, puerperal sepsis was a significant cause of maternal death and remains so in the developing world.

Pulmonary embolism is more likely to occur in the first few days after delivery than in the first 24 hours, particularly in women who are slow to mobilise after surgery (Caesarean section) and/or other complications (e.g. severe pre-eclampsia, wound haematoma, physical disability).

Although very rare (3–4 cases/100 000 pregnancies per year), ischaemic stroke is more common in the first 2–3 weeks postpartum than in non-pregnant women. Interestingly, pregnant women are less likely to have stroke than non-pregnant women, presumably because of the generalised vasodilatation that occurs in pregnancy. In the puerperium, the increase in clotting factors persists while the vascular system rapidly returns to normal.

Women at risk are those with pre-existing vascular disease of any cause (atherosclerosis, systemic lupus erythematosus), haematological disorders (antiphospholipid syndrome, disseminated intravascular coagulation) or cardiac causes of emboli (cardiomyopathy, endocarditis). Substance abuse (amphetamines, cocaine or heroin) is also associated with an increased risk of stroke. Although not typically causing collapse, there may be a loss of consciousness with strokes, and a careful history and examination may reveal a persistent neurological deficit. An urgent CT scan is required to look for intracranial causes and blood tests to detect predisposing conditions, e.g. thrombophilia, pre-eclampsia (see Collapse in pregnancy).

As described previously, eclampsia can occur after delivery, but becomes less likely with the passage of each subsequent day.

■ Conclusion

Collapse in the puerperium is more common than during pregnancy, primarily due to postpartum haemorrhage. In this situation, the diagnosis is usually evident, and most clinicians involved in maternity care should be skilled in the assessment and management of postpartum haemorrhage. However, collapse may be due to other causes and is equally as frightening as it is in pregnancy. Once again resuscitation should begin immediately and the diagnosis made while resuscitation is taking place.

CTG ABNORMALITIES

Dilip Visvanathan

■ Introduction

A cardiotocograph (CTG) is a non-invasive method of recording the fetal heart rate and maternal contractions, and became commercially available in the 1960s. A retrospective study done in the late 1970s[1] showed that fetal heart monitoring in labour reduced the incidence of cerebral palsy and perinatal mortality, although this was not confirmed on a subsequent meta-analysis of randomised controlled trials.[2] These have shown no reduction in cerebral palsy, neonatal encephalopathy or perinatal mortality. Furthermore it has also shown that using fetal heart monitoring in labour is associated with an increase in obstetric intervention.

The overall incidence of cerebral palsy, neonatal encephalopathy and perinatal mortality is low. Intrapartum contributions to these conditions are even less frequent. The high false-positive rates of an abnormal CTG to predict these conditions, therefore, explain the increased maternal intervention rates. It is for this reason that attempts are being made for a second line of non-invasive monitoring in the event of an abnormal CTG. Many units today use the STAN (ST wave analysis on the fetal electrocardiogram) machine for this reason. It is important, therefore, to confirm fetal compromise with acid–base analysis of a fetal blood sample prior to offering a mother a Caesarean section for a non-acute abnormal CTG.

Governing bodies like the National Institute for Health and Clinical Excellence (NICE) and the Royal College of Obstetricians and Gynaecologists (RCOG) have now discouraged the use of CTG in the low-risk woman. CTG is only recommended in two situations: (1) where there is an increased risk of perinatal death, cerebral palsy or neonatal encephalopathy; and (2) where oxytocin is being used for induction or augmentation of labour.

■ Basis of the cardiotocograph

The fetal heart rate monitor recognises and processes fetal heart-rate pattern and identifies uterine contractions. Most monitors used in clinical practice include a transducer that uses ultrasound and the Doppler principle to detect fetal heart movements. These are processed and then displayed on a strip chart. The uterine contractions are detected by the change in maternal abdominal circumference.

■ The normal CTG

Baseline fetal heart rate: normal range 110–160 beats per minute

This is the mean level of the fetal heart rate (FHR) when this is stable but excludes accelerations and decelerations. Baseline FHR is determined over a time period of 5 or 10 minutes and is expressed in beats per minute (bpm; Fig. 1).

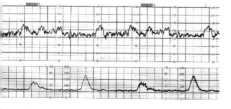

Figure 1 CTG showing a baseline fetal heart rate of 125 bpm, baseline variability of 7–8 bpm and accelerations. There are no decelerations. The frequencies of uterine contractions are ? per 10 minutes.

Baseline variability: normal range (5–15 bpm)

Baseline variability indicates the integrity of the autonomic nervous system and occurs as a result of beat to beat variation in the heart rate. It is measured by estimating the difference in beats per minute between the highest peak and lowest trough of fluctuation in a 1-minute segment of the trace between contractions.

Acceleration

An acceleration would be defined as a transient increase in FHR of 15 bpm or more from baseline lasting 15 seconds or more (Fig. 2). A reactive trace is when there are at least two accelerations in a 20-minute period. It is accepted that the presence of accelerations indicates a vigorous and healthy fetus that will be born with normal blood gases. The significance of no accelerations on an otherwise normal CTG is unclear.

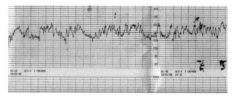

Figure 2 CTG showing accelerations. The presence of accelerations is considered to be a good sign of fetal health and shows that the mechanisms responsible for fetal heart reactivity are intact.

■ Baseline changes in the CTG

Baseline changes in the fetal heart pattern

The baseline FHR is mainly controlled by the autonomic nervous system via the vagus nerve. Baroreceptors are found in the arch of the aorta and the carotid sinus at the junction of the internal and external carotid arteries. When stretched, it causes a bradycardia. Stimulation of the chemoreceptors found in the aortic and carotid bodies cause tachycardia.

Fetal tachycardia

A fetal tachycardia occurs when the baseline FHR is higher than 160 bpm (Fig. 3). It can be moderate (161–180 bpm) or abnormal (>180 bpm).

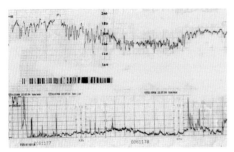

Figure 3 CTG showing a baseline tachycardia secondary to a very active fetus.

The sympathetic system matures earlier than the vagus and hence the baseline FHR tends to fall as gestation advances. One of the compensatory responses to hypoxia is an increase in the baseline FHR. It is important, therefore, to note changes in the baseline rate as labour progresses. The causes of fetal tachycardia are summarised in Box 1.

Fetal bradycardia

A baseline fetal heart rate of less than 110 bpm is considered as a fetal bradycardia (Fig. 4). It may be moderate (100–109 bpm) or abnormal (<100 bpm). It can be physiological in the post term fetus owing to continuing development of the vagus. It could also occur owing to head compression. A sustained fetal bradycardia is an obstetric emergency and causes, such as placental abruption, uterine rupture, uterine hyperstimulation and cord prolapse, must be considered. The causes of fetal bradycardia are outlined in Box 2.

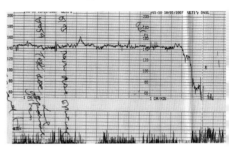

Figure 4 CTG showing a fetal bradycardia secondary to maternal hypertension. Note the epidural top up that was given previously.

Box 1 Causes of fetal tachycardia

Physiological
- Active fetus
- Fetal prematurity
- Maternal anxiety and stress
- Maternal tachycardia

Pharmacological
- Anticholinergic drugs (atropine)
- Sympathomimetics (ritodrine, terbutaline)

Pathological
- Maternal pyrexia
- Hyperthyroidism
- Fetal hypoxia
- Maternal/fetal anaemia
- Chorioamnionitis
- Fetal tachyarrhythmia

Box 2 Causes of fetal bradycardia

Physiological
- Post maturity
- Cord compression
- Rapid descent
- Vigorous vaginal examination
- Normal variation

Pharmacological
- Epidural and spinal anaesthesia
- Paracervical block
- Benzodiazepines
- Substance abuse (cocaine)

Pathological
- Uterine hyperstimulation
- Maternal seizure
- Maternal hypothermia
- Fetal heart block
- Fetal hypoxia

Reduced baseline variability

A reduced baseline variability is less than 5 bpm (Fig. 5). It is non-reassuring baseline if it lasts for more than 40 but less than 90 minutes. If the reduced baseline variability lasts for more than 90 minutes, it is abnormal (see Table 1).

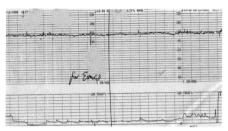

Figure 5 CTG demonstrating a baseline variability of less than 5 bpm.

The presence of normal baseline variability requires an intact cerebral cortex, midbrain, vagus nerve and a cardiac conduction system. Normal baseline variability indicates that the fetus does not suffer from cerebral asphyxia. A gradual reduction of the baseline variability in the presence of other patterns of fetal hypoxia indicates that the fetal compensatory mechanism to maintain cerebral oxygenation is being lost. The causes of reduced baseline variability are summarised in Box 3.

Sinusoidal pattern

A regular oscillation of the baseline long-term variability that resembles a sine wave is called a sinusoidal pattern (Fig. 6). This smooth undulating pattern, lasting at least 10 minutes, has a relatively fixed period of 3–5 cycles per minute, and amplitude of 5–15 bpm above and below the baseline. Another distinguishing feature is that baseline variability is absent. The pattern was first described in infants with severe rhesus alloimmunisation and fetal anaemia. It is considered an abnormal finding and associated with a poor fetal outcome.

Periodic changes in the fetal heart pattern
Decelerations

Transient episodes of slowing of the FHR below the baseline level measuring 15 bpm or more, and lasting 15 seconds or more are known as

> ### Box 3 Causes of reduced fetal baseline variability
>
> #### Physiological
> Quiet sleep state
>
> #### Pharmacological
> - Narcotics, e.g. morphine, diazepam
> - Magnesium sulphate
> - Vagal blockade – atropine or scopolamine
> - Substance abuse, e.g. heroin
>
> #### Pathological
> - Fetal cerebral hypoxia
> - Fetal heart block
> - Congenital neurological abnormality e.g. anencephaly
> - Other, e.g. *in utero* infection, asphyxial event
> - Fetal anaemia

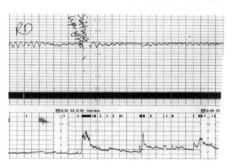

Figure 6 CTG showing sinusoidal pattern. The baby was born by Caesarean section and had severe anaemia.

decelerations. Uterine activity needs to be monitored accurately in order to classify the different decelerations as management depends on the type of the deceleration.

Early decelerations Early decelerations are characterised by uniform, repetitive, periodic slowing of the FHR with onset early in the contraction and a return to baseline at the end of the contraction (Fig. 7). These are usually persistent and occur with each contraction. The causes of early decelerations are physiological – head compression resulting in increased vagal tone – not pathological.

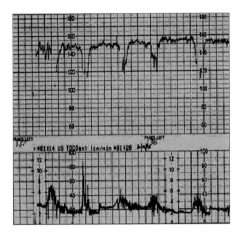

Figure 7 CTG demonstrating early decelerations.

Late decelerations   Late decelerations are characterised by uniform, repetitive, periodic slowing of the FHR with an onset in the mid to end part of the contraction and a nadir more than 20 seconds after the peak of the contraction, and ending after the contraction (Fig. 8). In the presence of a non-accelerative trace with baseline variability <5 bpm, the definition would include decelerations <15 bpm. Late decelerations are thought to occur owing to a decreased blood flow (associated with a uterine contraction) beyond the capacity of the fetus to extract oxygen. The causes of late decelerations are given in Box 4.

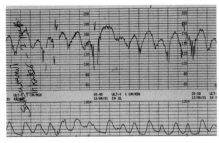

Figure 8 CTG showing a baseline fetal tachycardia with late decelerations secondary to uterine hyperstimulation from intravaginal prostaglandin gel.

Variable decelerations

Typical variable decelerations   These are characterised by intermittent periodic variable slowing of FHR with rapid onset and recovery (Fig. 9).

Box 4 Causes of late decelerations

Reduction in placental perfusion provoked by uterine contractions

Pre-existing placental dysfunction
- Pre-eclampsia
- Intrauterine growth restriction
- Diabetes
- Chronic hypertension
- Post-term pregnancy

Maternal condition
- Diabetic ketoacidosis
- Uterine hyperstimulation
- Maternal hypotension

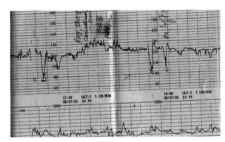

Figure 9 CTG showing variable decelerations. It is important to check the baseline features. Here the baseline rate is 130 bpm, with a baseline variability of 10–15 bpm, and there are accelerations.

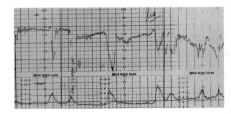

Figure 10 CTG showing shouldering variable decelerations. There is, however, a baseline tachycardia and reduced baseline variability. This would then be classified as atypical variable decelerations.

Time relationships with a contraction cycle are variable and they can occur in isolation. Sometimes they resemble other types of deceleration patterns in timing and shape. The causes of

Table 1 Categories of features in fetal heart trace patterns

Feature	Baseline (bpm)	Variability	Decelerations	Accelerations
Reassuring	110–160	⩾5	None	Present
Non-reassuring	100–109	<5 for >30 minutes but <90 minutes	Early	The absence of accelerations in an otherwise normal trace is of uncertain significance
	161–180		Variable	
			Single Prolonged deceleration <3 minutes	
Abnormal	<100	<5 for ⩾90 minutes	Atypical variable decelerations	
	>180		Late decelerations	
	Sinusoidal pattern ⩾10 minutes		Single prolonged deceleration >3 minutes	

Table 2 Classification of fetal heart trace patterns

Normal	A cardiotocograph where all four features fall into the reassuring category
Suspicious	A cardiotocograph whose features fall into one of the non-reassuring categories and the remainder of the features are reassuring
Pathological	A cardiotocograph whose features fall into two or more non-reassuring categories, or one or more abnormal categories

variable decelerations are umbilical cord compression generally in the first stage of labour and substantial head compression during the active phase of the second stage of labour. Both these events cause activation of the vagus nerve with a subsequent reduction in the FHR.

Atypical variable deceleration In addition to the features described, variable decelerations are said to be atypical if they have any of the following characteristics (Fig. 10):

- loss of primary or secondary rise in baseline rate;
- slow return to the baseline FHR after the end of the contraction;
- prolonged secondary rise in the baseline rate;
- biphasic deceleration;
- loss of variability during deceleration;
- continuation of the baseline rate at lower level.

These features indicate that the fetus is mounting a compensatory response to hypoxia, which it will develop if the condition persists over a period of time. It is, therefore, important

to ensure that both types of variable decelerations, especially atypical ones, are recognised and appropriate action taken. That action may be fetal blood sampling or delivery, depending on the overall clinical situation.

Categories of fetal heart trace pattern

It has been recommended by NICE and the RCOG that CTGs should be classified into three groups – normal, suspicious or pathological depending on the features that are present. These are outlined in Tables 1 and 2.

References

1. Shenker L, Post RC, Seiler JS. Routine electronic monitoring of fetal heart rate and uterine activity during labor. *Obstet Gynecol* 1975; **46:** 185–9.
2. Prentice A, Lind T. Fetal heart rate monitoring during labour – too frequent intervention, too little benefit? *Lancet* 1987; **2:** 1375–7.

EPIGASTRIC PAIN IN PREGNANCY

Ana Ignjatovic and Margaret Myszor

■ History

A full history of the presenting complaint is extremely important, as are any associated symptoms. The history must be interpreted with reference to the gestational age, as aetiologies change throughout pregnancy.

Specific questions that may aid diagnosis include the following.

■ Did the pain start gradually or suddenly?
■ Is it dull, aching and constant, or is it sharp and stabbing?
■ Is it associated with meals?
■ Is it well localised and has there been any change?
■ Are there any associated features, e.g. nausea and vomiting?
■ Are there any obvious relieving or exacerbating factors?

■ Physical examination

■ Clinical findings may be less obvious and more difficult to elicit in pregnancy than in non-pregnant women with the same disorder.
■ Peritoneal signs are often absent in pregnancy as a result of lifting and stretching of the anterior abdominal wall. This means that any underlying inflammation is not in direct contact with the peritoneum, thus reducing guarding.
■ To help distinguish extrauterine tenderness from uterine tenderness, examination of the patient in a lateral decubitus position may be useful. This manoeuvre displaces the uterus to one side.

■ Laboratory investigations

Commonly used laboratory tests have different ranges in pregnancy (see Appendix) and, therefore, can be of limited use in aiding diagnosis.

■ Radiological investigations

■ Ultrasound scanning is the most commonly used investigation for investigating a pregnant abdomen. It is safe, and the gallbladder, liver, pancreas and kidneys can be evaluated easily.
■ Ionising radiation that produces exposures <0.05 Gy (=50 rad) have not been associated with fetal abnormalities or pregnancy loss. However, there is a possible association between prenatal radiation exposure and childhood cancer.
■ Ionising radiation should only be used when absolutely indicated medically, and other imaging options have been considered and rejected.
■ Magnetic resonance imaging (MRI) is not recommended in the first trimester and not all MRI contrast agents are approved for use in pregnancy. It has been used in later pregnancy to exclude morbidly adherent placentae. It must be remembered that the duty of care of any attending doctor is primarily to the mother as the fetus has no legal standing whilst *in utero*.

■ Conditions with increased frequency in pregnancy

The following conditions occur more frequently in pregnant women compared with non-pregnant women:

■ gastro-oesophageal reflux/oesophagitis;
■ biliary colic;
■ acute cholecystitis.

■ Conditions due to pregnancy

The following conditions occur as a result of pregnancy:

■ rupture of the rectus abdominis muscles;
■ acute fatty liver of pregnancy;
■ HELLP (haemolysis, elevated liver enzymes and low platelets);
■ spontaneous rupture of the liver (due to HELPP).

■ Conditions incidental to pregnancy

These are:

■ non-ulcer dyspepsia;
■ gastric and duodenal ulceration;
■ gastritis and duodenitis;
■ acute and chronic pancreatitis.

Gastro-oesophageal reflux disease

This condition is common in non-pregnant women and almost universal to some degree in pregnancy. It is due to an increased intra-abdominal pressure from a gravid uterus and leads to dysfunction of the lower oesophageal sphincter (Fig. 1). This is also aggravated by increased serum progesterone levels, which cause relaxation of involuntary muscle. There is also delayed clearance of the reflux leading to increased acid exposure times.

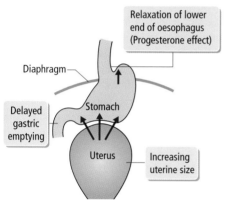

Figure 1 Diagram of factors affecting acid reflux.

Clinical features include:

- heartburn (retrosternal pain related to meals, posture and exercise);
- waterbrash (excess salivation, especially during an episode of pain);
- regurgitation of acid and bile, which can, rarely, give rise to nocturnal sore throat or indeed asthma.

Treatment

General measures include elevation of the head of the bed, small frequent meals and avoiding anything that obviously exacerbates the symptoms. Patients should be advised to avoid eating just prior to lying down. Alginates can be very useful for symptomatic relief of mild symptoms. Although there is no conclusive evidence for the safety of H2 blockers and proton-pump inhibitors in pregnancy, both have been widely used for symptomatic relief of refractory symptoms.

Biliary colic and acute cholecystitis

Asymptomatic gallbladder disease occurs in 3–4 per cent of pregnant women. It is estimated that acute cholecystitis occurs in 1:1130 to 1:12 890 pregnancies.

Clinical features

- Pain is usually moderately severe and constant in both acute cholecystitis and biliary colic. It is most commonly felt in the right upper quadrant but can be epigastric radiating to the back.
- Vomiting occurs in 50 per cent of patients and fever is common in cholecystitis.
- Ultrasound scanning is diagnostic and safe.
- Blood tests are of limited value as both leucocytosis and raised alkaline phosphatase levels are observed in healthy pregnancies.
- Transient increases in amylase can occur in 30 per cent of those with biliary colic but markedly raised levels suggest pancreatitis.

Treatment

Conservative treatment with intravenous fluids and analgesia, particularly pethidine, is the initial approach. Broad-spectrum antibiotics should be included if systemic symptoms are prominent. Surgery may be necessary but timing is controversial, with advocates of both surgery postpartum and during pregnancy. Ideally this should be undertaken during the second trimester, which minimises the risks for premature delivery. Laparoscopic cholecystectomy is safe in pregnancy, although caution must be observed owing to potential pressure on the inferior vena cava as well as the increasing size of the uterus.

Acute pancreatitis

This occurs most commonly secondary to gallstones and is associated with a fetal loss of 10–20 per cent. In these cases, endoscopic retrograde cholangiopancreaticogram and sphincterotomy have been performed safely in pregnant patients with gallstone pancreatitis or obstructive jaundice. In such cases, the uterus must be protected with a lead shield.

Gastric ulcer

This is a very rare condition in this age group. It presents with epigastric pain after eating, and is often associated with anorexia and weight loss. It is commonly caused by *Helicobacter pylori* and diagnosed endoscopically. If this condition is suspected during pregnancy in an *H. pylori*-positive individual, then blind treatment without an endoscopy would be appropriate.

■ Duodenal ulcer

There is a decreasing incidence of this condition in the Western world owing to the declining incidence of *H. pylori*. Almost all cases are caused by this organism or the use of non-steroidal anti-inflammatory agents. The clinical features in this condition include epigastric pain before meals. As with gastric ulceration, blind treatment may be indicated during pregnancy in an *H. pylori*-positive patient.

■ Gastritis, duodenitis and non-ulcer dyspepsia

These conditions can present with dyspeptic symptoms of mild to moderate epigastric discomfort and a feeling of fullness after meals. Endoscopy is not usually necessary in a young age group if symptoms are relieved by antacids, H2 blockade or proton-pump inhibition.

■ Conclusions

1 The site of pain in the pregnant woman may be different to that seen in the non-pregnant state.

2 Laboratory investigations may not help because of the change in their normal range found in pregnancy.

3 Radiological investigations are generally contraindicated during pregnancy unless there are extremely good reasons for using them. Ultrasound is widely used and is safe in pregnancy.

4 Gastro-oesophageal reflux disease is very common in pregnancy and is the commonest cause of epigastric pain.

5 Other conditions include biliary colic, cholecystitis, pancreatitis and peptic ulceration, which may need a different management plan in pregnancy.

6 There are rare causes of epigastric pain that only occur in pregnancy. These include HELPP (haemolysis, elevated liver enzymes and low platelets) with spontaneous rupture of the liver, and pre-eclampsia with subcapsular haemorrhage of the liver.

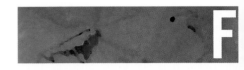

FEVER, POSTOPERATIVE (GYNAECOLOGICAL)

Urvashi Prasad Jha and Swasti

■ Introduction

Postoperative fever is a common problem seen after surgery. It is important to evaluate the patient carefully in order to identify those who may require a 'wait-and-see' approach, those who require investigations, and those who need urgent assessment and intervention. Fever may even be a sign of serious significance prior to the onset of systemic inflammatory response syndrome and multiorgan dysfunction syndrome. On the other hand, if fever continues for 2–3 weeks with no cause diagnosed despite repeated clinical and laboratory assessments, the patient is provisionally diagnosed to have 'fever of unknown origin'.

In order to increase the cost effectiveness of investigating postoperative fever, aggressive investigations could be targeted in some patient groups. These include those with a high fever, moderately increased white cell count, an increased number of febrile days, patients who have had bowel surgery or surgery for malignancy, and those who look ill.

■ Definition of fever

'Fever is the rise of normal core temperature of an individual that exceeds the normal daily variation and occurs in connection with an increase in the hypothalamic set point.'[1]

The mean oral temperature of healthy individuals 18–40 years of age is 36.8° ± 0.4°C (98.2° ± 0.7°F). It has a diurnal variation with low levels of 37.2°C (98.9°F) at 6 am and higher levels of 37.7°C (99.9°F) between 4 to 6 pm.[1] An am temperature of >37.2°C (98.9°F) or a pm temperature exceeding 37.7°C (99.9°F) is defined as fever.[1]

Clinically significant postoperative fever is defined as the presence of a temperature $\geq 38°C$ (100.4°F) on two occasions at least 4 hours apart, excluding the first 24 hours after surgery, or one temperature greater than 38.6°C (101.5°F) and persisting for two postoperative days.[1,2]

The incidence of postoperative fever as published in the literature varies widely from 14 to 91 per cent.[3] This may be infectious or non-infectious in origin. Many patients with postoperative fever do not have an underlying infectious cause. A total of 80–90 per cent of patients with fever on the first postoperative day usually have no infection, whereas 80–90 per cent of patients who develop fever on or after the fifth postoperative day commonly have an identifiable infection.[3,4] Infection is more likely to be present in a patient who develops fever after 2 days of surgery.[5]

Manifestations of fever[6]

These are:

- shivering;
- chills – these may alternate with feeling hot;
- general malaise;
- somnolence;
- anorexia;
- arthralgia, myalgia, skin sensitivity to touch;
- absence of sweating;
- increased blood pressure and heart rate.

Time-related causes of postoperative fever[7]

The time at which the fever begins will suggest its origin. It should be borne in mind that these time-related causes are guidelines and do not serve as absolute rules. There are no rigid demarcations between the time frames described since, on many occasions, there is a temporal overlap in the causes described (see Fig. 1).

Intraoperative causes of postoperative fever are:

- pre-existing sepsis;
- intraoperative septicaemia;
- transfusion reaction;
- heat stroke;
- *malignant hyperthermia*.

Miscellaneous causes of postoperative fever

Although not common in the general population, the following should be borne in mind, since a select group of patients may be at risk from these causes:

- sinusitis (prolonged nasogastric intubation);
- pharyngitis;
- infected central catheters;
- ventilator-associated pneumonia;
- nosocomial infections;
- infected haematoma;
- acute gout or flare-up;
- acute alcohol withdrawal;
- hyperthyroidism/thyrotoxicosis/thyroid storm;
- adrenal insufficiency;
- phaeochromocytoma;
- myocardial infarction;
- pulmonary embolism;
- neuroleptic malignant syndrome;
- intracranial pathologies;
- meningitis;
- medications (anaesthesia or other);
- drug fever associated with skin rash and/or eosinophilia, e.g.
  - antiepileptics – phenytoin;
  - antibiotics – beta-lactam antibiotics, sulphonamide antibiotics, piperacillin, tazobactam;
  - anti-inflammatory agents – indomethacin;
  - intraoperative drugs – succinylcholine.

The causes of fever in the postoperative period are traditionally remembered using a simple mnemonic of five Ws. The five Ws of causes of postoperative fever according to postoperative day (POD) of fever are shown in Table 1.

Life-threatening causes of early postoperative fever

Malignant hyperthermia is a rare, dominantly transmitted, genetic disorder that is triggered intraoperatively by the administration of succinyl choline. It occurs within 30 minutes after onset of general anaesthesia but may even present 10 hours after anaesthesia. Tachycardia develops and the blood pressure is unstable. The fever is life

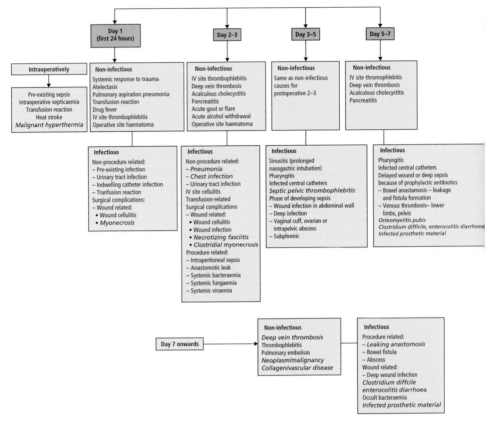

Figure 1 Causes of fever according to time of onset postoperatively.

Table 1 The five Ws of causes of postoperative fever according to postoperative day (POD)

POD 1–2	*Wind* (respiratory) – atelectasis occurs within 24–48 hours, aspiration pneumonia, ventilator-associated pneumonia
POD 3–5	*Water* – cystitis and urinary tract infection, especially in catheterized patients
POD 4–6	*'W(V)eins'/wings/walking* – deep vein thrombosis, intravenous (IV) site phlebitis from all sites of vascular access IVs
POD 5–7	*Wound* – check for wound infection (Fig. 2). Treatment is drainage, and excision and removal of sutures in some situations. It is essential to diagnose serious problems such as necrotizing fasciitis and peritonitis owing to an intestinal leak (internal wound)
POD7 +	*Wonder drugs* – drug reactions (uncommon), including drugs received preoperatively, antibiotics, intraoperative drugs, transfusion products, anti-inflammatory agents

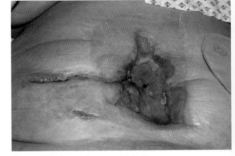

Figure 2 Postoperative wound infection.

threatening and may shoot up to 41–42°C (105–107°F). Muscle rigidity develops with acidosis, hypoxia and cardiac arrhythmias. The treatment is to stop all anaesthetic drugs, hyperventilate the patient with oxygen, give dantrolene sodium and procainamide, initiate cooling and diuresis to prevent precipitation of myoglobin.

Adrenal insufficiency typically occurs in patients who have been on long-term steroids owing to iatrogenic suppression of the hypothalamic–pituitary–adrenal axis. Fever and refractory hypotension may develop; steroid supplementation in time is life saving.

Pulmonary embolism usually presents as a postoperative patient with sudden haemodynamic instability and collapse. Fever, although uncommon, may be present.

Alcohol withdrawal frequently presents with fever. Prompt recognition and treatment prevents excessive morbidity and mortality.

Myonecrosis is commonly due to wound infection with *Clostridium* species or group A streptococci. It is a surgical emergency in which the patient presents with shock, tachycardia, fever and severe septicaemia in the first 24 hours postoperatively. The diagnosis is easily made if the dressing is opened and the wound examined. Thin, brownish, copious, malodorous discharge is present. The skin may be discoloured and there may be crepitations and bullae formation. The patient is usually in severe pain and restless. If not treated in time, vascular collapse, renal failure, haemoglobinuria and jaundice develop. Radical debridement of all the involved devitalised tissue and prompt initiation of high doses of penicillin or tetracyclines is mandatory. The rare differential diagnosis is metastatic myonecrosis from adenocarcinoma of the bowel.

Necrotizing fasciitis: if the diagnosis and treatment of this condition is delayed, overwhelming sepsis may occur, as it is a rapidly progressing potentially life-threatening bacterial infection.

It results from wound infection with polymicrobes – haemolytic streptococci, staphylococcus, anaerobes or mixed bacteria – resulting in necrosis of the superficial fascia that characteristically spares the underlying muscle. The toxicity is worse than the associated fever and leucocytosis with hyperthermia or hypothermia, hypotension, tachycardia and lethargy. Locally the wound has dusky faded skin with subcutaneous oedema, induration, crepitations, hyperaesthesia and cutaneous bullae formation, and the lesion undermines the skin. Haemoconcentration,

hypocalcaemia, haemolysis, hyperbilirubinaemia, and hepatic, renal and pulmonary insufficiency, and septic shock develop. The patient should be treated aggressively as one with major burns.

Predisposing risk factors include diabetes mellitus, trauma, alcoholism, an immunocompromised state, hypertension, peripheral vascular disease, intravenous drug abuse and obesity. A wide excision of the involved wound with debridement and redebridement, if necessary, is performed. Total parenteral nutrition is started via a central line with adequate replacement and correction of calcium, fluids, electrolytes and calories. Broad-spectrum antibiotics need to be started and changed according to the culture reports once they become available.

Intestinal leak with peritonitis can occur from either an early or delayed leaking anastomotic site or intestinal perforation following intraabdominal or intrapelvic surgery, where inadvertent enterotomy may have occurred. Early diagnosis depends on a high degree of suspicion with an urgent exploratory laparotomy to repair the leak, perform a peritoneal toilet lavage, start appropriate antibiotics and resuscitate the patient with fluids, electrolytes and multivitamins. Ketoacidosis is prevented by ensuring adequate total parenteral nutrition until such time as the patient is permitted oral intake.

■ Approach to a patient with fever in the post-operative period

A careful history, elaborate physical examination and necessary investigations are the keys to successfully diagnosing the cause of postoperative fever. An early and timely accurate diagnosis can help the physician to manage the patient appropriately and minimise morbidity.

The presence of a non-infectious cause of fever does not necessarily exclude the presence of an infective cause, as the two can coexist.

■ History
Complaints

A thorough history with details of the pattern and degree of the fever; of concomitant symptoms pertaining to various systems, including respiratory, gastrointestinal, genito-urinary, neurological and cardiac, is critical to an early correct diagnosis. For example, *Clostridium difficile*-associated enterocolitis may present with fever associated with diar-rhoea and abdominal pain; calf pain points to deep vein thrombosis (DVT); cough with sputum and breathlessness indicates a pulmonary origin; urinary frequency, dysuria, haematuria, urgency, suprapubic or loin pain suggest cystitis or pyelonephritis.

The site of any pain helps localise the wound, intravenous catheter site infections or inflam-mation. Intense pain with restlessness in a patient is ominous and warrants urgent exclu-sion of clostridial myonecrosis. On the other hand, a patient who presents with fever and delirium must have acute alcohol withdrawal high on the list of the differential diagnosis.

Atelectasis may be associated with rigors, altered mentation and hypotension.

First suspicion of wound infection in the first 3–4 postoperative days is when there is increas-ing wound pain, erythema, oedema and low-grade fever. Over the next 1–3 days, a spiking pattern develops with more obvious signs of wound infection. Frequent inspection of the wound (i.e. daily) should be carried out in those patients who complain of wound pain.

Pre-operative conditions and coexisting diseases

A detailed past history should be obtained with regards to any previous pyrexial illness, family history of malignant hyperpyrexia, hyper-thyroidism, obesity, use of tobacco, intravenous drugs or alcohol, prior transfusions, drug aller-gies or hypersensitivities.

Patients with certain conditions are more susceptible to infection, such as those with obesity, diabetes, malnutrition, debilitating dis-eases, malignancy, renal insufficiency, hyper-tension and advanced age. Pre-existing medical conditions likely to predispose to fever include urinary tract infections, thoracic infections, e.g. empyema, chronic bronchitis, moderate and severe kyphoscoliosis, cardiac valvular diseases amongst others. A high risk of suspicion for an infectious cause in these patients can prevent undue prolongation of morbidity.

The presence of pre-operative bacterial vaginosis is a high risk factor for developing postoperative fever in women undergoing gynaecological surgery.[8] All these women should be treated pre-operatively with intravaginal and/or oral clindamycin or metronidazole.

Details of the surgery

The following aspects of the surgery need to be considered in arriving at a provisional diagnosis:

- the date of surgery;
- its type and the duration of the procedure performed;
- use of pre-existing or implanted prostheses;
- type and time of perioperative antibiotic prophylaxis used;
- onset of symptoms;
- existence of symptoms prior to surgery;
- any complications with the surgery;
- history of prolonged postoperative ventilation;
- prolonged hospital stay.

■ Targeted examination

Noting all the vital signs is relevant. The pulse rate is an important sign. It is an ominous sign if the degree of tachycardia is out of proportion to the temperature rise, in which case severe sepsis should be suspected. This is also true when there is an associated hypotension or oliguria. Tachypnoea usually points to a pulmonary aetiology.

The temperature can be taken orally or rec-tally, but the site used should be consistent. Oral temperature is 0.5°C less than rectal tempera-ture and 0.5°C higher than the axillary tempera-ture recorded. The pattern and trend of fever should be noted from the temperature chart.

The general condition of the patient may provide clues to the cause of fever. This may range from normality to evidence of mild sys-temic toxicity to a poor general condition with hypotension and systemic vascular collapse.

A detailed examination of the surgical incision site should always be made even in the absence of localizing symptoms to exclude silent wound dehiscence. The presence of cellulitis, abscess, necrotizing fasciitis or gas gangrene is usually locally symptomatic. Examination of the wound should include inspection of the colour of the peri-incisional skin (whether dusky, erythematous, necrotic, blue or black), the associated induration, oedema and tenderness, and the presence of hyperaesthesias, crepitation, cutaneous bullae and spreading erythematous streaks.

In the early stages of a wound infection, there is increasing tenderness and periwound oedema. Later, erythema may develop with elevated skin temperature and fluctuation. There are more local signs with staphylococcal infections than with enteric organisms, when the tenderness is increased but the erythema may be minimal. Other signs of infection, such as tachycardia, malaise, chills and leucocytosis, may develop.

The depth of any wound dehiscence should be assessed to see which structures are affected and whether any necrotic tissue needs to be excised. The nature, colour and smell of any discharge provide indicators to the nature of the wound infection. The lymph nodes draining the area should also be examined for any evidence of involvement.

All intravenous puncture sites with or without indwelling cannulae plus drain sites should be examined for overt skin erythema and tenderness as well as for underlying swelling, infection and collection of pus.

The chest should be examined carefully with auscultation for evidence of collapse, pneumonia, pleural effusion or empyema.

The abdomen should be examined for features of peritonitis, localised infection and subphrenic or pelvic abscess, if any abdominal or pelvic surgery has been performed. Lower abdominal tenderness, rebound tenderness, tenderness on rectal and vaginal examination with or without the presence of a pelvic mass and vaginal discharge may indicate pelvic cellulitis, infection or a pelvic abscess.

Tenderness over the kidneys, bladder and prostate may be present with any urinary tract infection.

Infective processes in the bone in the early stages may have tenderness only over the infected area but with progression there will be swelling, empyema and ultimately discharge of pus.

If, on examination of the central nervous system, neck stiffness, photophobia and altered consciousness are present, then meningitis and infection of the central nervous system may need to be excluded.

■ Laboratory and radiological investigations[6]

The following tests would need to be performed where clinically indicated and appropriate.

- Urinalysis.
- Haematological assessment:
  - complete blood count with total and differential white cell count and peripheral smear;
  - depressed white cell counts are seen in severe sepsis, immunocompromised or malnourished patients;
  - platelet count is elevated as a response to stress but decreases with disseminated intravascular coagulopathy;
  - erythrocyte sedimentation rate/C-reactive protein;
  - coagulation screen is important in patients with severe sepsis;
  - immunological tests are essential in transfusion reactions.
- Serum biochemistry:
  - urea, electrolytes and creatinine;
  - liver function tests;
  - glucose;
  - arterial blood gases – metabolic acidosis is one of the earliest signs of developing septic shock;
  - myocardial enzymes;
  - serum amylase.
- Bacteriological assessment – this should be directed as appropriate and samples taken as indicated in the individual case. Identification of a causative organism and its antibiotic sensitivities should always be attempted prior to starting antibiotics in patients suspected to have an infection as the cause of the fever. The following samples may be required:
  - blood culture;
  - sputum, pleural or peritoneal aspirate;
  - urine, skin and wound swab of discharge or needle aspiration;
  - cerebrospinal fluid (by lumbar puncture);
  - intravascular catheters;
  - aspiration of tissue fluid from spreading edge of cellulitis should be performed and sent for

culture on removal of the intravenous catheter or drain;
- stool.
■ Radiographic imaging:
- chest X-ray;
- abdominopelvic X-ray – displacement of air-filled organs by a mass is seen in the presence of pelvic abscess;
- ultrasound and Doppler help detect venous thrombosis, abscesses and hematomas;
- computerised tomography and magnetic resonance imaging scanning can identify abscesses, haematomas and other lesions;
- bone scans detect osteomyelitis.
■ Electrocardiograms (ECGs) and echocardiography are helpful in myocardial ischaemia, intracardiac thrombosis and pulmonary embolism.

■ Summary of routine infection screen

1 Chest examination, chest X-ray, sputum for culture, ECG.
2 Wound examination, swab for culture.
3 Urinary symptoms, urine for culture and sensitivity.
4 Examine for DVT.
5 Examine intravenous sites (phlebitis), catheter sites (epidural) and drain sites.
6 Examine pressure areas.
7 In children, examination of ears and mouth.
8 Total leucocyte count, differential leucocyte count.
9 Blood cultures, if cause of infection is uncertain.

■ Management

The treatment of postoperative fever in a surgical patient is directed at the cause.

General therapy requires the replacement of fluid losses and calorie requirements, which increase with fever. Sensible losses like sweating increase by 250 mL/degree rise of fever per day and insensible losses of evaporation from skin and lungs increase by 50–75 mL/degree rise of fever per day.

Children, elderly and cardiac patients should have their fever treated primarily by antipyretics and sponge baths with tepid water. Antipyretics, such as paracetamol, non-steroidal anti-inflammatory drugs (NSAIDs) and aspirin, are indicated only when the temperature is more than 39°C. They also help reduce the systemic symptoms of associated myalgias, arthralgias and headache. Aspirin and NSAIDs have the disadvantage of lowering platelet count, gastrointestinal irritation and haemorrhage, and Reye's syndrome in children.

In patients suspected to have an infection, the elimination of the source of infection is one of the main principles of management after identification of the site and the offending organism. Appropriate selection of systemic antibiotics is essential. If the patient is acutely ill and has septicaemia, intravenous broad-spectrum antibiotics are started without waiting for cultures. These can be changed if necessary after the availability of the sensitivity report.

Surgical intervention may be required in the form of wound debridement, excision of infected wound or diseased organ to eliminate the source of infection and drainage of pus. Swabs and tissue should be sent for Gram stain, culture and sensitivity at this point even if ent earlier, followed by saline-soaked dressings. Correction of lesions causing obstruction of the hollow organs and elimination of spaces in which infection may develop are necessary.

Septic pelvic thrombophlebitis may develop 2–4 days postoperatively. The clinical signs may be unreliable and so are best confirmed by Doppler ultrasound or venography. A tender cord may be palpable in the uterine cornua or parametrium. This requires immediate anticoagulation with heparin therapy plus broad-spectrum antibiotics. If there is no response to treatment, then bilateral ovarian ligation may be required.

In patients with severe systemic sepsis, fluid resuscitation should be initiated early. Ionotropes and vasoactive agents may need to be started to address the myocardial depression associated with systemic infections. In seriously ill patients, respiratory support with oxygen may be required and they may also need to be transferred to an intensive therapy unit.

■ References

1. Mackowiak PA. Fever. In: Mandell GL, Bennett JE, Polin R, eds. *Principles and*

Practice of Infectious Diseases, 5th edn. Philadelphia: Churchill Livingstone, 2000: 604–21.

2. Ahya SN, Flood K, Paranjothi S. *The Washington Manual of Medical Therapeutics*, 30th edn. Philadelphia: Lippincott Williams and Wilkins, 2001.

3. Fanning J, Neuhoff RA, Brewer JE, Castaneda T, Marcotte MP, Jacobson RI. Frequency and yield of postoperative fever evaluation. *Infect Dis Obstet Gynecol* 1998; **6**: 252–5.

4. Garibaldi RA, Brodine S, Matsumiya S, Coleman M. Evidence for the non-infectious etiology of early postoperative fever. *Infect Control* 1985; **6**: 273–7.

5. Pile JC. Evaluating postoperative fever: a focused approach. *Cleve Clin J Med* 2006; **73**: S62–66.

6. Biddle C. The neurobiology of the human febrile response. AANA Journal course. Update for nurse anesthetists. *AANA J* 2006; **74**: 145–50.

7. Dellinger EP. Approach to the patient with postoperative fever. In: Gorbach SL, Bartlett JG, Blacklow NR, eds. *Infectious Diseases*, 3rd edn. Philadelphia: Lippincott Williams and Wilkins, 2004: 817.

8. Bacterial vaginosis a major culprit in postoperative fever. *Ob/Gyn News* 1999; Nov 15.

9. Sikora C, Embil JM. Fever in the post-operative patient: a chilling problem. Presented at 'Bug Day 2003', Health Sciences Centre, Winnipeg (October 2003). *Can J Contin Med Educ* 2004; May: 93–8.

FEVER, PUERPERAL

Dilip Visvanathan

Definition of puerperal pyrexia

Puerperal pyrexia is commonly defined as a temperature elevation of 38°C on two occasions after the first 24 hours postpartum.[1]

History

Puerperal fever was one of the commonest causes of maternal death before the concept of antisepsis and introduction of antibiotics. The use of unsterile instruments, repeated vaginal examinations in labour and physicians examining patients without washing their hands were contributing factors. It was only in 1847 that Ignaz Semmelweis, a Hungarian physician working in the Vienna General Hospital discovered that hand washing could significantly reduce the incidence of puerperal sepsis.

Today deaths from infection of the genital tract after delivery are fortunately rare in the developed world. However, the principles of antisepsis are as important in practice as they were in the past owing to the rising incidence of hospital-acquired infection.

Aetiology

The commonest cause of puerperal pyrexia remains infection of the genital tract and this is a common problem in the developing world. However, infections at other sites as a consequence of the delivery or concurrent infection also need to be considered. Non-infective causes include venous thromboembolism, which must be excluded, as it is now the commonest direct cause of maternal death in the UK. The causes of puerperal pyrexia are summarized in Fig. 1.

Uterine infection

Endometritis is one of the most common serious complications of the puerperium and is a major cause of maternal morbidity[2]. Major risk factors for developing postpartum uterine infection include pre-existing chorioamnionitis and lower segment Caesarean section (LSCS), as well as a history of prolonged rupture of membranes and repeated vaginal examinations for cervical assessment. It is commonly caused by *E. coli*, or group A or B streptococcus.[3–5]

Cardinal symptoms of a uterine infection are the presence of a foul-smelling discharge and a fever of 38°C or more, together with a tender uterus on examination. It is usually due to a

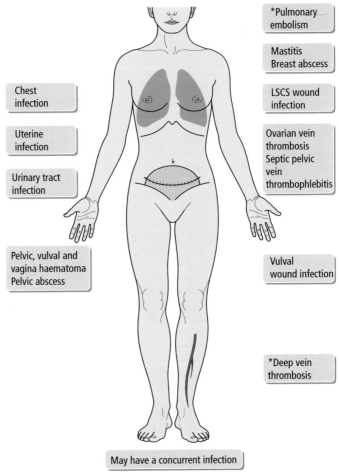

Figure 1 Causes of puerperal pyrexia (* denotes non-infective causes). LSCS, lower segment Caesarean section.

combination of organisms and consequently responds to broad-spectrum antibiotics. Early involvement of microbiologists can be invaluable in seriously ill patients and in those who fail to respond to conventional antibiotics. Endometritis in the presence of retained products of conception on ultrasonography warrants timely uterine evacuation. Intravenous antibiotics are continued until the patient has been afebrile for at least 24 hours.[1,6] Most units give prophylactic antibiotic therapy at Caesarean section, which reduces the infection risk by approximately 60 per cent.[7] Prophylactic antibiotics are also given to women with prolonged rupture of membranes.

■ Infection of abdominal wounds and vulval wounds (LSCS and episiotomy)

Lower segment caesarean section wound

Inspection of the abdominal wound for swelling, discharge and cellulitis is important in the postpartum period. In cases of discharge from the wound, swabs for bacterial culture should be undertaken followed by the commencement of broad-spectrum antibiotics. In one study, risk factors for postoperative fever, endometritis and wound infection were analysed in 761 consecutive Caesarean sections.[8] Postoperative fever was observed in 12 per cent, endometritis in 4.7 per cent and wound infection in 3 per cent of cases. Wound infections were less frequent in cases with a history of previous Caesarean section(s) and after elective Caesarean sections, but was increased if the duration of operation was greater than one hour, if there had been a preceding induction of labour or puerperal endometritis had developed.

Perineal wound

Examination of the perineum and wound swabs before antibiotic therapy in women with puerperal pyrexia is equally important. The common organisms in both sites are likely to be staphylococci, streptococci or *E. coli*, and this should be reflected in the spectrum of antibiotics prescribed.

■ Urinary tract infection

Urinary tract infection (UTI) is the most frequent infection in the puerperium. Contamination by catheterisation, urinary retention and symptomatic bacteriuria all contribute to cystitis. An uncontaminated catheterized specimen that shows pyuria and bacteriuria will establish the diagnosis. Treatment with antibiotics will result in prompt resolution of the infection in most cases.[1,9]

Stray-Pdersen et al. studied 6803 women in the postpartum period and screened them for bacteriuria by culture of voided mid-stream urine (MSU).[9] A significant growth was found in 8.1 per cent. The urine was recollected in this group by suprapubic aspiration and bacteriuria was confirmed in 52 per cent, corresponding to an incidence of bladder bacteriuria of 3.7 per cent. A history of previous urinary tract infection, bacteriuria in pregnancy, operative delivery, epidural anaesthesia and bladder catheterization increased the risk of postpartum urinary tract infection. Only 21 per cent of the women complained of dysuria; this symptom occurred significantly more often after operative delivery and in patients with previous urinary tract infection. The lack of urinary symptoms suggests that all women with postpartum pyrexia should have an MSU sent for culture and sensitivity.

■ Breast disease

In the puerperium, breast problems range from relatively minor ones, such as sore nipples, milk stasis and mastitis, to more serious conditions, such as abscesses and, rarely, inflammatory neoplasms. They may cause significant pyrexia as a presenting problem. Inflammatory changes are easily treated with frequent breast emptying; infectious processes require antibiotics. The symptoms of mastitis include fever, erythema, pain and malaise. The patient is usually several weeks postpartum when the condition develops. *Staphylococcus aureus* and *Staphylococcus epidermidis* are commonly isolated organisms. Breast abscess need to be ruled out in patients not responding to antibiotic treatment.[1,10]

Breast abscesses typically develop in lactating women. The standard treatment is surgical incision, breaking down loculi and drainage of pus. Benson suggested an alternative approach of curettage and primary obliteration of the cavity under antibiotic cover;[11] this gave equally good results with reduced morbidity.

■ Septic pelvic vein thrombophlebitis

Septic pelvic vein thrombophlebitis (SPVT) is an uncommon but serious postpartum complication occurring in about 1 in 2000 pregnancies. It is characterized by pain, antibiotic-resistant fever and tachycardia. Clinically, the patient appears well with little tenderness and no obvious localising signs. SPVT usually becomes evident 4–8 days postpartum after the signs of the initiating endometritis have resolved. The use of contrast-enhanced computerised tomography (CT) increases the diagnostic certainty. Treatment is by heparin and broad-spectrum antibiotics. If there is no resolution of the fever after a week of therapeutic heparin, further investigations to exclude a pelvic abscess or haematoma are required so that surgical drainage may be carried out.[12,13]

■ Ovarian vein thrombosis

Ovarian vein thrombosis is a rare but potentially serious complication following childbirth. The incidence is about 1 in 6000 deliveries. The majority of patients present during the first week postpartum, with fever and right lower quadrant abdominal pain. This condition can mimic an appendicular abscess with leucocytosis on haematological investigation.

Colour Doppler sonography is the favoured diagnostic procedure, CT scan being a supplementary tool. Treatment consists of anticoagulants and antibiotics. A high index of suspicion is crucial to diagnose and treat this condition in order to avoid serious consequences.[14,15]

■ Vulval, vaginal and pelvic haematoma

Puerperal, vulval and vaginal haematomas are uncommon complications of childbirth with the potential for serious morbidity and possible mortality. Prevention, using good surgical technique with attention to haemostasis in the repair of lacerations and episiotomies, should limit the occurrence of these complications. It is important to diagnose these haematomas early so that early prompt treatment may be carried out. Management includes correcting hypovolaemia and intervention with active surgical management, if the haematoma is large or expanding. The use of surgical drains may be a beneficial adjunct to the management.[16,17]

A pelvic ultrasound is often performed in the evaluation of patients with fever following a Caesarean section. Under these circumstances, a bladder-flap or a subfascial haematoma is occasionally demonstrated and the fever is attributed to these findings.[18–21]

In a study by Gemer et al., the incidence of bladder flap haematomas following Caesarean section was 9 per cent but was not significantly associated with febrile morbidity.[22] In contrast, subfascial haematomas were diagnosed in 4.5 per cent of the patients and nearly all were associated with postoperative fever.

A subfascial haematoma also has the potential for significant spread and its volume is difficult to estimate. Thus proper recognition of a subfascial haematoma, and its distinction from a superficial haematoma and bladder-flap haematoma is important.[23]

■ References

1. James DK, Steer PJ, Carl P, Gonik WB. *High Risk Pregnancy – Management Options*, 2nd edn. Philadelphia: WB Saunders.

2. Arulkumaran S, Symonds MI, Fowlie A. *Oxford Handbook of Obstetrics and Gynaecology*. Oxford: Oxford University Press, 2004.

3. Sweet RL, Ledger WJ. Puerperal infections morbidity: a two-year review. *Am J Obstet Gynecol* 1973; **117:** 1093–100.

4. Goldenberg RL, Klebanoff MA, Nugent R, Krohn MA, Hiller S, Andrews WW. Bacterial colonization of the vagina during pregnancy in four ethnic groups. *Am J Obstet Gynaecol* 1996; **174:** 1618.

5. Cunnigham FG, McDonald PC, Gant NF. *Williams Obstetrics*, 20th edn. Stamford, Connecticut: Appleton & Lange, 1997: 549.

6. Hamadeh G, Dedmon C, Mozley PD Postpartum fever. *Am Fam Physician* 1995; **52:** 531–8.

7. French L. Prevention and treatment of postpartum endometritis. *Curr Womens Health Rep* 2003; **3:** 274–9.

8. Sunio S, Saarikoski S, Vohlonen I, Kauhanen O. Risk factors for fever, endometritis and wound infection after abdominal delivery. *Int J Gynaecol Obstet* 1989; **29:** 135–42.

9. Stray-Pdersen B, Blakstad M, Bergan T. Bacteriuria in the puerperium. Risk factors, screening procedures, and treatment programs. *Am J Obstet Gynecol* 1990 ;**162:** 792–7.

10. Oslen CG, Gordon RE Jr. Breast disorders in nursing mothers. *Am Fam Physician* 1990; **41:** 1509–16.

11. Benson EA. Management of breast abscesses. *World J Surg* 1989; **13:** 753–6.

12. Keogh J, MacDonald D, Kelehan P. Septic pelvic thrombophlebitis – an unusual treatable postpartum complication. *Aust NZ J Obstet Gynaecol* 1993; **33:** 204–7.

13. Duff P, Gibbs RS. Pelvic vein thrombophlebitis – diagnostic dilemma and

therapeutic challenge. *Obstet Gynaecol Survey* 1983; **38:** 365–73.

14. Prieto-Nieto MI, Perez-Robledo JP, Rodriguez-Montes JA, Garci-Sancho-Martin L. Acute appendicitis-like symptoms as initial presentation of ovarian vein thrombosis. *Ann Vasc Surg* 2004; **18:** 481–3.
15. Hakim FA, Khan NN, Qushmaq KA, Al-Shami SY. An unusual presentation of postpartum ovarian vein thrombosis. *Saudi Med J* 2007; **28:** 273–5.
16. Ridgway LE. Puerperal emergency. Vaginal and vulval hematomas. *Obstet Gynecol Clin North Am* 1995; **22:** 275–82.
17. Zahn CM, Hankins GD, Yeomans ER. Vulvovaginal haematoma complicating delivery. Rationale for drainage of the haematoma cavity. *J Reprod Med* 1996; **41:** 569–74.
18. Baker ME, Bowie JD, Killam AP. Sonography of post cesarean-section bladder-flap hematoma. *AJR* 1985; **144:** 757–9.
19. Winsett MZ, Fagan CJ, Deepak GB. Sonographic demonstration of bladder-flap hematoma. *J Ultrasound Med* 1986; **5:** 483–7.
20. Baker ME, Kay H, Mahony BS, Cooper CJ, Bowie JD. Sonography of the low transverse incision, cesarean section: a prospective study. *J Ultrasound Med* 1988; **7:** 389–93.
21. Herzberg BS, Bowie JD, Kliewer MA. Complication of cesarean section: role of transperineal US. *Radiology* 1993; **188:** 533–6.
22. Gemer O, Shenhav S, Segal S, Harari D, Segal O, Zohav E. Sonographically diagnosed pelvic hematomas and postcesarean febrile morbidity. *Int J Gynaecol Obstet* 1999; **65:** 7–9.
23. Wiener MD, Bowie JD, Baker ME, Kay HH. Sonography of subfacial hematoma after cesarean section. *AJR* 1987; **148:** 907–10.

FITS IN PREGNANCY

Peter Muller

The onset of seizures in pregnancy can be classified into two groups:

- *obstetric* – eclampsia; and
- *non-obstetric* – medical condition
  - primary seizure disorder
  - cerebrovascular accident
  - neoplasia
  - infection
  - rare conditions.

Eclampsia

Diagnosis

Eclampsia is defined as:[1,2]

- a new-onset, grand mal seizure in a woman with pre-eclampsia;
- a new-onset, grand mal seizure that cannot be attributed to other causes.

Eclampsia should be the primary initial diagnosis in all cases of new-onset, pregnancy-related, grand mal seizures and these patients should be managed accordingly. Maternal morbidity and mortality are increased in pre-eclamptic patients who develop eclampsia, and there is a widely accepted successful approach to the initial management of an eclamptic fit with the use of magnesium sulphate.[3] Maternal risks associated with eclampsia include abruptio placentae, disseminated intravascular coagulopathy, pulmonary oedema, acute renal failure, aspiration pneumonia and cardiopulmonary arrest.[4] The diagnosis of eclampsia can be confirmed by the presence of hypertension and proteinuria along with the typical timing. However, the signs and symptoms can be very varied.[3]

Hypertension

Eclampsia occurs more frequently with severe hypertension (diastolic blood pressure >110 mmHg; 54 per cent) than mild hypertension (diastolic blood pressure of 91–109 mmHg; 30 per cent). However, 16 per cent of eclamptic women initially have a normal blood pressure. Eclampsia occurring before 32 weeks' gestation is more commonly associated with severe hypertension.[4]

Proteinuria

Some degree of proteinuria is usually present in women who develop eclampsia. A significant amount of proteinuria, greater or equal to 3+, is found in nearly half (48 per cent) of the cases, although it may be absent in a significant number (14 per cent).[4]

Oedema

Oedema is generally not helpful in the diagnosis as it is so common in pregnancy and it may be completely absent in a quarter of the cases (26 per cent).[4]

Timing

Eclampsia can develop antepartum, intrapartum or postpartum, with reported frequencies of 38–53 per cent, 18–19 per cent and 28–44 per cent, respectively.[4,5] Current antepartum and immediate postpartum therapies appear to be shifting the percentage of eclampsia cases to the later postpartum period.[6] In recent surveys, over half of the postpartum cases of eclampsia occur beyond 48 hours postpartum[4,6,7] and there are reported cases of eclampsia as late as 23 days after delivery.[3] Patients with these 'atypical' eclamptic seizures commonly present to accident and emergency clinicians who may have less awareness of this obstetric problem.[6] A majority of cases occur after 28 weeks (91 per cent) with few occurring prior to 20 weeks (1.5 per cent).[4]

Clinical signs and symptoms

Occipital or frontal headaches, visual changes, such as blurred vision and photophobia, and right upper quadrant pain can be experienced prior to the onset of eclampsia. Headache is the most common antecedent symptom with 50–70 per cent of women describing headaches of some nature. Visual changes are seen in 19–30 per cent and right upper quadrant pain is present in 12–19 per cent of cases.[5,6] At least one of these symptoms will be present in 59–75 per cent of patients with eclampsia.[3] It is important to realise that approximately 20 per cent of

women who develop eclampsia do not have any pre-convulsion signs or symptoms.[3] Severe unremitting headaches are commonly used to assess risk of impending eclampsia, as criteria in classifying severe pre-eclampsia,[2] and in directing management such as the initiation of magnesium sulphate and need to expedite delivery. Unfortunately, headaches have only limited discriminatory benefit on whether a patient with pre-eclampsia will develop eclampsia[8] (see Headache in pregnancy).

Hyperreflexia is commonly seen in women who develop eclampsia and should be part of any initial and ongoing surveillance examination of a woman with pre-eclampsia. However, it must be remembered that seizures do occur in women without hyperreflexia and uncomplicated pregnancies have evidence of hyperreflexia. Consequently, attention to patient's deep tendon reflexes is included in the thorough evaluation in patients with pre-eclampsia, but its use in the prediction of eclampsia remains limited.[9]

The initial seizure activity is a generalised tonic–clonic convulsion, most often self-limited to approximately a minute. However, if left untreated, seizure activity can resume quickly, one after another.[10] Focal neurologic findings are rare, unless there is another neurologic complication, such as a cerebrovascular accident.

Initial evaluations

Initial evaluations are required to help confirm the diagnosis, to assess the maternal morbidities associated with eclampsia,[11] and to prepare for a safe and expedited delivery. The emergent aspect of eclampsia, however, requires proceeding with direct management well before the test results are complete.

Laboratory

Laboratory investigations should include:

- haemoglobin, haematocrit;
- platelet count and coagulation studies;
- creatinine;
- serum uric acid;
- serum transaminase levels and lactic dehydrogenase
- serum urea and electrolytes, and glucose levels.

Pulse oximetry should be considered to evaluate for aspiration pneumonia or pulmonary oedema, seen in 2–3 per cent and 3–5 per cent of cases, respectively. If pulse oximetry is below 92 per cent, arterial blood gases are required.[3]

Radiological

A chest X-ray may be required if maternal hypoxaemia is present and/or pulmonary examination is abnormal. Routine neuroimaging has not been advocated for women with eclampsia.[3,12] The clinician, on the other hand, should have a low threshold in ordering neuroimaging to women with an 'atypical' presentation of convulsions and where the diagnosis may be in doubt.

Fetal assessment

Maternal hypoxaemia occurs during the convulsion and can lead to fetal heart rate alterations, such as bradycardia, transient late decelerations, decreased variability and tachycardia. In a majority of cases, these fetal heart alterations are transient as the maternal hypoxaemia resolves post-convulsion. For those cases where these fetal heart rate findings persist for 15–20 minutes despite maternal resuscitation therapies, the diagnosis of abruptio placentae should be considered.

Management of eclampsia

Eclampsia is an obstetric complication requiring an efficient and organised management protocol. The aims of the initial management are to reduce maternal morbidity and prevent further convulsions. An important priority is to obtain the input of the most senior personnel available, namely medical, midwifery and nursing.

Airway

The mother needs to be protected from injuring herself and obstructing her airway. In order to achieve these objectives, plus reducing the risk of aspiration and excessive hypoxia, guard rails should be used and the patient should be turned on their side into the recovery position. Supplemental oxygen should be commenced by mask or nasal prongs. The insertion of a padded tongue blade to prevent maternal injury has been advocated.[3] However, many clinicians refrain from using the tongue blade, as it commonly institutes a gag reflex, is difficult to introduce during the primary convulsion, delays other primary therapies and is unlikely to prevent an oral injury that occurs at the onset of the primary convulsion.

Fits

The next priority of the clinical team is to institute therapy to prevent recurrent convulsions. After much early debate, magnesium sulphate has become the primary therapy to prevent such recurrent convulsions. The Collaborative Eclampsia Trial demonstrated that magnesium sulphate reduces the recurrence of convulsions by >50 per cent when compared to diazepam and phenytoin.[13] In this large study, there was, in addition, a significant decrease in maternal mortality, incidence of pneumonia, need for mechanical ventilation and intensive care admissions.

Standard magnesium protocols have included 4 or 6 g IV loading dose over 15–20 minutes, followed by 1 to 2 gram/hour intravenous (IV) infusion. Recurrent convulsions still occur in approximately 9–10 per cent of women treated with magnesium sulphate.[14] A second IV loading dose of 2 g usually controls these episodes. Magnesium sulphate should be continued for 24 hours post delivery. Magnesium sulphate is renally excreted, thus oliguria (<30 mL/h) should lead the clinician to reduce or even discontinue (in cases of anuria) the infusion. Surveillance of deep tendon reflexes are generally sufficient to gauge magnesium toxicity, where loss of patellar and ankle reflexes occurs at levels of 9–12 mg/dL; however, obtaining serum magnesium levels in patients with severe oliguria, where serum levels can rise quite quickly, may be prudent.

Blood pressure

Antihypertensive therapy should be instituted for severe hypertension when systolic blood pressure is above 160 mmHg and/or diastolic blood pressure is above 105–110 mmHg. The commonly used drugs include nifedipine, hydralazine and labetalol, usually according to departmental protocols.

Delivery of the baby is indicated for all cases of eclampsia once the mother's condition is stable. The assessment will include evaluation of coagulation, renal, liver, respiratory and neurologic function. Blood pressure should be well controlled and anaesthesia consultation should be sought. Regional anaesthesia, unless specific contraindications are present (i.e. coagulopathy) is generally favoured for both Caesarean section and labour.[2] Eclampsia is not a contraindication for a normal vaginal birth, which in many cases may proceed rapidly if the cervix is favourable. However, mode of delivery will depend on gestational age, reassuring fetal heart rate and cervical favourability.

Prevention

Ideally, maternal and neonatal risks would be reduced if we were able to prevent the eclamptic fit. Despite this fact, prophylactic use of magnesium sulphate is not commonly prescribed for patients with pre-eclampsia during the peripartum period.

A recent review of randomised trials on the prophylactic use of magnesium sulphate demonstrated that magnesium sulphate reduces eclampsia by greater than 60 per cent.[11] The Magpie Trial,[15] the largest of these trials comparing magnesium sulphate to placebo, demonstrated a 58 per cent reduction in eclampsia, a 46 per cent reduction in abruptio placentae and a non-significant trend in reduced maternal mortality. Unwanted side effects were more common in those patients receiving magnesium sulphate, but there was no significant difference in serious maternal morbidity. The number of patients needed to be treated to prevent one case of an eclamptic fit is 63 women with severe pre-eclampsia and 109 with mild pre-eclampsia. For those patients with clinically 'imminent' eclampsia and no clinically 'imminent' eclampsia, the numbers needing to be treated were 36 and 129, respectively.

Some clinicians have used these data to develop management protocols where the use of prophylactic magnesium sulphate should be initiated only in those patients with symptoms of impending eclampsia. However, many women develop eclampsia without any antecedent signs or symptoms.[3] The Magpie Trial did demonstrate that the number of women needing to be treated to prevent one case in developed nations was relatively high at 385. However, selective magnesium prophylaxis has resulted in an overall increased incidence of eclampsia in women with non-severe disease.[16] For these reasons, there is debate on the use of prophylactic magnesium in women in developed nations with mild pre-eclampsia. Despite this controversy, the evidence does support the use of magnesium sulphate prophylaxis in the peripartum period for women with severe pre-eclampsia.

■ Non-eclampsia medical conditions

The clinician must consider *non-obstetric* medical conditions, when the primary convulsion presents in an atypical fashion. Atypical presentations would include convulsions that:

- occur more than 48 hours after delivery;
- occur prior to 24 weeks' gestation;
- occur without evidence of hypertension and/or proteinuria;
- are unresponsive to magnesium sulphate;
- have prolonged mental status changes;
- develop focal neurological symptoms;
- have an associated cardiopulmonary arrest.

Differential diagnosis

The differential diagnosis for non-eclampsia convulsions will include:

- primary seizure disorder – first episode;
- cerbrovascular accident
  - intracranial haemorrhage
  - subarachnoid haemorrhage
  - cerebral venous thrombosis
  - arterial embolism or thrombosis;
- hypertensive encephalopathy;
- hypoxic encephalopathy
  - neurogenic vasovagal syncope;
- neoplastic cranial mass;
- infection
  - viral or bacterial meningitis/encephalitis
  - malaria;
- rare conditions
  - thrombotic thrombocytopenic purpura
  - hyponatraemia.

Evaluations

The significant adverse maternal outcomes and different strategies for the above diagnosis mandates early radiological assessment for cases with atypical presentations. Computerised tomography (CT) scanning is reasonable for those emergent cases where an early diagnosis of an intracranial haemorrhage, subarachnoid haemorrhage or intracranial neoplastic mass will dictate early management. CT scanning is readily available in most acute services hospitals and requires shorter scanning time, which reduces artefact from patient movement. If readily available in the institution, a magnetic resonance imaging (MRI) scan is commonly preferred by our radiology colleagues for the stable patient to review most intracranial pathologies. MRI is more sensitive for diagnosing cerebral venous thrombosis than non-contrast CT, but is not as sensitive as CT in assessing acute intracranial haemorrhage.[17]

If clinical examination suggests maternal central nervous system infection (fever and nuchal rigidity), the primary method for diagnosis of meningitis is lumbar puncture.

For those patients with new onset of seizures that are not consistent with eclampsia and no pathologic finding is seen on neuroimaging, referral to the neurology laboratory for electroencephalography testing may assist in the diagnosis of a primary seizure disorder.

Management

The management depends *solely* on the underlying pathology.

Conclusion

Eclampsia should be the primary initial diagnosis in all cases of new-onset, pregnancy-related, grand mal seizures. Ongoing treatment should be directed initially towards this obstetric complication. However, the clinician must be cognizant of other significant maternal medical conditions that also require intensive, but different, evaluations and treatments. Attention to the varying presentations will assist the clinician in differentiating eclampsia from the other maternal medical conditions.

References

1. Report of the National High Blood Pressure Education Program Working Group on High Blood Pressure in Pregnancy. *Am J Obstet Gynecol* 2000; **183**: S1–S22.
2. ACOG practice bulletin. Diagnosis and management of preeclampsia and eclampsia. Number 33, January 2002. *Obstet Gynecol* 2002; **99**: 159–67.
3. Sibai BM. Diagnosis, prevention, and management of eclampsia. *Obstet Gynecol* 2005; **105**: 402–10.
4. Mattar F, Sibai BM. Eclampsia. VIII. Risk factors for maternal morbidity. *Am J Obstet Gynecol* 2000; **182**: 307–12.
5. Douglas KA, Redman CW. Eclampsia in the United Kingdom. *BMJ* 1994; **309**: 1395–400.
6. Chames MC, Livingston JC, Ivester TS, Barton JR, Sibai BM. Late postpartum eclampsia: a preventable disease? *Am J Obstet Gynecol* 2002; **186**: 1174–7.
7. Katz VL, Farmer R, Kuller JA. Preeclampsia into eclampsia: toward a new paradigm. *Am J Obstet Gynecol* 2000; **182**: 1389–96.
8. Witlin AG, Saade GR, Mattar F, Sibai BM. Risk factors for abruptio placentae and eclampsia: analysis of 445 consecutively managed women with severe preeclampsia and eclampsia. *Am J Obstet Gynecol* 1999; **180**: 1322–9.
9. Sibai BM, McCubbin JH, Anderson GD, Lipshitz J, Dilts PV Jr. Eclampsia. I. Observations from 67 recent cases. *Obstet Gynecol* 1981; **58**: 609–13.
10. Lindheimer FRJMCG. *Chesley's Hypertensive Disorders in Pregnancy*, 2nd edn. Stamford, Connecticut: Appleton and Lange, 1999.
11. Sibai BM. Magnesium sulfate prophylaxis in preeclampsia: evidence from randomized trials. *Clin Obstet Gynecol* 2005; 48: 478–88.
12. Witlin AG, Friedman SA, Egerman RS, Frangieh AY, Sibai BM. Cerebrovascular

disorders complicating pregnancy – beyond eclampsia. *Am J Obstet Gynecol* 1997; **176:** 1139–45.

13. Which anticonvulsant for women with eclampsia? Evidence from the Collaborative Eclampsia Trial. *Lancet* 1995; **345:** 1455–63.

14. Witlin AG. Prevention and treatment of eclamptic convulsions. *Clin Obstet Gynecol* 1999; **42:** 507–18.

15. Altman D, Carroli G, Duley L, *et al.* Do women with pre-eclampsia, and their babies, benefit from magnesium sulphate? The Magpie Trial: a randomised placebo-controlled trial. *Lancet* 2002; **359:** 1877–90.

16. Alexander JM, McIntire DD, Leveno KJ, Cunningham FG. Selective magnesium sulfate prophylaxis for the prevention of eclampsia in women with gestational hypertension. *Obstet Gynecol* 2006; **108:** 826–32.

17. Mettler FA. *Essentials of Radiology,* 2nd edn. Philadelphia: Saunders, 2005.

GENITALIA, AMBIGUOUS (INCLUDING CONGENITAL ANOMALIES)

Kausik Banerjee

It is estimated that genital anomalies occur 1 in 4500 live births. The birth of a child with ambiguous genitalia is a social emergency. The first encounter of the parents with the health professional in the delivery room may have a lasting impact on parents and their relationship with their infant. The neonate should be referred as 'your baby' or 'your child', and not 'he', 'she' or 'it'. It is best not to attempt a diagnosis or offer gender assignment at the first encounter. It is

important to emphasise that the infant with genital anomaly has the potential to become a functional member of society. Genital anomaly is not shameful. It should be explained to the parents that, although the best course of action may not initially be clear, the health care professionals will work with the family to reach a decision that is best suited in the particular circumstances.

There has been significant progress in diagnosis, understanding the pathology, improvement in surgical techniques, understanding the psychosocial issues and accepting the place of patient advocacy. Terms such as intersex, pseudohermaphroditism, hermaphroditism and sex reversal are all controversial, and are perceived by parents as potentially stigmatising and confusing. The European Society for Paediatric Endocrinology (ESPE) and its American counterpart, the Lawson Wilkins Pediatric Endocrine Society (LWPES) have jointly published a consensus statement on the management and nomenclature of intersex disorders. The new nomenclature for this condition is disorders of sex development (DSD). DSD is defined by congenital conditions in which development of chromosomal, gonadal or anatomical sex is atypical. The proposed changes in nomenclature are outlined in Table 1.

Table 1 Proposed revised nomenclature for intersex conditions

Previous	Proposed
Intersex	Disorders of sex development (DSD)
Male pseudohermaphrodite: undervirilisation or undermasculinisation of an XY male	46, XY DSD
Female pseudohermaphrodite: overvirilisation or masculinisation of an XX female	46, XX DSD
True hermaphrodite	Ovotesticular DSD
XX male or XX sex reversal	46, XX testicular DSD
XY sex reversal	46, XY complete gonadal dysgenesis

It is helpful to examine the child in the presence of the parents to demonstrate the precise abnormalities of genitalia. One should emphasise that the genitalia of both sexes develop from the same fetal structures and either overdevelopment and underdevelopment is possible, the abnormal appearance can be rectified and the child will be raised either as a boy or a girl. It is also important not to encourage the parents to name the child or register the birth until the sex of rearing is established.

■ Normal genital development

Undifferentiated gonadal tissue with potential to develop into either a male or female genital structure is present in the fetus as early as 6 weeks' gestation. The presence or absence of genetic and hormonal influences, which are responsible for the active process of male differentiation, dictate the genital appearance of the neonate. An abnormality along the male pathway that interferes with masculinisation or, in the case of a genetic female, the presence of virilising influences on the female embryo results in an intersex condition.

The sex-determining region in the Y chromosome (*SRY*) gene situated on the short arm of Y chromosome is responsible for male sex differentiation. Undifferentiated gonad forms a testis under the influence of *SRY*. Testosterone from the testes stimulates maturation of Wolffian structures (vas deferens, epididymis and seminal vesicles) and anti-Müllerian hormone suppresses the Müllerian structures (fallopian tubes, uterus and upper vagina). Peripheral conversion of testosterone to dihydrotestosterone in the skin of external genitalia is responsible for masculinisation of genital structures. The major part of male differentiation is complete by 12 weeks' gestation. Penile growth and testicular descent progress throughout the pregnancy.

Female sexual differentiation occurs in the absence of *SRY*.

■ Clinical findings in a neonate with suspected DSD

Apparent male

- Severe hypospadias with separation of scrotal sacs.
- Hypospadias with undescended tesis.
- Bilateral impalpable testes with or without micropenis in a term neonate (Fig. 1).

Apparent female

- Foreshortened vulva with single opening.
- Inguinal hernia containing a palpable gonad.
- Clitoral hypertrophy (Fig. 2).

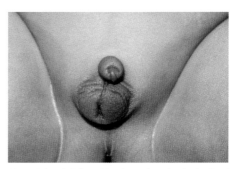

Figure 1 A male infant with micropenis and underdeveloped scrotum.

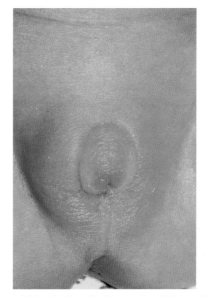

Figure 2 A female infant with clitoromegaly and fullness of the labia. Congenital adrenal hyperplasia is the underlying diagnosis.

Indeterminate

- Ambiguous genitalia.

■ Causes of genital abnormality in a neonate

Conceptually, it is simpler to think of the causes in terms of histology of the gonads, which dictates the prognosis with regard to fertility. This is outlined in Table 2.

Table 2 Causes of genital anomaly according to gonadal tissue

Gonadal	Cause of genital anomaly tissue
Ovary	1. Congenital adrenal hyperplasia (CAH)
	2. Maternal source of virilisation (luteoma, exogenous androgens)
	3. Placental aromatase deficiency
Testis	1. Luteinising hormone receptor defect: Leydig cell hypoplasia/aplasia
	2. Androgen biosynthesis defect: 17-OH steroid dehydrogenase deficiency, 5α-reductase deficiency, StAR (steroidogenic acute regulatory protein) mutations
	3. Defect in androgen action: complete/partial androgen insensitivity syndrome (CAIS/PAIS)
	4. Disorders of anti-Müllerian hormone (AMH) and AMH receptor: persistent Müllerian duct syndrome
Ovary and testis	True hermaphrodite
Dysgenetic gonads	1. Gonadal dysgenesis (Swyer syndrome)[a]
	2. Denys–Drash syndrome[b]
	3. Smith Lemli Opitz syndrome[c]
	4. Camptomelic dwarfism[d]
Other	1. Cloacal exstrophy
	2. MURCS (Müllerian, renal, cervicothoracic somite abnormalities)

[a]*Gonadal dysgenesis* (Swyer syndrome): a phenotypic female with 46, XY karyotype who does not have any functional gonads to induce puberty.

[b]*Denys–Drash syndrome*: a rare disorder consisting of the triad of (1) congenital nephropathy, (2) Wilms tumour, and (3) genital anomaly resulting from mutation in the Wilms tumour gene (WT1) situated on chromosome 11 (11p 13).

[c]*Smith Lemli Opitz syndrome*: a rare disorder caused by defect in cholesterol synthesis; it is autosomal recessive in inheritance. Affected individuals have multiple congenital anomalies: intrauterine growth restriction, dysmorphic facial features, microcephaly, low-set ears, cleft palate, genital anomaly, syndactyly, mental retardation.

[d]*Camptomelic dwarfism* (bent limbs): this has an autosomal dominant inheritance and is caused by mutations in *SOX9* (a sex-determining region in the Y chromosome-related gene located at the long arm of chromosome 17). Features include short stature, hydrocephalus, anterior bowing of the femur, tibia, talipes and poor masculinisation.

■ Clinical evaluation

A detailed obstetric history is vital to determine the possibility of maternal endocrine disturbances and/or any exposure to drugs or hormonal agents. A positive family history of unexplained neonatal death, abnormal genital development, abnormal pubertal development or infertility should be determined, as well as a history of consanguinity. This may point to an autosomal recessive disorder.

Physical examination includes examination of the phallus, the extent to which urogenital sinus has closed and the position of urethral meatus. Fullness and rugosity of labioscrotal folds should be noted, and an attempt should be made to palpate any gonads in these folds or the inguinal region. This may require considerable patience.

To make a definitive diagnosis based solely on physical findings would be unwise, as the appearance of external genitalia can be extremely variable even in the same clinical condition. The only conclusion that can be made from a palpable gonad is that the diagnosis is not a genetically female infant with congenital adrenal hyperplasia (CAH).

■ Investigations

The commonest cause of genital anomaly in a neonate is CAH. Hence a biochemical screen for this disorder is indicated in all infants with signs of virilisation and non-palpable gonads. 21-Hydroxylase deficiency is the commonest enzyme deficiency (95 per cent) responsible for CAH. An elevated 17-hydroxyprogesterone is suggestive of CAH secondary to 21-hydroxylase deficiency; however, a more extensive biochemical panel is advised for the rarer form of CAH. The infant's electrolytes should be monitored closely as hyponatraemia (low sodium) and hyperkalaemia (raised potassium) often manifests from 48 hours onwards, and demands appropriate intervention (treatment of hypovolaemia and circulatory collapse, provision of sodium and hydrocortisone).

A karyotype (chromosome analysis) is also done as an initial investigation. A fluorescent *in situ* hybridisation for the Y chromosome can be obtained within 48 hours in most places; however, a detailed karyotype (with G banding) often takes up to a week.

An ultrasound scan by an experienced person can identify the presence of ovaries and a uterus relatively quickly, and can be suggestive of a female sex.

Further investigations are needed if the CAH screen is negative and the gonad(s) are palpable. A genitogram (preferably by a paediatric radiologist experienced in children's urological anomalies) is required to identify a vagina, a uterine canal and fallopian tube(s) or the vasa deferentia. Appropriate biochemical tests will be required to identify any testosterone biosynthetic defect, 5α reductase activity or androgen sensitivity. These investigations are best undertaken in a tertiary centre, which has expertise in dealing with this condition.

A summary of these investigations is shown in Fig. 3 and Fig. 4 outlines the adrenal steroid hormone synthesis.

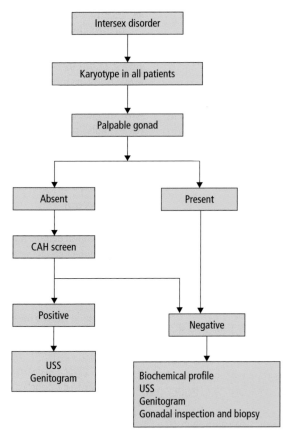

Figure 3 Laboratory and imaging studies in newborns with genital anomaly. CAH, congenital adrenal hyperplasia; USS, ultrasound scan.

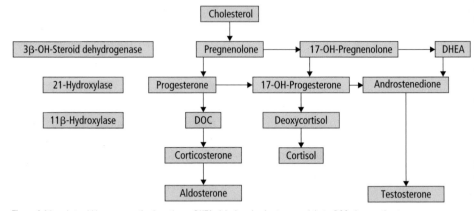

Figure 4 Adrenal steroid hormone synthesis pathway. DHEA, dehydroepiandrosterone sulphate; DOC, deoxycorticosterone.

■ Deciding the sex of rearing

This is based on a number of considerations:

- fertility potential;
- capacity for normal sexual function;
- endocrine status;
- potential for malignant change;
- availability of corrective surgical procedures and timing of surgery.

Long-term management of these children requires significant expertise and involvement of a multidisciplinary team consisting of:

- paediatrician/paediatric endocrinologist;
- paediatric urologist;
- psychologist;
- geneticist;
- gynaecologist (depending on the underlying condition).

■ Further reading

American Academy of Pediatrics, Committee on Genetics. Evaluation of the newborn with developmental anomalies of the external genitalia. *Pediatrics* 2000; **106:** 138–42.

Hughes IA, Houk C, Ahmed SF, Lee PA, LWPES1/ESPE2 Consensus Group. Consensus statement on management of intersex disorders. *Arch Dis Child* 2006; **91:** 554–63.

Hyun G, Kolon TF. A practical approach to intersex in the newborn period. *Urol Clin North Am* 2004; **31:** 435–43.

Rangecroft L. Surgical management of ambiguous genitalia. *Arch Dis Child* 2003; **88:** 799–801.

■ Useful websites (for parents and professionals)

www.bsped.org
www.cah.org.uk
www.hopkinsmedicine.org/pediatricen-docrinology/cah
www.magicfoundation.org
www.medhelp.org/www/ais

GLYCOSURIA OF PREGNANCY

Rina Davison

Most women will demonstrate glycosuria at some time during their pregnancy owing to a fall in the renal tubular threshold for glucose. Consequently, glycosuria is not a reliable diagnostic tool for diabetes. Any suspicion of diabetes must be confirmed by blood glucose measurement.

There are three main types of diabetes in pregnancy:

- pre-existing type 1 diabetes;
- pre-existing type 2 diabetes;
- gestational diabetes, which is hyperglycaemia first recognised in pregnancy.

Interpretation of the oral glucose tolerance test (OGTT) leads to the definitions shown in Table 1.

Table 1 Definitions of type of diabetes mellitus from oral glucose tolerance test results

Type 1 and 2	Gestational
Fasting 2 hours $\geqslant$7 mmol/L	Fasting $\geqslant$6 mmol/L
2-hour value $\geqslant$11.1 mmol/L	2 hours $\geqslant$7.8 mmol/L

■ Pre-exisiting diabetes

In European women, the incidence of diabetic pregnancy is relatively low (about 1 in 300 of all pregnancies) but this depends on the local prevalence of both type 1 and type 2 diabetes in women of child-bearing age. There are marked ethnic and national differences, e.g. there is a tenfold greater incidence of type 1 diabetes in women aged 15–40 years in Northern European countries compared to Southern Greece. Owing to the younger age of onset observed in type 2 diabetes in Oriental, Middle Eastern, Hispanic American, African, South Asian and Caribbean women, the prevalence of diabetes may be as high as one in ten pregnancies in some of these communities. Pregnancy in a diabetic mother carries a greater risk to both mother and the offspring than pregnancy in the general obstetric population.

Effect of pregnancy on diabetes

Physiologically, normal pregnancy is associated with an increase in maternal insulin production and insulin resistance. Therefore, maternal insulin dosage requirements increase as pregnancy progresses – up to 2–3 times pre-pregnancy doses. Maternal renal disease and proliferative retinopathy may accelerate during and after pregnancy, thereby making regular review essential.

Effect of pre-existing diabetes on pregnancy outcome

Recent data confirm that women with poorly controlled diabetes have an increased rate of miscarriage and pre-eclampsia. These women have a higher incidence of preterm labour and a >60 per cent Caesarean section rate. Perinatal, stillbirth and neonatal mortality rates are all 5–10-fold higher than in non-diabetic pregnancies. Congenital abnormalities are up to three times higher than the background rate, particularly neural tube defects and congenital heart disease. Over half of singleton babies have a birth weight over the 90th centile for their gestational age and one-third of term babies are admitted to neonatal units for problems such as hypoglycaemia (Box 1).

Box 1 Obstetric and perinatal complications of pre-existing diabetes

Maternal	Fetal
Pre-eclampsia	Congenital abnormalities:
	■ HbA_{1c} <8–5% risk
	■ HbA_{1c} >10–25% risk
Increase in Caesarean section rate	Macrosomia – prolonged labour, prematurity, birth trauma
Premature labour	Intrauterine growth restriction
	Neonatal hypoglycaemia (8–60% prevalence)
Long-term risk of type 2 diabetes	Respiratory distress syndrome
	Hypocalcaemia
	Intrauterine death – fasting >5 mmol/L in the last 4–8 weeks' gestation
	Later risk of obesity and diabetes

Management of pre-existing diabetes

The essential basis of treatment is good metabolic control, beginning most importantly, before conception (see Box 2).

Box 2 Pre-conception management of pre-existing diabetes

- Patient education regarding benefits of tight diabetic control to improve pregnancy outcome
- Contraception advice
- Review of drug therapy for pregnancy
- Ophthalmology review
- Serum creatinine and urine, microalbumin
- Optimised diabetic control, i.e. HbA_{1c} <6.5%
- Switch type 2 diabetic patients on to insulin; stop oral hypoglycaemia agents
- *Start* pre-conceptual folic acid 5 mg daily

Pregnant women should be managed in a joint pregnancy diabetic clinic by obstetricians and physicians with expertise in the care of such women. Dieticians, midwives and specialist diabetes nurses should also be an essential part of the multidisciplinary team.

First trimester management

Accurate dating of the pregnancy is an obstetric imperative and is best confirmed by ultrasound examination at 8–10 weeks. Patients should be reviewed regularly in the antenatal diabetic clinic for discussion of blood glucose self-monitoring results and advice on increasing insulin requirements. Nuchal scanning is also beneficial from 11 weeks onwards.

Second and third trimester management

The keystone of management is achieving maternal normoglycaemia. Increasing maternal insulin resistance necessitates an increased insulin dose. The target capillary blood glucose should be 4–5 mmol/L fasting and 4.5–7 mmol/L postprandially. All pregnant diabetic women should be on a strict, low-sugar, low-fat, high-fibre diet and a four times daily basal bolus regime, i.e. three premeal injections of fast-acting insulin and one nocturnal injection of intermediate-acting insulin.

Obstetric supervision by a specialist midwife and obstetrician should be more frequent than for uncomplicated pregnancy. Ultrasound examination of the fetus every 4 weeks will allow detection of intrauterine growth restriction and evolving macrosomia (>4 kg) and hydramnios. The risk of late unexplained fetal death may be less when blood glucose control is good. Many units use biophysical tests for fetal viability regularly with the possibility of early delivery in mind. A detailed ultrasound of the fetus at 18–20 weeks' gestation with particular assessment of the fetal heart is necessary. The timing and mode of delivery has to balance the risk of prematurity with its associated complications against the risk of late intrauterine death and macrosomia with its attendant complications. Most obstetricians plan delivery between 38 and 39 weeks.

■ Gestational diabetes

Gestational diabetes (GDM) may be asymptomatic but can have serious consequences for the mother and baby if it remains undetected. The incidence of GDM in the UK is about 1 in 20. It usually develops in the second or third trimester induced by changes in carbohydrate metabolism and decreased insulin sensitivity. It is 11 times more common in women of Asian background and three times more common in black women compared to European women. Therefore, all pregnant women should have a test for glycosuria at every antenatal visit and, if positive, laboratory glucose should be checked as a confirmatory test.

A random laboratory blood glucose measured at booking and again at 28 weeks will pick up undiagnosed diabetes early in pregnancy and gestational diabetes later in pregnancy. The diagnosis of gestational diabetes will require a 75 g oral glucose tolerance test (see Table 1 for diagnostic criteria). Certain women are at high risk of developing gestational diabetes and may need an OGTT before 28 weeks for diagnosis, e.g. 20–24 weeks (Box 3).

Box 3 High-risk groups for gestational diabetes

- Obese women, body mass index >30 at booking
- First-degree relative with diabetes
- A history of polycystic ovarian syndrome
- Gestational diabetes in a previous pregnancy
- Macrosomia in a previous pregnancy
- A previous unexplained stillbirth or neonatal death
- Women who have glycosuria on two or more occasions in the current pregnancy
- Age >40
- A history of hypertension

The reason for diagnosing as early as possible is that GDM is associated with increased perinatal morbidity and macrosomia in the same way as pre-existing diabetes.

Management

Diet, education and frequent blood glucose monitoring at home is essential. At present, basal bolus insulin treatment is advised for all mothers with gestational diabetes whose venous plasma glucose despite diet remains >5.8 mmol/L fasting or 8 mmol/L postprandially. It may be that even lower criteria will be shown to decrease the prevalence of fetal macrosomia. Regular ultrasound assessment for fetal growth is needed to influence timing and mode of delivery.

Pre-pregnancy counselling for women at risk of GDM

In women who have a high risk of gestational diabetes, a pre-pregnancy educational programme on nutrition and lifestyle will reduce the number who require active treatment. Previous gestational diabetes is very likely to recur and often the woman remains diabetic. Women identified as having GDM have a greatly increased risk (up to 50 per cent) of developing type 2 diabetes within 10–15 years and hence lifestyle modification is essential for both pregnancy and the long-term non-pregnant state.

■ Management of diabetes during active labour

Insulin infusion regimes for women with established diabetes and women with gestational diabetes who are on insulin are standard. For women with gestational diabetes treated with diet alone, blood glucose levels should be monitored during labour, and intravenous insulin and dextrose infusion should only be started if the blood monitoring stix are persistently above 8.

■ Management after delivery

Women with established type 1 diabetes

Dextrose and insulin infusions should be continued until the women are eating and drinking normally. Once eating and drinking, they should return to their pre-pregnancy insulin doses immediately after delivery.

Women with established type 2 diabetes

This is the same as for type 1 diabetes but, once eating and drinking, they can usually return to their pre-pregnancy oral medication.

Women with gestational diabetes treated with insulin

The insulin should be *stopped immediately after delivery*, once these women are eating and drinking.

It is important to remember that all women who have gestational diabetes require a further OGTT 6–10 weeks after delivery to ensure type 2 diabetes has not developed.

HAEMATEMESIS IN PREGNANCY

Oliver Brain and Margaret Myszor

■ Key points in management

Definitions

- *Haematemesis* is the vomiting of red blood.
- *Coffee-ground vomiting* is the vomiting of small amounts of altered blood.
- *Melaena* is the passage of black tarry stool (altered blood) and occurs if blood loss is >50 mL.

Presentation

- Haematemesis with or without melaena.
- There may be symptoms of dizziness, abdominal or retrosternal pain.
- There may be signs of shock or cardiovascular compromise.

Management of a haematemesis

This includes the following.

1 Full blood count, clotting, urea and electrolytes, liver function tests (± cross-match)
2 Large-bore intravenous access, if moderate or severe.
3 Intravenous fluid resuscitation (crystalloid or colloid); blood if severe.
4 Nil by mouth, if moderate or severe.

5 Give appropriate antacid medication.
6 Gastroenterologist review, if moderate or severe (Table 1).

Common causes in pregnancy

These are as follows:

- Mallory–Weiss tear;
- oesophagitis;
- gastric or duodenal ulceration or erosions.

■ Introduction

Haematemesis is the vomiting of blood caused by haemorrhage from the upper gastrointestinal tract (oesophagus, stomach or duodenum). If severe enough, the bleeding may also give rise to melaena – the passage of black tarry stools. Most commonly the haemorrhage is due to significant disruption of the mucosa and underlying blood vessels, e.g. an ulcer, but occasionally disordered haemostasis will cause a minor defect to bleed enough to cause haematemesis or melaena. Vomiting of small amounts of altered blood ('coffee-ground' vomit) is common but rarely of any significance. Coffee-ground haematemesis will occur with gradual blood loss as the stomach acid converts haemoglobin to haematin. 'Fresh' haematemesis will occur if a medium–large vessel is eroded and this is often accompanied by cardiovascular compromise.

The causes of haematemesis to be considered in a pregnant woman are the same as for the general population. However, there are certain diagnoses one should consider more likely in pregnancy, e.g. hyperemesis leading to a Mallory–Weiss tear, and these have been highlighted in the text and

Table 1 Severity of haematemesis

Severity	Haemoglobin	Pulse rate	Blood pressure	Endoscopy
Mild	Normal	Normal	Normal	Not indicated
Moderate	>10 g/dL	>100 bpm	Normal	Elective endoscopy, if possible, within 24 hours
Severe	<10 g/dL	>100 bpm	Systolic BP <100 mmHg	Urgent, if evidence of ongoing bleeding despite resuscitation

BP, blood pressure; bpm, beats per minute.

NB: Poor prognosis in upper gastrointestinal bleeds is almost invariably related to significant co-morbidities or advancing age of the patient. As pregnancy necessarily occurs in the young, generally free of co-morbidities, severity is most usefully based on the degree of haemodynamic compromise.

the table with italics. Likewise, some common causes of acute haemorrhage, such as non-steroidal anti-inflammatory drugs (NSAIDs) or acute alcohol use, should be less frequent in pregnancy, but should always be considered.

In most cases of haematemesis, the history and examination will give the most likely source of the haemorrhage. If vomiting occurred before the haematemesis, it may be due to a Mallory–Weiss tear. Significant reflux symptoms may point towards oesophagitis with or without an associated hiatus hernia. Those with chronic peptic ulceration (a diminishing number due to the treatment of *Helicobacter pylori*) will sometimes give a long history of dyspepsia or previous ulceration. A history of alcoholism or physical signs of cirrhosis may indicate varices, although fertility will be reduced in such patients.

All patients with a moderate or severe haematemesis should have an endoscopic examination, once adequately resuscitated. Historically there was some reluctance to use endoscopy during pregnancy. However, it is now understood to be safe in pregnancy,[1] and should not only provide a definitive diagnosis but may also allow effective endoscopic therapy.

■ Causes of haematemesis

The causes of haematemesis within the general population are illustrated in Table 2. Rare causes

Table 2 Causes of haematemesis by anatomical site and incidence in an unselected population

Site	Common	Less common <5%
Oesophagus	Mallory–Weiss tear 10% Oesophagitis 5–10%	Oesophageal varices
Stomach	Gastric ulcer 20% Gastric erosion	Gastritis Tumour
Duodenum	Duodenal ulcer 35% Duodenal erosion	Duodenitis
Disordered haemostasis	Warfarin Heparin	Chronic liver disease
Miscellaneous		Swallowed blood from nose, mouth or throat

include angiodysplasia, Dieulafoy's lesion, portal hypertensive gastropathy, thrombocytopenia, disseminated intravascular coagulation/coagulopathy, Osler–Weber–Rendu syndrome and scurvy.

Swallowed blood

Bleeding from the nose, mouth or throat can be swallowed and later vomited, masquerading as blood loss from further down the gastrointestinal (GI) tract. Except in epistaxis (which can be heavy), this would usually be a small volume. Careful questioning and examination will often elucidate the source and prevent the need for endoscopy.

Pregnancy is associated with *gingivitis* and bleeding gums, but this would rarely be severe enough to cause haematemesis.

Oesophagus
Hiatus hernia and reflux oesophagitis

Hiatus hernia is a common finding (see Epigastric pain in pregnancy). Owing to the increased intra-abdominal pressure and the effect of increased progestogens on smooth muscle during pregnancy, the incidence of both hernias and of associated *reflux oesophagitis* is increased. This will normally cause retrosternal burning and waterbrash, but also occasionally haematemesis. Treatment is appropriate acid suppression.

Mallory–Weiss tear (Fig. 1)

A mucosal tear at the oesophagogastric junction due to forceful vomiting can result in haematemesis. The tears are usually linear. Nausea and vomiting occurs in 70–85 per cent of pregnancies,[1] but will not normally cause further problems. Hyperemesis gravidarum, however, causes intractable vomiting, which usually occurs at 8–12 weeks' gestation and has an incidence of 0.5–2 per cent[1] (see Vomiting in pregnancy). Owing to the sustained nature of the vomiting, there is an increased risk of developing *Mallory–Weiss tears*.

Treatment is to control the vomiting, and occasionally Mallory–Weiss tears will need injection sclerotherapy at endoscopy. There is some evidence linking hyperemesis with *H. pylori* infection,[2] so eradication, if found at endoscopy, would be warranted.

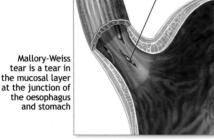

Mallory-Weiss tear is a tear in the mucosal layer at the junction of the oesophagus and stomach

✿ADAM.

Figure 1 Mallory–Weiss tear. Reproduced with permission from A.D.A.M., Inc.

In the general population, Mallory–Weiss tears are often associated with excess alcohol use.

Oesophageal varices (Fig. 2)

Varices develop as a result of portal hypertension, most commonly due to cirrhosis (and in the West alcoholic cirrhosis) but portal vein thrombosis should be considered in pregnancy. Bleeding from varices is often brisk, requiring prompt resuscitation and endoscopic therapy (banding or injection). There may be physical signs of chronic liver disease (jaundice, spider naevi, palmar erythema, ascites), but their absence does not exclude portal hypertension and varices.

The physiological changes that occur during pregnancy may exacerbate the pathophysiological changes that occur in portal hypertension[3] and make variceal haemorrhage more likely. To avoid complications, known cirrhotics should be prepared for pregnancy with endoscopic eradication of varices, more so because beta-blocker therapy is relatively contraindicated during pregnancy.

Oesophageal ulcer

Oesophageal ulcer is an infrequent cause of haematemesis and is usually benign in this age group. It may be associated with hiatus hernias and reflux oesophagitis, which are relatively common during pregnancy.

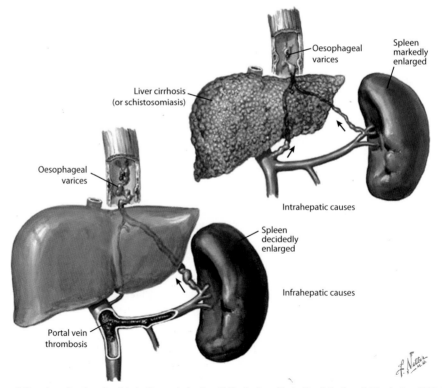

Oesophageal varices

Spleen markedly enlarged

Liver cirrhosis (or schistosomiasis)

Oesophageal varices

Intrahepatic causes

Spleen decidedly enlarged

Infrahepatic causes

Portal vein thrombosis

Figure 2 Oesophageal varices. Reprinted with permission from Netter Anatomy Illustration Collection, © Elsevier Inc. All Rights Reserved.

Stomach

Gastric ulcer

There is no particular association between gastric ulcers and pregnancy. Symptoms prior to haematemesis include epigastric pain, often soon after eating, and there may be associated anorexia; however, symptoms are variable and often non-specific. There is an association with NSAIDs, and also with *H. pylori* (approximately 60 per cent of benign, non-NSAID-induced, gastric ulcers are associated with *H. pylori*).

Acute gastritis

In acute gastritis, bleeding can occur from small erosions/minute ulcers and, therefore, the haemorrhage is normally small. The patient will often complain of epigastric pain, nausea and vomiting.

NSAIDs are the most common cause of bleeding from erosive gastritis, but they should be avoided during pregnancy. Other causes include ingestion of alcohol or irritant foods. Ingestion of corrosive liquids, such as strong acids or alkalis, is rare but serious – look for ulcerated oral mucosa and enquire about depressive illness. Acute tropical infections leading to gastritis include dengue, yellow fever, blackwater fever and variola.

Rarities

- Angiodysplasia – idiopathic, or associated with aortic stenosis or Osler–Weber–Rendu syndrome (autosomal dominant inheritance, characterised by angiodysplastic lesions in mucosal membranes).
- Dieulafoy's lesion – bleeding vessel with no surrounding ulceration.

Duodenal disorders

There are no particular associations between pregnancy and duodenal disease.

Duodenal ulcer

Duodenal ulcers are often asymptomatic before bleeding occurs owing to the ulcer eroding a vessel. Classically the pain, if present, is epigastric, radiates to the back and is worse some hours after eating. As with gastric ulcers, bleeding can be massive and initial management should be effective resuscitation followed by endoscopy. The majority of duodenal ulcers are associated

with *H. pylori* infection (73–95 per cent),[4,5] and they should therefore be treated with eradication therapy. Unlike gastric ulcers, repeat endoscopy to assess healing is unnecessary.

H. pylori infection in the developed world is becoming increasingly uncommon in the child-bearing age group. Advice on treatment, if found, should be sought from the endoscopist, but will include a proton pump inhibitor and two antibiotics for 1 week.

Duodenitis

Inflammation of the duodenum can also lead to haematemesis, but is less severe. Once again *H. pylori* should be excluded.

Portal hypertension

Portal vein obstruction

The aetiology of portal vein thrombosis is unknown in around 8–15 per cent of cases, but it can complicate pregnancy (especially in eclampsia). In unselected patients, the other causes include malignancy, systemic infection and myeloproliferative disorders.

Portal vein thrombosis can present with haematemesis from oesophageal varices or, alternatively, with right upper quadrant pain and hepatomegaly, or splenomegaly. As the liver retains normal synthetic function and clotting remains unaffected, variceal bleeding may be better tolerated when compared with cirrhotic bleeds. Moreover, there is not the same risk of developing encephalopathy. Treatment is endoscopic ablation of varices.

Cirrhosis/chronic liver disease

As previously discussed (see section on Oesophageal varices), this can lead to haematemesis from oesophageal or gastric varices. The haemorrhage is often made worse by the associated thrombocytopenia or coagulation abnormalities.

Disordered haemostasis

Many medical conditions can lead to disordered haemostasis, some of which are associated with pregnancy. Generally, by far the most common cause of deranged clotting encountered is iatrogenic via coumarin use (warfarin) or heparins.

However, warfarin is teratogenic and heparin in pregnancy (either unfractionated or low molecular weight) is only used in a small number of circumstances (e.g. for pulmonary embolism).

Thrombocytopenia

Low platelets are found in 7–8 per cent of pregnancies,[6] but most of these will be due to gestational thrombocytopenia (mild) and will not cause GI haemorrhage. Even in the HELLP syndrome (haemolysis, elevated liver enzymes, low platelets; see Jaundice and liver disease in pregnancy), the thrombocytopenia is usually moderate and haematemesis would be an unusual presentation.

Severe thrombocytopenia ($<50\,000\,mL$) causing GI haemorrhage during pregnancy is rare and will usually be due to a concomitant unrelated illness, e.g. leukaemia. Alternatively, it can occur as part of disseminated intravascular coagulation (see later).

Disseminated intravascular coagulation

In disseminated intravascular coagulation (DIC), there is widespread activation of the clotting cascade leading to platelet and clotting-factor consumption. Obstetric causes include placental abruption, amniotic fluid embolism and postpartum haemorrhage; however, haematemesis is a very uncommon complication in pregnancy-associated DIC, especially as DIC is usually short-lived in such situations.

Chronic liver disease

Liver disease may result in a number of defects in haemostasis owing to thrombocytopenia, reduced clotting factor synthesis, vitamin K deficiency and functional abnormalities of platelets. Chronic liver disease is uncommon in pregnancy and may well have a significant impact on fertility in any case.

Inherited haematological conditions

Von Willebrand's disease can be autosomal dominant or recessive. It leads to defective platelet function and thus epistaxis, bruising and bleeding after minor trauma. However, haematemesis or GI haemorrhage would be rare.

Drugs

These are covered above (NSAIDs and anticoagulants).

Miscellaneous causes

Scurvy, a rare cause of haematemesis, is due to vitamin C deficiency, and would normally cause bleeding, swollen gums, anaemia and cutaneous haemorrhages.

■ References

1. ACOG (American College of Obstetrics and Gynecology) Practice Bulletin: nausea and vomiting of pregnancy. *Obstet Gynecol* 2004; **103**: 803–14.
2. Jacoby EB, Porter KB. *Helicobacter pylori* infection and persistent hyperemesis gravidarum. *Am J Perinatol* 1999;**16**: 85–8.
3. Duke J. Pregnancy and cirrhosis: management of hematemesis by Warren shunt during third trimester gestation. *Int J Obstet Anesth* 1994; **3**: 97–102.
4. Tytgat G, Langenberg W, Rauws E, Rietra P. Campylobacter-like organism (CLO) in the human stomach. *Gastroenterology* 1985; **88**: 1620.
5. Ciociola AA, McSorley DJ, Turner K, Sykes D, Palmer JB. *Helicobacter pylori* infection rates in duodenal ulcer patients in the United States may be lower than previously estimated. *Am J Gastroenterol* 1999; **94**: 1834–40.
6. Burrows RF, Kelton JG. Incidentally detected thrombocytopenia in healthy mothers and their infants. *N Engl J Med* 1988; **319**: 142–5.

HAEMATURIA (BLOOD IN THE URINE)

Tony Hollingworth

This condition is defined as the presence of red blood cells in the urine, and should not be confused with haemoglobinuria, in which the

Box 1 Causes of haematuria in women

- Physiological
  - Menstruation
  - Caruncle – eversion of urethral meatus
- Infection
- Pyelonephritis
- Cystitis
- Urethritis
- Tuberculous infection of kidneys and bladder
- Trauma
  - Renal injury
  - Foreign body in bladder including urinary catheter
  - Foreign body in urethra
- Inflammatory/autoimmune
  - Glomerulonephritis
  - Polyarteritis nodosa
  - Chronic interstitial nephritis
  - Irradiation changes to renal tract
- Stones
  - Renal,ureteric or vesical
- Tumours – benign and malignant
  - Renal
  - Ureteric
  - Bladder
  - Urethral
- General
  - Drugs, including anticoagulants
  - Bleeding disorders.

pigment alone is filtered through the kidneys. It can be divided into:

- *microscopic haematuria*, where blood is found on 'dipstick' testing; and
- *macroscopic haematuria* or *frank haematuria*, which is an unusual symptom to present to the gynaecologist.

The causes will vary with age and also in the presence of absence of a pregnancy.

In pregnancy, the urine is checked with a 'dipstick' at each visit. It is unusual to find frank haematuria without other obvious symptoms.

In most cases, the cause of the haematuria is infection. Any urinary infection may be associated with some symptoms of frequency, dysuria and offensive urine, although not invariably so.

In non-pregnant women, haematuria may occur as a result of contamination from menstrual blood flow. In younger women, the causes are usually benign, including urinary tract infection, stones and insertion of a catheter for any length of time.

In postmenopausal women, the complaint may be of blood in the urine when in actual fact it is due to postmenopausal bleeding for whatever cause. Bladder carcinoma may also present with haematuria and this diagnosis should be considered in women over the age of 40 years.

In gynaecology, the investigations may be limited to sending a midstream specimen of urine for microbiological investigation, an ultrasound scan of the renal tract and possible cystoscopy. Usually these patients will be referred on to an urologist. Many countries have adopted guidelines for the investigation of haematuria, e.g. American Urological Association and the European Association of Urologists guidelines. More recently, guidelines from the National Institute for Health and Clinical Excellence (NICE) have recommended referral to exclude a possible malignancy.

Box 1 gives a list of causes of haematuria for completeness. The classification can be either anatomical, starting from the kidney and working down the tract, or by type of condition.

■ **Useful website**

www.nice.org.uk/CG027

HEADACHE IN PREGNANCY

Greg Davis

Although headache in pregnancy is common, the literature on this condition in pregnancy is surprisingly sparse. In their lifetime, 99 per cent of women will experience headaches and about one-third of women will get headaches while pregnant, particularly in the second trimester. The majority of headaches (>95 per cent) in pregnancy are benign (primary headaches) but fear of a serious intracranial cause will often lead pregnant women to present with the symptom. Of those pregnant women with primary headaches, about two-thirds will have migraine and one-third tension-type headaches.

The pain of headaches is thought to arise in a widespread network of sensory fibres that surround intracranial blood vessels. These sensory fibres originate in the trigeminal ganglia and are found in the adventitial layer of all major cerebral blood vessels. Headache may result from direct stimulation of these fibres, causing pain, or secondary to the inflammatory effects of vasoactive neuropeptides released after stimulation of the sensory fibres. Because of this complex interaction, there are a number of potential points for intervention with treatment. This also explains why there are a variety of pharmacological agents with differing actions that are effective in treating some headaches but not others.

Reproductive hormones and, in particular, oestrogen, influence this system directly and indirectly by modifying cerebral blood flow and concentrations of neurochemicals. For example, prior to puberty, males and females are equally affected by migraine, but there is a 3 to 1 ratio in favour of females after puberty.

■ Classification

The 2004 International Headache Society Classification divides headaches into primary (e.g. migraine or tension), where headache is the dominant symptom, and secondary, where it is usually part of a systemic condition (e.g. preeclampsia, trauma) (Box 1). Although not specific to pregnancy, this classification is also useful considering headaches in pregnancy.

After excluding headache due to preeclampsia, the vast majority of headaches in pregnancy will be either migraine or tension-type headaches, and most women presenting with headache in pregnancy will not need extensive investigation. However, because of the possibility of serious underlying pathology, the clinical

---

Box 1 International Headache Society Classification of headaches (2004) with examples relevant to pregnancy

Primary headaches
- Migraine
- Tension-type headache
- Cluster (uncommon in pregnancy)
- Other primary headaches (cough, exertional)

Secondary headaches
- Post head or neck trauma
- Vascular disorders (subarachnoid haemorrhage, imminent eclampsia, acute ischaemic stroke)
- Non-vascular intracranial disorder (idiopathic intracranial hypertension, postdural puncture, tumours)
- Substance use or withdrawal (alcohol, cocaine, caffeine withdrawal, medication overuse)
- Disorders of homeostasis (hypoglycaemia, hypoxia)
- Disorders of cranial structures (sinusitis, jaw pain, tooth abscess)
- Psychiatric disorder (depression, anxiety)
- Neuralgias (trigeminal, Bell's palsy)

---

significance of the presenting symptoms must be assessed with a careful history and appropriate examination. In general, a sudden onset of pain or change in the pattern of chronic headache makes a serious cause more likely (see Box 2). Likewise, associated features, such as fever or neck stiffness, focal neurological signs or hypertension, are indications for thorough investigation.

■ Clinical assessment

As with any pain, when assessing headache, the quality, location, severity, time course, and exacerbating and relieving factors should be fully explored. The woman should be questioned about any neurological symptoms associated with the headache, such as numbness, tingling, loss of or alteration in sensation or movement, and systemic disturbance, such as fever, anorexia or skin rashes. A complete medication history should be taken to rule out medication overuse in chronic headache and to assess what has been helpful in alleviating the headache. Simple analgesics such as paracetamol are not likely to relieve significant headaches due to underlying pathology.

Examination should begin with blood pressure measurement and a brief general physical examination with particular attention to any system of interest, e.g. throat and sinuses, if an upper respiratory tract infection is suspected. A more detailed examination will not usually be necessary in pregnancy. However, if there are focal neurological symptoms, a neurological screening examination should be performed comparing the affected with the non-affected side.

The family or companions should be questioned on any changes in personality, loss of consciousness or alteration in mental state in the pregnant woman. The level of consciousness and cognitive ability can be assessed during history-taking and clinical examination. The optic fundi should be inspected for papilloedema (blurring of the optic discs). The pupils, visual fields and the presence of extraocular movements should also be assessed. The motor system should be examined with finger–nose testing, observing for the drift of outstretched hands, and heel–toe

walking. The deep tendon reflexes and plantar responses should be elicited, and the presence of clonus assessed.

■ Investigations

If, after appropriate history and neurological examination and in the absence of any of the warning features in Box 2, the woman has no persistent neurological symptoms or signs, and the headache resolves, she can be followed clinically without performing further investigations. Diagnostic testing is required if there is a suspicion of an underlying cause for the headache. The purpose of testing is to make the diagnosis, exclude other causes of headache, and to rule out diseases that might complicate headache or its treatment e.g. diabetes and pre-eclampsia. The nature and extent of the investigations will be determined by the clinical possibilities after history-taking and examination.

As discussed before, pre-eclampsia is the most common cause of secondary headache in pregnancy and must always be excluded first. After pre-eclampsia, cerebral thrombosis, vascular anomaly or intracranial bleeding are the most likely serious diagnostic possibilities requiring exclusion in women presenting with new-onset headache in pregnancy. Spontaneous thrombosis in pregnancy is more likely if there is an underlying hypercoagulable state, such as pre-eclampsia or thrombophilia. Blood should be taken for complete blood count, liver function tests, urea and electrolytes, creatinine, prothrombin time, partial thromboplastin time and thrombophilia screen, if a secondary cause is suspected.

Lumbar puncture

Lumbar puncture is necessary in a number of clinical situations:

- severe headache with suspicion of infection (meningitis) or subarachnoid haemorrhage;
- severe, rapid-onset, recurrent headache;
- a progressive headache (increasing headache with little or no remission);
- or an atypical headache disorder.

This should be delayed until after neuroimaging, if raised intracranial pressure is suspected (if papilloedema is detected), unless meningitis is the likely cause, in which case it should be performed as soon as possible.

Radiological studies

Non-contrast computerised tomography (CT) is recommended as the first-line investigation, particularly after trauma or if there is possible intracranial haemorrhage. It is superior to magnetic resonance imaging (MRI) for the assessment of bony structures and detection of acute intracranial haemorrhage (subarachnoid, subdural following head trauma, intraparenchymal), but its sensitivity declines with time from the initial haemorrhage. For all other indications, including angiography, MRI is preferred but should be performed after consultation with a neurologist (Fig. 1). Although there is no evidence of harmful effect, MRI is not recommended in the first trimester of pregnancy. It is likely that this recommendation will change with more experience with its use in pregnancy.

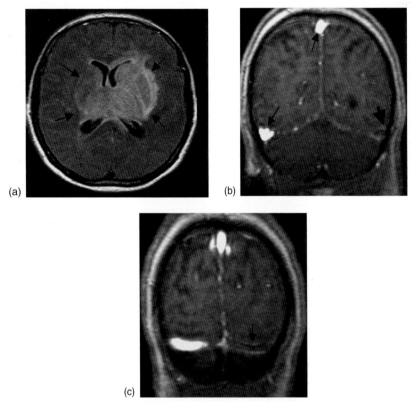

Figure 1 This 39-year-old woman with a history of antiphospholipid syndrome presented with severe, constant headache and focal neurological signs two weeks postpartum. (a) This FLAIR* image shows bithalamic venous ischaemia (area marked by arrows) owing to occlusion of the internal cerebral veins by thrombus. (b) On time-of-flight magnetic resonance venography, increased signal confirming blood flow is seen in the superior sagittal sinus (arrowed at the top of the image) and the right transverse sinus (arrowed at 7 o'clock), but there is thrombus visible in the left transverse sinus (large arrow at 4 o'clock). (c) A similar image more posteriorly in the brain to that in (b) confirms these findings and demonstrates clot in the left transverse sinus (dark line arrowed). *FLAIR, fluid-attenuated inversion recovery (This is a heavily T2-weighted sequence. The cerebrospinal fluid is black, which allows for optimal visualisation of periventricular and cortical signal changes.)

With all radiological investigations in pregnancy, both parents and health workers will be concerned about the effects on the fetus. It is believed that fetal exposure up to 5 rad does not result in miscarriage, anomalies or impaired growth. The exposure to the uterus from a standard head or cervical spine CT is less than 1 mrad and MRI does not use ionizing radiation. While concern for fetal welfare is appropriate, in this clinical setting the importance of an accurate diagnosis outweighs the minimal potential for fetal harm.

■ Primary headaches

Migraine

Migraine is a usually a severe, unilateral and throbbing headache aggravated by activity with associated nausea, vomiting, photophobia, phonophobia (sensitivity to sound) and sometimes, but not always, an aura. Migraines last from hours to days and often develop in a crescendo pattern. The nausea and vomiting may be severe and more debilitating than the headache. Migraines without an aura are more common (common migraine) and usually more disabling than those with an aura (classic migraine). The aura is a neurological symptom(s), typically visual change with scotomata (an area of loss or impairment of visual acuity surrounded by a field of normal or relatively well preserved vision) or, less commonly, visual field loss, sensory changes (numbness or tingling) or speech changes. The symptoms of the aura develop over 15–20 minutes and precede the headache by less than 1 hour. Migraines are often preceded by neck stiffness, fatigue and nausea, but these symptoms do not constitute an aura.

To establish the diagnosis of migraine, the woman must experience five or more similar episodes. In addition, considerable improvement in, or disappearance of, migraine is reported by 70–80 per cent of women in pregnancy, probably as a result of the sustained rise in oestrogen levels. In women with a history of migraine, improvement occurs early in pregnancy, is maintained through pregnancy and recurs in the first week postpartum in 60 per cent of these women. Therefore, the diagnosis of new-onset migraine in pregnancy, especially with aura, must be made with great caution and only after exclusion of more serious causes of headache with transient neurological symptoms. If there are persisting neurological signs, or the headache becomes progressive or recurrent, then further investigation is necessary.

Tension-type headaches

In comparison to migraines, tension-type headaches have few characteristic features. They are not affected by activity, are often diffuse and bilateral, and may be localised to either head or neck. There is no associated nausea or vomiting, but there may sometimes be photophobia or phonophobia. They may develop in association with neck or back pain, or with facial neuralgias. Typical descriptions include 'a tight band around my head' or 'my head in a vice'. They are worse in the evenings and with stress, and may last from hours to days. If they are present for more than half the month, they are termed chronic.

Tension-type headaches have not been studied extensively in pregnancy. There have been reports both of improvement and no differences in pregnancy in retrospective studies.

■ Secondary headaches

Head trauma

In pregnancy, this is most likely to occur after vehicular accident and is usually the result of a direct injury to the head. It should also be suspected where domestic violence has occurred and it is important to realize that domestic violence is reported to increase 3–4-fold in pregnancy.

Vascular disorders

Hypertension in pregnancy

The headache associated with pre-eclampsia and eclampsia is thought to be due to cerebral arterial vasospasm. This leads either to ischaemia or hypertensive encephalopathy, both of which may be associated with headache. It is usually bilateral, throbbing, and worsened by activity and rising blood pressure. It may be associated with blurred vision, flashing lights and/or scotomata and, as such, is a warning of imminent eclampsia, suggesting an urgent need for seizure prophylaxis.

Brain haemorrhage

The classic presentation of subarachnoid haemorrhage is the sudden onset of severe incapacitating headache, neck stiffness and collapse. However, at least 50 per cent will have a less dramatic onset with a progressive, severe, unremitting headache. It is caused by the rupture of either an arteriovenous malformation, or a saccular or berry aneurysm. It is a widely held belief that subarachnoid haemorrhage is more common in pregnancy but this has been questioned in more recent studies. Subarachnoid haemorrhage accounts for 50 per cent of cerebral haemorrhages in pregnancy occurring in 1 in 10 000 pregnancies with a 50 per cent maternal mortality.

Intracerebral haemorrhage is a rare event that may be more common in pregnancy. It also presents with sudden severe headache, often accompanied by rapidly progressive neurological signs. In pregnancy it is most often seen with a hypertensive disorder, usually eclampsia, although it is also associated with cocaine and alcohol abuse.

Brain CT is the preferred diagnostic modality if brain haemorrhage is suspected. However, the deteriorating clinical state of the mother often requires rapid neurosurgical intervention and delivery of the baby because of the risks to the mother and baby. If the mother is clinically stable, the diagnostic work-up should begin immediately with a brain CT. If this is not helpful, lumbar puncture should be performed looking for blood in the cerebrospinal fluid.

Cerebral venous thrombosis

Although still rare, the risk of stroke in young women increases 13-fold in pregnancy with the most common cause being cerebral venous thrombosis. It is thought to be more common in hypercoagulable states, such as underlying thrombophilia or pre-eclampsia. The usual presentation is with focal neurological symptoms and signs, but thrombosis of the superior sagittal sinus is reported to cause severe progressive headache without focal signs. It may be associated with the development of hypertension, which can delay the diagnosis because the neurological condition is incorrectly attributed to pre-eclampsia.

Benign intracranial hypertension

Benign intracranial hypertension is ten times more common in obese women of childbearing age compared to the general population. Women with the condition may become pregnant or it may develop anew during pregnancy. It is a syndrome with the symptoms and signs of raised intracranial pressure without a cause detectable on CT or MRI. It may be due to increased production or impaired resorption of cerebrospinal fluid. It presents with a global headache that may be worse lying down, and progressive diplopia and visual loss if untreated. There is a 10 per cent risk of permanent visual impairment in this condition, but this risk is not affected by pregnancy and there is no increased risk to the mother or fetus in pregnancy.

On testing, diplopia and papilloedema will be present and there may be impairment of visual fields and acuity. Other causes, most commonly cerebral venous thrombosis with this presentation, need to be excluded by brain MRI. If the diagnosis is still not clear, lumbar puncture will be necessary to demonstrate an abnormally raised opening pressure.

Brain tumour

Although most pregnant women who present with severe and/or new-onset headache will fear that they have a brain tumour, only half of brain tumours are associated with headache and the headache is often mild. Pregnancy does not increase the risk of developing a brain tumour; however, it may worsen symptoms from vascular tumours like meningiomas or acoustic neuromas.

Postpartum headache

About 40 per cent of women develop headache in the first week postpartum. The cause is uncertain but, given that women with pre-existing migraine may experience an improvement in pregnancy, it is likely to be due to the rapid drop in oestrogen.

Another major cause of postpartum headache is inadvertent dural puncture, which occurs in about 1–2 per cent of women during lumbar epidural insertion. About 15 per cent of women will also complain of headache following obstetric spinal anaesthesia. The headache is similar in both instances and is usually tolerable when the woman is lying down. However, it is often severe on standing and this may necessitate treatment so that the woman may care for her baby. The dramatic effect of posture in the context of a history of spinal or epidural anaesthesia/analgesia usually makes the diagnosis straightforward. If the diagnosis is not clear, other rarer complications, which may cause headache in this setting, such as subdural haematoma and septic meningitis need to be excluded.

Systemic and other conditions

Headache can occur in a variety of other medical conditions in pregnancy. Examples are hypoglycaemia with the treatment of diabetes and fever due to any intercurrent infection. Other substances can cause headache in both pregnant and non-pregnant women, e.g. monosodium glutamate ('Chinese restaurant headache'), nitrates in processed meats ('hot-dog headache') and alcohol soon after ingestion (in contrast to a hangover). Chocolate and cheese can cause headaches both in migraineurs and others. Headaches are also seen with the use of and withdrawal from illicit drugs, e.g. amphetamines, cocaine, barbiturates and opiates.

Other demands of pregnancy

Finally, it is important to remember that pregnancy is often a time of profound change in a woman's and/or a couple's life. This may cause emotional stress and 'broken' sleep may cause tiredness, both of which can contribute to headache development. This can be especially problematic when the woman has difficulty in sleeping owing to her increasing abdominal size and discomfort, or the presence of young children in the family.

HEARTBURN DURING PREGNANCY

Dilip Visvanathan

■ Introduction

The prevalence of heartburn in the normal population is around 7 per cent. In pregnancy, however, 45–85 per cent of women report gastro-oesophageal reflux disease (GORD) and heartburn.[1] This increase is thought to be due to the relaxation of the lower gastro-oesophageal sphincter secondary to circulating levels of progesterone. Progesterone is also thought to reduce the peristaltic activity of the stomach. The situation is compounded by the increasing size of the gravid uterus causing pressure on the stomach and, therefore, symptoms usually worsen in the third trimester of pregnancy.

Heartburn is associated with diseases other than GORD as illustrated in Box 1. *Helicobacter pylori* infection does not have a direct relationship with heartburn.

Box 1 Causes of heartburn

- Gastro-oesophageal reflux disease (GORD)
- Gastritis
- Peptic ulceration
- Achalasia
- Cancer of the gastro-oesophageal junction
- Gallstones

Many women present with heartburn for the first time in pregnancy. The typical symptoms of heartburn and GORD are given in Box 2. The majority of women present with these symptoms and the diagnosis can be made with confidence without need for specific investigation. Further investigation is warranted very rarely in women who have ALARM and atypical symptoms as described in Box 3. Upper gastrointestinal tract endoscopy can be safely performed with conscious sedation and careful monitoring of the mother and fetus.

Box 2 Heartburn and symptom variation with gastro-oesophageal reflux disease (GORD)

Typical symptoms of GORD
- Heartburn
  - Retrosternal chest pain originates in epigastrium and radiates to the neck
  - Exacerbated after meals
  - Exacerbated by changes in posture, such as lying down and bending forwards
- Regurgitation

Symptoms associated with GORD
- Epigastric pain
- Nausea and bloating
- Abdominal discomfort

Box 3 Symptoms that require further investigation of heartburn

---

Symptoms that may be due to gastro-oesophageal reflux disease but need exclusion of other disease
- ALARM – odynophagia, dysphagia, anaemia and weight loss
- Atypical symptoms – angina-like chest pain, chronic cough, hoarseness and asthma

In pregnant women with GORD, symptoms usually resolve with delivery of the baby. However, GORD can cause significant morbidity not only due to the pain but also due to disturbances in sleep. In most women, explanation and reassurance of the temporary nature of GORD in pregnancy with lifestyle modification is all that is required. This includes using an extra pillow at night, avoiding large meals and spicy hot food, wearing loose-fitting clothes and avoiding stooping.

Cabbage, broccoli and lettuce, are all high in raffinose, a sugar that produces gas in the stomach. This may aggravate symptoms and should only be taken in moderation. As the stomach empties to the right side, sleeping on the right side (rather than on the left) in itself can sometimes help. A drug history should be taken and non-steroidal anti-inflammatory drugs stopped. Other drugs that aggravate GORD, such as calcium antagonists, should be avoided and alternatives used if required. Many women find relaxation techniques, herbal medicines, acupuncture, acupressure, aroma therapy and homeopathy useful.

If these measures do not alleviate symptoms, then drug therapy is required. The benefits and risks of drug treatment should be discussed as none of the drugs used in the treatment of GORD have been evaluated in pregnancy by large randomised controlled trials. Fetal safety has been extrapolated from animal study data and cohort studies. Use of the smallest dose to achieve symptom control is, therefore, the therapeutic aim.

Drug treatment should follow a step-up algorithm. Antacids or sucralfate are considered as first-line drug therapy. They have little systemic absorption and, therefore, do not pose much risk to the fetus. Over-the-counter remedies for neutralising stomach acid can be helpful, but using them too often and for too long can cause constipation (if they contain aluminium) or diarrhoea (if they contain magnesium). Alginates are used for the symptomatic treatment of heartburn and oesophagitis, and appear to act by a unique mechanism that differs from traditional antacids. Gaviscon is an alginate, which in the presence of gastric acid precipitate, forms a gel. Both *in vitro* and *in vivo* studies have demonstrated that alginate-based rafts can entrap carbon dioxide, thus providing a relatively pH-neutral barrier. Several studies have demonstrated that the alginate rafts can preferentially move into the oesophagus in place, or ahead, of acidic gastric contents during episodes of gastro-oesophageal reflux; further-more, they can act as a physical barrier to reduce reflux episodes.[2]

If symptom control is still not obtained, then second-line treatment includes histamine receptor blockade (ranitidine is preferred because of its documented efficacy and safety profile in pregnancy, even in the first trimester) and prokinetics (metoclopramide). Proton pump inhibitors (PPIs) are not recommended in pregnancy and should be reserved for intractable symptoms or complicated reflux disease. Lansoprazole may be the preferred PPI because of its safety profile in animals and case reports of safety in human pregnan-cies. Most drugs are excreted in breast milk and only the H_2-receptor antagonists (with the exception of nizatidine) are safe to use in lactation.[3]

■ References

1. Anton C, Anton E, Drug VL, Stanciu C. Hormonal influence on gastrointestinal reflux during pregnancy. *Rev Med Chir Soc Med Nat Iasi* 2003; **107:** 798–801.
2. Lindow SW, Regnell P, Sykes J, Little S. An open-label, multicentre study to assess the safety and efficacy of a novel reflux suppressant (Gaviscon Advance) in the treatment of heartburn during pregnancy. *Int J Clin Pract* 2003; **57:** 175–9.
3. Richter JE. Review article: the manage-ment of heartburn in pregnancy. *Aliment Pharmacol Ther* 2005; **22:** 749–57.

HIRSUTISM/VIRILISM

Anne Clark

Hirsutism is defined as excessive body hair growth in women where it is not normally found, usually with a central body distribution. In about 10–15 per cent of hirsute women, hormone levels are in the normal range and a diagnosis of 'idio-pathic hirsutism' is made.[1] Excessive facial and body hair caused by excess androgen production is usually associated with anovulatory ovaries and loss of cyclical menstrual function.

The more severe state of virilism (clitoro-megaly, deepening of the voice, balding, increased muscle mass and changes to a male-like body habitus) is rarely seen and is usually secondary to adrenal hyperplasia, androgen-producing tumours of adrenal or ovarian ori-gin, or exogenous steroid use. Nearly every woman with hirsutism will have increased pro-duction of testosterone and androstenedione.[2] Table 1 shows the sources and incidences of conditions that result in increased androgens, which can result in hirsutism/virilism.

There are two types of hair that grow in adults:

■ vellus hair – the downy unpigmented hair associ-ated with the prepubertal years; and
■ terminal hair – the coarse pigmented hair that grows on various parts of the body during the adult years.

Hirsutism occurs when resting vellus hairs are transformed to terminal hairs following expo-sure of the hair follicle to increased androgen levels. Androgens, particularly testosterone, ini-tiate growth and increase the diameter and pig-mentation of hair. *Oestrogens essentially act in the opposite way to androgens, and progestins have minimal direct effects on hair.* Once the transfor-mation from vellus to terminal hair occurs, the terminal growth pattern persists, even if the increased androgen levels stop.

It is also important to note that a woman's total number of hair follicles is determined by 22 weeks' gestation and thereafter no new follicles

Table 1 Differential diagnoses and incidence of hirsutism/virilism

Polycystic ovary syndrome (PCOS)	10% of all women
Idiopathic hirsutism	10–15% of hirsute women
Ovarian	
Benign tumours: the vast majority of ovarian androgen-secreting tumours are benign. The most common in premenopausal women is a Sertoli–Leydig tumour; others include cystic teratomas and luteinised thecomas	<1% of all ovarian tumours of which 75% are benign. Usually occur in the younger age group
Malignant tumours: these can arise from the hilus, Leydig cells or sex cords (Sertoli and granulosa cell) or epithelial cells	25% of all these types of tumour are malignant (i.e. 25% of the 1% above)
Adrenal	
Tumours (benign and malignant)	2/1 000 000 per year
Congenital adrenal hyperplasia, atypical form	1–5% of hirsute women
Cushing's syndrome (excessive cortisol secretion)	Overall incidence of 1 per 100 000 per year
Pituitary adrenocorticotrophic hormone (ACTH) overproduction – the most common diagnosis	Female to male ratiois 5:1 with a peak incidence 30–50 years of age
ACTH, cortisol or corticotrophin-releasing hormone production by a tumour	
Increased adrenal cortisol secretion	
Exogenous drug related	
Anabolic steroid use	Usually athletes or body builders[3]
Overdose of androgens	Usually postmenopausal women on hormone replacement therapy
Hair-stimulating drugs – phenytoin, diazoxide, danazol, cyclosporine, minoxidil	
Pregnancy	
Luteoma	Unilateral in 45% of cases, associated with a normal pregnancy
Theca–lutein cysts	Bilateral, associated with trophoblastic disease or multiple pregnancy
Ovarian cancer	Solid, unilateral ovarian lesions

will be produced *de novo*. The concentration of hair follicles laid down per unit area of facial skin differs little between men and women, but does differ between races and ethic groups. For example, Asian women with androgen-secreting tumours are rarely hirsute because of their low concentration of hair follicles per unit skin area.

The diagnosis of hirsutism/virilisation may seem daunting, but a basic history, examination, transvaginal ultrasound scan of the ovaries and a few laboratory investigations will give you the diagnosis in the majority of cases. The diagnostic evaluation of hirsutism/virilism is shown in Fig. 1.

■ Medical history

The focus should be on the onset and duration of the symptoms of hirsutism/virilisation, menstrual and medication history. Hirsutism associated with a history of menstrual irregularity since the teenage years, early 20s or increased body weight with a long gradual worsening of the condition is polycystic ovary syndrome (PCOS) until proved otherwise. Box 1 gives the revised diagnostic criteria of polycystic ovaries and PCOS,[4] the commonest cause of hirsutism.

If there is a history of sudden onset and rapid progression of androgen excess leading to

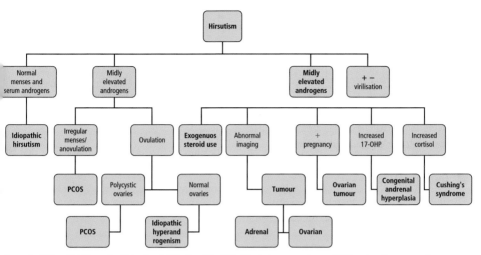

Figure 1 Differential diagnosis of hirsutism/virilisation. 17α-OHP, 17α-hydroxyprogesterone; PCOS, polycystic ovary syndrome.

Box 1 Revised diagnostic criteria of polycystic ovary syndrome (2003 Rotterdam PCOS Consensus)

Revised 2003 criteria (2 out of 3)

1 Oligo- or anovulation
2 Clinical and/or biochemical signs of hyperandrogenism
3 Polycystic ovaries[a]

and exclusion of other aetiologies (congenital adrenal hyperplasia, androgen-secreting tumours, Cushing's syndrome)

---

[a]Using ultrasound criteria, polycystic ovaries are defined by the presence of 12 or more follicles in each ovary, each measuring 2–9 mm in diameter, and/or increased ovarian volume (>10 mL).

---

which is not a true tumour but an exaggerated reaction of the ovarian stroma to normal levels of chorionic gonadotrophin. The solid lesion is unilateral in 45 per cent of cases, causes virilisation in 35 per cent of women and regresses postpartum. Signs of masculinisation occur in 80 per cent of female fetuses. The other virilising condition that occurs in pregnancy, theca–lutein cyst, occurs when high levels of human chorionic gonadotrophin are present as a result of trophoblastic disease or multiple pregnancy; 30 per cent of women will have virilisation.

■ **Physical examination**

The purpose of the physical and laboratory evaluations are to rule out adrenal and ovarian tumours, assess the severity of androgen excess and evaluate the source of the hyperandrogenism (ovarian vs. adrenal). The presence or absence of the following should be assessed.

■ signs of androgen excess:
  ● degree of hirsutism – this was traditionally quantified by the Ferriman–Gallwey scoring system, but it is now of little practical use clinically;
  ● acne;
  ● if anovulatory, also assess breasts for galactorrhoea.

virilisation, it must always be considered to be related to a tumour until proved otherwise, particularly if the woman develops hirsutism later than the age of 25 years. Ovarian tumours are more common than adrenal tumours.

If the woman is pregnant, then development of virilisation is most likely due to a luteoma,

- Signs of increased insulin levels:
  - acanthosis nigricans – this grey–brown velvety discoloration of the skin is found at the neck, groin, axillae and vulva.
- Signs of an ovarian lesion on pelvic examination – unilateral or bilateral.
- Signs of Cushing's syndrome:
  - moon facies, buffalo hump, abdominal striae, centripetal fat distribution, hypertension.

■ Investigations

The investigations will include blood tests and imaging designed to look for the underlying diagnosis.

- Blood tests for androgen excess. There is no absolute level that is pathognomonic for a tumour and no minimum androgen level that excludes a tumour:
  - total testosterone;
  - dehydroepiandrosterone sulphate (DHEAS);
  - unbound testosterone (measure sex hormone binding globulin);
  - 17α-hydroxyprogesterone, if congenital adrenal hyperplasia suspected;
  - testosterone/epitestosterone (T/E) ratio, if exogenous testosterone suspected.
- Blood tests if anovulatory in addition to androgen testing:
  - prolactin levels;
  - thyroid function.
- Blood tests if acanthosis nigricans or insulin resistance suspected:
  - 2-hour glucose and insulin levels after a 75 g glucose load.
- Blood tests if ovarian tumour suspected:
  - ovarian tumour markers – Ca-125, inhibin and Müllerian-inhibiting substances (sex cord tumours).
- Tests if excessive cortisol secretion (Cushing's syndrome) suspected:
  - single-dose overnight dexamethasone test – initial test of choice;
  - confirm an abnormal result with a 24-hour urinary free cortisol excretion.
- Transvaginal ultrasound scan of ovaries:
  - polycystic ovary pattern;
  - ovarian tumour or cysts.

- Computed tomography is preferable as it gives better resolution than magnetic resonance imaging, if an adrenal tumour is suspected.
- Retrograde venous catheterization may be required to determine the location (ovary vs. adrenal) and site (left vs. right) of the excess hormone production.

In any differential diagnosis, it should be remembered that the important conditions are the ones that are common and the ones that kill people.

■ References

1. Azziz R, Carmina E, Sawaya ME. Idiopathic hirsutism. *Endocr Rev* 2000; **21:** 347–62.
2. Speroff L, Fritz M. *Clinical Gynaecologic Endocrinology and Infertility*, 7th edn. Lippincott, Williams & Wilkins, 2005.
3. Dickinson B, Goldberg L, Elliot D, *et al.* Hormone abuse in adolescents and adults: a review of current knowledge. *Endocrinologist* 2005; **15:** 115–25.
4. Revised 2003 consensus on diagnostic criteria and long-term health risks related to polycystic ovary syndrome. *Fertil Steril* 2004; **81:** 19–25.

HOT FLUSHES

Urvashi Prasad Jha and Swasti

■ Introduction

Most women in their perimenopausal and postmenopausal years have hot flushes (described as 'flashes' in the USA) as a result of oestrogen deficiency and withdrawal. However, it is important to remain aware of the other causes of flushing. Reviewing the differential diagnosis will help in appropriate patient management and avoid unnecessary administration of hormone replacement therapy (HRT) in those in whom the aetiology is different – a case in point for 'the eyes will not see what the mind does not know'. This section outlines the approach to a patient with hot flushes.

■ Definition

Flushing describes episodic attacks of redness of the skin together with a sensation of warmth or burning of the face, neck and, less frequently, the upper trunk and abdomen. It is the transient nature of the attacks that distinguishes flushing from the persistent erythema of photosensitivity or acute contact reactions. Repeated flushing over a prolonged period of time can lead to telangiectasis and occasionally to classical rosacea of the face.[1]

A typical hot flush begins with a sensation of warmth in the head, scalp and face, followed by facial flushing that may radiate down, progressing towards the neck and to other parts of the body towards the feet. It may be followed by a chill. A hot flush is associated with an increase in core temperature body and pulse rate, and followed by a decline in temperature and profuse perspiration over the area of flush distribution. Visible changes occur in about 50 per cent of women. Each hot flush may last for a few seconds or for up to 5 minutes. It may occur as frequently as every hour to several times per week or just occasionally.

■ Differential diagnosis of hot flushes

1 *Physiological flushing or blushing* is seen from anger, embarrassment, or as a result of having hot drinks or being in an overheated environment.

2 *Menopausal flushing* in perimenopausal and postmenopausal women. This may or may not be associated with sweats or chills. Palpitations may also be present as a part of the vasomotor symptomatology. The mechanism is due to the pulsatile secretion of follicle-stimulating hormone (FSH) in increased amounts. FSH will cause the peripheral vasodilatations, especially in the skin.

3 Flushes may be seen as a symptom of an *underlying systemic disorder*, which has not currently been diagnosed. These diseases include the following.
   - Carcinoid syndrome.
   - Mastocytoses – benign proliferative disorders of reticuloendothelial system owing to a hyperplastic

rather than a neoplastic process. Clinically, patients with mastocytoses present with episodic bright-red flushing, which may be accompanied by headache, dyspnoea and wheezing, palpitations, abdominal pain, diarrhoea and syncope. The flushing of cutaneous mastocytosis typically lasts more than 30 minutes, unlike the typical carcinoid flush, and that associated with menopause, which last <10 minutes.
   - Basophilic chronic granulocytic leukaemia.
   - Pancreatic cell tumours – insulinoma and VIPoma [a pancreatic endocrine tumour producing vasoactive intestinal peptide (VIP)].
   - Pheochromocytoma – flushing, although rare, may be seen.
   - Renal cell carcinoma.
   - Medullary carcinoma of the thyroid.
   - Hyperthyroidism/thyrotoxicosis.
   - Diabetes.
   - Panic disorders.
   - Hyperhidrosis.
   - Obesity.
   - POEMS (polyneuropathy, organomegaly, endocrinopathy, monoclonal proteinaemia and skin changes).
   - Male hypogonadism (pseudocarcinoid syndrome).

4 *Gustatory flushing* – flushes may be associated with eating certain foods and food additives. This may be seen when the following are ingested.
   - Alcohol intake in those with an aldehyde dehydrogenase deficiency (see section 6 below).
   - Hot beverages.
   - Spicy or sour foods.
   - Red pepper.
   - Monosodium glutamate.
   - Sodium nitrate.
   - Nitrites.
   - Sulphites (additives in food).
   - Scomboid fish poisoning (from ingesting spoiled tuna, mackerel).

5 Hot flushes are associated with the *intake of certain drugs/vitamins* including the following.
   - Vasodilators – nitroglycerine, prostaglandins.
   - All calcium channel blockers.
   - Nicotinic acid (not nicotinamide).
   - Selective serotonin reuptake inhibitors.
   - Cholinergic drugs (metrifonate, antihelminthic drugs).
   - Cephalosporins.

- Anti-oestrogens – selective oestrogen receptor modulators tamoxifen, clomiphene.
- Danazol
- 4-Hydroxyandrostenedione.
- Luteinizing hormone-releasing hormone agonists or antagonists.
- Aromatase inhibitors.
- Niacin.
- Chlorpropamide.
- Glucocorticoids (with epidural or intra-articular injection), oral triamcinolone.
- Cortisol/corticotrophin-releasing hormone.
- Bromocriptine.
- Thyrotrophin-releasing hormone.
- Rifampicin.
- Doxorubicin.
- Cyclosporine.
- Sildenafil citrate.
- Systemic use of morphine and other opiates.

6 Flushing reactions *related to alcohol*.
- Drugs:
  - disulfiram
  - chlorpropamide
  - phentolamine
  - griseofulvin
  - metronidazole
  - ketoconazole
  - chloramphenicol
  - quinacrine
  - cephalosporin antibiotics (cefamandole, cefoperazone and moxalactam).
- Eating *Coprinus* mushrooms.
- Fermented alcoholic beverages (beer, sherry), which may contain tyramine or histamine.
- Occupational 'degreaser's' flush in workmen drinking beer after exposure to industrial solvents (trichloroethylene vapour, carbon disulphide, xylene, etc.).
- Genetic susceptibility in Asian and Native American populations.
- Carcinoid flushing (induced by alcohol).
- Mastocytosis flushing

7 *Dumping syndrome*, which usually follows gastric outflow surgery.

8 *Auriculotemporal nerve syndrome* (Frey's syndrome) as seen after parotid surgery, trauma, infection or facial Herpes zoster.

9 *Harlequin syndrome* – this consists of hemifacial flushing and sweating with or without warmth and anhidrosis (lack of sweating) of the contralateral limbs. It may be associated with lung cancer, Pancoast's syndrome, which is apical lung cancer affecting the adjacent structures, and Horner's syndrome.

10 *Neurological flushing* may be seen in patients with the following conditions.
- Spinal cord injury.
- Migraine.
- Parkinson's disease.
- Brain tumours – secondary to rapid rise in intracranial pressure.
- Emotional flushing and somatic stress-related disorders (e.g. anxiety).
- Climacteric flushing.
- Cholinergic erythema.

11 *Familial monoamine oxidase* (MAO) *deficiency.*

12 Women on *anticancer treatment* particularly cytotoxics.

13 Men who have undergone *androgen ablation*.

14 Rosacea is seen in those patients with *persistent flushing of long standing*, so that it is an effect rather than a cause.

■ Diagnostic approach to a patient with hot flushes

The following clinical details need to be ascertained during the initial evaluation of a patient with hot flushes.

1 *Character of the flush*. Determine the frequency and severity of the hot flushes, whether patchy/confluent, the colour of the flush, and whether it is associated with cyanosis or pallor. It is important to ascertain the effect on an individual's function and quality of life, work, sleep and/or recreation. At this point, if menopausal hot flushes are high on the differential diagnosis, it is appropriate to determine contraindications to HRT and any reservations the patient may have against HRT.

2 *Determination of provocative or palliative factors*. A number of factors precipitate flushes in patients with carcinoid syndrome and these are listed in Box 1. Hot flushes are also precipitated by alcohol in patients with mastocytosis and medullary thyroid

Box 1 Factors that can precipitate flushing in the carcinoid syndrome[2]*

- Foods and beverages
  - hot food/beverage
  - spicy food
  - chocolate
  - cheeses
  - tomatoes
  - avocados
  - red plums
  - walnuts
  - eggplant
  - alcohol
- Emotional stress
- Valsalva manoeuvre
  - straining
  - vigorous coughing
- Sudden direct pressure on a large carcinoid tumour

carcinoma. Gustatory sweating occurs in auriculotemporal nerve syndrome after eating any food. It also follows certain foods and emotions in patients with familial MAO deficiency. Exercise induces sweating in patients with Harlequin syndrome. Menopausal sweating may be worsened with any of these factors in addition to a hot or humid environment and confined spaces.

3 *Determine if there are any concomitant and associated features.* Ask if sweating and palpitations occur with hot flushes. Enquire regarding any respiratory symptoms, gastrointestinal symptoms (such as nausea, diarrhoea, vomiting), hypertension, hypotension, headache, urticaria or facial oedema to exclude systematic and other causes of hot flushes.

4 *Exclude common dietary causes.* When the diagnosis remains obscure after evaluation of a 2-week diary, the patient should be given an exclusion diet listing foods high in histamine, foods and drugs that affect urinary 5-hydroxyindoleacetic acid

(5-HIAA) tests, and foods and beverages that cause flushing. If the flushing reactions disappear completely, restoring the excluded items individually can identify the causative agent. However, if the hot flushes reactions continue unchanged, then a further metabolic work-up should be undertaken.[2]

■ Diagnostic or metabolic work-up

Levels of FSH indicate ovarian reserve. FSH values of >10 IU/L are indicative of declining ovarian function. FSH values >20 IU/L are diagnostic of ovarian failure in women in the perimenopausal age group with hot flushes even in the absence of cessation of menstruation. Serum pooled prolactin levels are useful in differentiating hyperprolactinaemia from menopause. After 1–3 years of cessation of menstruation (menopause), luteinising hormone levels reach to over 30 IU/L.

Although, as mentioned, there are multiple different aetiologies for hot flushes apart from menopause, carcinoid syndrome is one that is essential to suspect and exclude given the underlying association with malignancy. A brief discussion of the diagnosis of carcinoid syndrome follows.

Clinically, carcinoid syndrome may be suspected in those patients where flushing episodes are associated with systemic symptoms of diarrhoea, wheezing, weight loss and hepatomegaly. Symptoms may be precipitated by a number of factors (see Box 1).

Biochemical testing includes the following.

1 Urinary excretion of 5-HIAA. The normal range of excretion of 5-HIAA in urine in 24 hours is 2–10 mg (10–50 μmol). Values above 30 mg (150 μmol)/24 hours are confirmatory of carcinoid in all such patients except in those with inability to convert serotonin to HIAA. Numerous factors, however, may interfere with this assay (see Box 2).

2 Serum levels of serotonin should be measured after receiving a diet free of substances that may confound the results.

3 Plasma chromogranin-A, substance P, neurokinin A are other tests useful in differentiating the non-endocrine causes of flushing.

Box 2 Factors that interfere with determination of urinary 5-hydroxyindoleacetic acid[3]*

Foods that produce false-positive results	Drugs that produce false-positive results	Factors that produce false-negative results
		Drugs
Avocados	Acetaminophen	Corticotropin
Bananas	Acetanilid	p-Chlorophenylalanine
Eggplants	Caffeine	Chlorpromazine
Pineapples	Fluorouracil	Heparin
Plums	Guaifenesin	Imipramine
Walnuts	Lugol's (iodine) solution	Isoniazid
	Melphalan	Methenaminemandelate
	Mephenesin	Methyldopa
	Methamphetamine	Monoamine oxidase inhibitors
	Methocarbamol	Phenothiazine
	Methysergide maleate	Promethazine
	Phenacetin	5-Hydroxyindoleacetic acid
	Phenmetrazine	
	Reserpine	

*This material is reproduced with permission from Wiley-Liss, Inc., a subsidiary of John Wiley & Sons, Inc.

Management of hot flushes

Menopausal hot flushes

The gold standard of treatment for menopausal hot flushes is oestrogen therapy. No other therapy has been approved by the Food and Drug Administration for the treatment of hot flushes. However, some women may be unsuitable for HRT, owing to contraindications; unwillingness to take HRT or inability to continue HRT owing to intolerable side effects. Table 1 provides specific doses/combinations of HRT.

The various options for managing hot flushes are detailed below.

Placebo

Placebo use may lead to a 20–50 per cent reduction in hot flushes after 4 weeks of treatment.

Hormonal therapy

The following hormones may be effective for the treatment of hot flushes:

- oestrogen;
- Femring;
- progestogens;
- androgens;
- tibolone;
- combinations of above.

Non-hormonal treatment

This includes use of the following drugs:

- antidepressants – venlafaxine (serotonin and norepinephrine reuptake inhibitors), paroxetine, fluoxetine;
- gabapentin-A – a GABA analogue used for seizure disorders as an anticonvulsant;
- evening primrose oil;
- veralapride;
- herbal remedies – black cohosh, red clover, dong quai;
- belladona is *not* advised now in view of its side effects;
- clonidine – an α-adrenergic agonist commonly used as an antihypertensive;
- cetrizine;
- nutraceuticals, such as vitamins – B complex, C and E;
- soy products.

Non-pharmacological treatments

These have been tried with variable success and include the following:

- behavioural interventions;
- relaxation training;
- cognitive behavioural intervention and diversion techniques;
- progressive muscle relaxation, or biofeedback or applied relaxation;
- hypnosis;
- acupuncture;
- deep breathing – paced abdominal respiration and muscle contraction relaxation of all muscle groups should be tried;
- a problem-solving approach should be used.

Lifestyle measures

Adopting certain lifestyle measures can decrease the intensity and frequency of hot flushes. It is recommended that all women with hot flushes be counselled regarding these options and encouraged to use them. They include:

- avoidance of triggering factors such as stress, caffeine, alcohol, spicy foods and beverages;
- avoidance of smoking;
- reduction of stress – practice meditation, yoga, massage, paced breathing;
- staying in a cold environment, avoiding warm places;
- keeping cool and the ambient temperature low, drinking cold drinks, bathing in cool water, using fans, using cotton sheets, wearing appropriate breathable cotton clothing, dressing in layers;
- exercise – undertake aerobic and weight-bearing exercises;
- weight loss

Treatment

Once the diagnosis has been established and the options have been discussed, the approach to a patient with hot flushes ultimately depends on the severity of symptoms, patient preferences and whether there are any contraindications to hormonal therapy.

1 If symptoms and effects on quality of life are mild, lifestyle modifications should be the first line of approach, then vitamin E may be tried.
2 If the hot flushes are more severe, then HRT/oestrogen therapy/progesterone therapy combinations may be initiated as appropriate.
3 If the patient is unwilling to take HRT or is unresponsive to it, then the following should be prescribed:
   - venlafaxine 37.5 mg/day for 1 week, then increased to 75 mg (watch for dystonia); or
   - paroxetine 10 mg/day for 1 week, then increased to 20 mg/day; or
   - gabapentin, if the above fail to relieve the flushes.

The symptoms will abate eventually even without treatment; the difficulty is not knowing how long they will persist. There has been reluctance in the UK recently to prescribe HRT owing to its potential problems but, on balance, it is extremely good in alleviating symptoms. However, rebound flushes can occur when the HRT is stopped.

Carcinoid-associated hot flushes

For the management of flushing associated with carcinoid syndrome, different drugs may be used depending on the site of the carcinoid tumour.

1 Corticosteroids, phenothiazines and bromocriptine are effective in patients with bronchial carcinoid tumours.
2 Cyprohepatidine, clonidine and α-interferons are used for hot flushes in patients with foregut carcinoid tumours.[24]
3 Somatostatins, and their analogues octreotide or lanreotide, are used for flushing associated with gastric and ileal carcinoids.[24–27] Adequate niacin supplementation as nicotinamide should be given.[28]
4 Antihistamines, such as H1 antihistamine hydroxyzine, cimetidine (H2 antagonist) and cromoglycate, are useful in patients with systemic mastocytosis.[29]
5 Sertraline is useful in patients with familial MAO deficiency.[30]

Table 1 Medication for hot flushes: dosages and effects

Drugs/preparations	Dose and route	Hot flush reduction % (active drug vs placebo)[4]	Comments
Oestrogens[5]			
Conjugated equine oestrogens (CEEs)	0.625 mg daily, 1.25 mg	70–90% vs. 40–60%	Oestrogen replacement therapy is the most effective medication that relieves hot flushes in women with oestrogen deficiency. It should be used with a progestogen and must not be used alone in women with a uterus. Very low doses of 0.325 mg CEE have also been used with success for hot flushes
Femring	Every 3 months		
Progestins			Need 20 days for effectiveness. Side effects include weight gain, breast tenderness
Megestrol[6]	20 mg orally twice daily	85% vs. 21%	
Medroxyprogesterone acetate[7]	20 mg orally once daily	73.9% vs. 25.9%	
Medroxyprogesterone acetate[8]	100 mg orally twice daily	86% vs. 33%	
Depot medroxyprogesterone acetate (DMPA)[9]	500 mg IM biweekly	86%	
Transdermal progesterone[10]	20 mg daily	83% vs. 19%	
Transdermal progesterone	32 mg daily	No significant effect	
Tibolone			Side effects include weight gain, fluid retention, vaginal bleeding, headache, facial growth
Combinations of oestrogen and progestogen			
Oestrogen + medroxyprogesterone			
Oestrogen + methyl testosterone			
Oral contraceptive pills			
Selective serotonin reuptake inhibitors (SSRIs)			
Venlaxafine[11]	75 mg orally daily	61% vs. 27%	Side effects include temporary nausea, dry mouth, anorexia, constipation, dystonia
Paroxetine[12]	12.5–25 mg orally daily	62.65% vs. 38%	Not to be taken with tamoxifen
Fluoxetine[13]	20 mg orally daily	50% vs. 36%	Side effects include insomnia, jitteriness, dry mouth, nausea, diarrhoea, headache, fatigue, sexual dysfunction
Citalopram[14]	10:20:30 mg orally daily	76% vs. 64%	

Drugs/preparations	Dose and route	Hot flush reduction % (active drug vs placebo)[4]	Comments
Dopamine antagonists (antidopaminergic)			
Veralipride[15]		63–80%	Useful in GnRH-induced flushing
Gabapentin[16]	900 mg daily in divided doses	50–100% vs. 29%	This is a γ-aminobutyric acid analogue. It is used for epilepsy and neurogenic pain. Side effects of dizziness, fatigue and peripheral oedema
Centrally acting α-adrenergic agonist decreases norepinephrine			
Clonidine[17]	0.1 mg orally daily	38–78% vs. 24–50%	Effective only after 4 weeks of treatment. Significant dose-related side effects such as insomnia, dry mouth, postural hypotension and constipation
Transdermal clonidine	0.1 mg daily as a weekly patch	20–80% vs. 36%	
Herbal formulations			
Soy[18]	25 mg soy protein diet	30–50% minor or nil improvement at 6 weeks, no significant difference at 60 days vs. 30%	
Black cohosh[19]	40–80 mg orally daily for only up to 6 months	No significant difference at 60 days	
Vitamin E[20]	400 IU orally twice daily	Minimal decrease of 1 hot flash/day vs. placebo	
Evening primrose oil[21]			Rich in γ- and δ linoleic acids (omega-3 and -6 fatty acids, respectively). It reduces night-time but not daytime hot flushes
Hesperidin[22]	900 mg daily		Derived from citrus fruits
Vitamin C[23]	1200 mg daily		

GnRH, gonadotrophin-releasing hormone; IM, intramuscular.

References

1. Greaves MW. Flushing and flushing syndromes, rosacea and perioral dermatitis. In: Champion RH, Burton JL, Burns DA, Breathnach SM, eds. *Rook/Wilkinson/Ebling Textbook of Dermatology*, Vol. 3, 6th edn. Oxford: Blackwell Scientific, 1998: 2099–104.
2. Cutaneous manifestations of disorders of the cardiovascular and pulmonary systems. In: Freedberg IM, Eisen AZ, Wolff K, Austen KF, et al., eds. *Fitzpatrick's Dermatology in General Medicine*, Vol. 2, 5th edn. New York: McGraw-Hill, 1999: 2064.
3. O'Toole D, Ducreux M, Bommelaer G, et al. Treatment of carcinoid syndrome: a prospective crossover evaluation of lanreotide versus octreotide in terms of efficacy, patient acceptability, and tolerance. *Cancer* 2000; **88:** 770–6.

4. AACE Menopause Guidelines Revision Task Force. American Association of Clinical Endocrinologists medical guidelines for clinical practice for the diagnosis and treatment of menopause. *Endocr Pract* 2006; **12**: 315–36.

5. MacLennan A, Lester S, Moore V. Oral estrogen replacement versus placebo for hot flashes. *Climacteric* 2001; **4**: 58–74.

6. Loprinzi CL, Michalak JC, Quella SK, *et al*. Megestrol acetate for the prevention of hot flashes. *N Engl J Med* 1994; **331**: 347–52.

7. Schiff I, Tulchinsky D, Cramer D, Ryan KJ. Oral medroxyprogesterone in the treatment of postmenopausal symptoms. *JAMA* 1980; **244**: 1443–5.

8. Aslaksen K, Frankendal B. Effect of oral medroxyprogesterone acetate on menopausal symptoms in patients with endometrial carcinoma. *Acta Obstet Gynecol Scand* 1982; **61**: 423–8.

9. Bertelli G, Venturini M, Del Mastro L, *et al*. Intramuscular depot medroxyprogesterone versus oral megestrol for the control of postmenopausal hot flashes in breast cancer patients: a randomized study. *Ann Oncol* 2002; **13**: 883–8.

10. Leonetti HB, Longo S, Anasti JN. Transdermal progesterone cream for vasomotor symptoms and postmenopausal bone loss. *Obstet Gynecol* 1999; **94**: 225–8.

11. Loprinzi CL, Kugler JW, Sloan JA, *et al*. Venlafaxine in management of hot flashes in survivors of breast cancer: a randomised controlled trial. *Lancet* 2000; **356**: 2059–63.

12. Stearns V, Beebe KL, Iyengar M, Dube E. Paroxetine controlled release in the treatment of menopausal hot flashes: a randomized controlled trial. *JAMA* 2003; **289**: 2827–34.

13. Loprinzi CL, Sloan JA, Perez EA, *et al*. Phase III evaluation of fluoxetine for treatment of hot flashes. *J Clin Oncol* 2002; **20**: 1578–83.

14. Suvanto-Luukkonen E, Koivunen R, Sundstrom H, *et al*. Citalopram and fluoxetine in the treatment of postmenopausal symptoms: a prospective, randomized, 9-month, placebo-controlled, double-blind study. *Menopause* 2005; **12**: 18–26.

15. David A, Don R, Tajchner G, Weissglas L. Veralipride: alternative antidopaminergic treatment for menopausal symptoms. *Am J Obstet Gynecol* 1988; **158**: 1107–15.

16. Guttuso T Jr, Kurlan R, McDermott MP, Kieburtz K. Gabapentin's effects on hot flashes in postmenopausal women: a randomized controlled trial. *Obstet Gynecol* 2003; **101**: 337–45.

17. Edington RF, Chagnon JP, Steinberg WM. Clonidine (Dixarit) for menopausal flushing. *Can Med Assoc J* 1980; **123**: 23–6.

18. Van Patten CL, Olivotto IA, Chambers GK, *et al*. Effect of soy phytoestrogens on hot flashes in postmenopausal women with breast cancer: a randomized, controlled clinical trial. *J Clin Oncol* 2002; **20**: 1449–55.

19. Jacobson JS, Troxel AB, Evans J, *et al*. Randomized trial of black cohosh for the treatment of hot flashes among women with a history of breast cancer. *J Clin Oncol* 2001; **19**: 2739–45.

20. Meydani SN, Meydani M, Blumberg JB, *et al*. Assessment of the safety of supplementation with different amounts of vitamin E in healthy older adults. *Am J Clin Nutr* 1998; 68: 311–18.

21. Chenoy R, Hussain S, Tayob Y, *et al*. Effect of oral gamolenic acid from evening primrose oil on menopausal flushing. *BMJ* 1994; **308**: 501–3.

22. Garg A, Garg S, Zaneveld LJ, Singla AK. Chemistry and pharmacology of the citrus bioflavonoid hesperidin. *Phytother Res* 2001; **15**: 655–69.

23. Smith CJ. Non-hormonal control of vasomotor flushing in menopausal patients. *Chic Med* 1964; **67:** 193–5.
24. Wilson JD, ed. *Williams Textbook of Endocrinology*, 9th edn. Philadelphia: W.B. Saunders, 1998.
25. O'Toole D, Ducreux M, Bommelaer G, *et al.* Treatment of carcinoid syndrome: a prospective crossover evaluation of lanreotide versus octreotide in terms of efficacy, patient acceptability, and tolerance. *Cancer* 2000; **88:** 770–6.
26. Larsen PR, ed. *Williams Textbook of Endocrinology*, 10th edn. Philadelphia: W.B. Saunders, 2003.
27. Rubin J, Ajani J, Schirmer W, *et al.* Octreotide acetate long-acting formulation versus openlabel subcutaneous octreotide acetate in malignant carcinoid syndrome. *J Clin Oncol* 1999; **17:** 600–6.
28. Fitzpatrick TB, Eisen AZ, *et al. Dermatology in General Medicine*, 4th edn. New York: McGraw Hill, 1993.
29. Greaves MW. Mastocytoses. In: Champion RH, Burton JL, Burns DA, Breathnach SM, eds. *Rook/Wilkinson/Ebling Textbook of Dermatology*, Vol. 3, 6th edn. Oxford: Blackwell Scientific, 1998: 2337–46.
30. Cheung NW, Earl J. Monoamine oxidase deficiency: a cause of flushing and attention deficit/hyperactivity disorder? *Arch Intern Med* 2001; **161:** 2503–4.

HYDROPS FETALIS

Mala Arora

Hydrops fetalis (Fig. 1) is defined as generalised fetal oedema or anasarca, which can be detected by an antenatal ultrasound scan (Figs 2 and 3). It can be a manifestation of a variety of underlying disorders. The condition is subdivided into immune or non-immune hydrops. The immune variety is more common in the developing countries while the non-immune variety is more common in the developed countries. Warsof

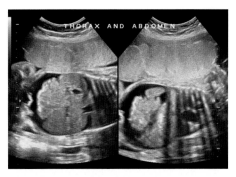

Figure 1 Hydrops fetalis.

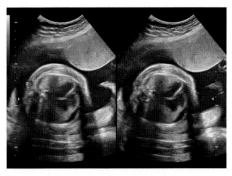

Figure 2 Ultrasound scan of hydrothorax.

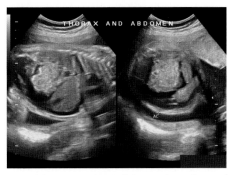

Figure 3 Transverse and sagittal ultrasound scan pictures of fetal ascites.

et al in 1986 reported a ratio of 9:1 of non-immune to immune cases.[1]

■ Immune

The best studied immunological cause of hydrops fetalis is pregnancy with a rhesus-positive fetus in a rhesus-negative mother who is already sensitised by either a previous pregnancy or blood transfusion. The immunoglobulin G (IgG) antibodies to the rhesus-positive red blood cells (RBCs) cross the placenta and destroy the fetal RBCs leading to fetal anaemia and hydrops. This was first reported by Levine in 1941.[2] The first pregnancy proceeds normally as the rhesus-negative mother is not sensitised. Fetomaternal haemorrhage occurs at placental separation and sensitises the mother.

Other procedures during pregnancy that can sensitise the mother are abruptio placentae, external cephalic version and amniocentesis. In subsequent pregnancies, the fetal red cells are destroyed by the maternal IgG antibody that can cross the placenta. In mild cases, the fetus has anaemia and haemolytic disease of the new-born, but in severe cases, it develops hydrops fetalis. If the antibody titres are high, hydrops will manifest at an earlier gestation.

Rhesus immunoglobulin was introduced in 1966. With careful immunisation of all rhesus-negative mothers after delivery and abortion, the incidence of immune hydrops has steadily declined in the last 40 years. However, rhesus isoimmunisation continues to be the single most common cause of immune hydrops fetalis in the developing countries.

Today, the mortality from immune hydrops is very low. This condition is managed with repeated cordocentesis, estimation of fetal haemoglobin and intrauterine transfusion of rhesus-negative blood.

Occasionally. immune hydrops may be due to other erythrocyte antigens apart from rhesus D antigen. These include the minor blood group antigens c, Kell, Fy, JK and Duffy, which can cause haemolysis.

In the UK, all pregnant women are screened for blood group disorders at the time of booking, and this may be repeated at 28 and 36 weeks' gestation. Likewise, antiD is given to non-immunised women throughout the pregnancy usually at booking, and at 28 and 36 weeks' gestation. If isoimmunisation occurs, then the titres of antibodies are monitored at appropriate intervals depending on the levels and the rapidity with which they are changing (either every 2 or 4 weeks).

Box 1 Causes of non-immune hydrops fetalis

Chromosomal
- Down's syndrome, other trisomies
- Turner syndrome
- Mosaicism
- Translocation 18q+, 13q−
- Triploidy

Cardiovascular
- Anatomic defects
- Tachyarrhythmia
- Congenital heart block
- Cardiomyopathy

Haematologic
- Alpha thalassaemia
- Arteriovenous shunts
- Vascular thrombosis
- Congenital leukaemia

Infections
- Parvovirus
- Cytomegalovirus
- *Toxoplasma*
- Syphilis
- Herpes
- Rubella
- Leptospirosis

Maternal
- Diabetes mellitus
- Pre-eclampsia
- Severe anaemia
- Hypoproteinaemia

Chondrodysplasias
- Thanatophoric dwarfism
- Osteogenesis imperfecta
- Achondrogenesis
- Hypophosphatasia

Twin pregnancy
- Twin-to-twin transfusion syndrome
- Acardiac twin

Congenital tumours
- Central nervous system, genitourinary, gastrointestinal, pulmonary, hepatic, placental
- Sacrococcygeal teratoma
- Tuberous sclerosis
- Neuroblastoma

Inborn errors of metabolism
- Mucopolysacharidosis Type VII
- Gaucher's disease
- Gangliosidosis
- Neuraminidase deficiency
- Fetal I cell disease
- Morquio's disease

■ Non-immune

Non-immune hydrops carries a higher fetal mortality rate. The causes are varied[3] and newer associations continually appear in literature. The causes are listed in Box 1.

Diagnoses for these conditions may include:

- serum screening of the mother for the underlying cause;
- ultrasound scanning looking for underlying anatomical defects;
- amniocentesis or cordocentesis as appropriate;
- in some cases, the diagnosis may only be made on postmortem examination and investigations.

Viral infections

A variety of viral infections during pregnancy will present as hydrops fetalis. The virus most often implicated is parvovirus B19. This is the only parvovirus that infects humans.

Parvovirus B19 infection was first reported as fifth disease in 1983[4] and was implicated as a cause of hydrops fetalis in 1984.[5] This rare viral infection is often asymptomatic in the mother, but may cause fever not exceeding 39°C, and/or arthralgias of fingers, knees or wrist. Replication of parvovirus occurs mainly in the erythroid precursors of the bone marrow. Hence it leads to haemolytic anaemia in the fetus, and occasionally

aplastic crisis. This will lead to fetal hydrops, which can be self-limiting. As the anaemia improves, so does the hydrops. In patients with decreased erythroid precursors, like sickle cell disease and thalassaemia, fetal deaths have been observed.

Prospective studies indicate that parvovirus B19 infection in the mother most often leads to delivery of a normal healthy fetus. Transplacental transmission is estimated to be in the range of 25–33 per cent and the incidence of fetal loss is 1.66–9 per cent.[6,7] The rate of infection is greater in pregnancies less than 12 weeks and lower in pregnancies greater than 20 weeks. Diagnosis is made by serological estimation of IgM and IgG antibodies in the mother. A positive IgM and a negative IgG result indicates recent infection. However, since the viraemia is transient and the hydrops may develop 3–12 weeks after maternal infection, the serology may be unhelpful. In these cases, the presence of the virus can be confirmed by nested polymerase chain reaction (PCR) studies on the amniotic fluid. In one study, the authors have compared the results of serology with PCR and/or in-situ hybridisation studies on maternal serum, cord blood or amniotic fluid.[8] As much as 95 per cent favourable fetal outcome has been reported with intrauterine blood transfusions.[9]

Other viral infections, such as measles, Coxsackie virus, cytomegalovirus, German measles, herpes and chickenpox, if associated with haemolysis, can also lead to hydrops.

Other pathogenic infections during pregnancy, such as syphilis, Toxoplasma and leptospirosis may also be associated with hydrops fetalis.

Red cell defects

Alpha thalassaemia[10] is a common cause of hydrops in the thalassaemic belt of South East Asia. The diagnosis is established by fetal blood sampling. The prognosis for alpha thalassaemia is not as good as for other causes of non-immune hydrops. Repeated fetal blood transfusion is the only option.

Congenital spherocytosis, elliptocytosis, sickle cell disease or any other red-cell defect that leads to haemolysis will cause hydrops fetalis. A rare genetic disorder of red cell protein has been described that presented as recurrent hydrops fetalis. This was a nucleotide substitution in the erythrocyte beta spectrin gene.[11,12] Other causes include aplastic anaemia and congenital leukaemias.

Cardiovascular disorders

Congenital cardiac defects that lead to poor tissue perfusion, as in Eisenmenger's syndrome, transposition of the great vessels, congenital heart block and cardiomyopathy, will lead to cardiac failure and hydrops fetalis.

Chromosomal abnormalities

Trisomy 21 (Down's syndrome), trisomy 18 (Edward's syndrome), trisomy 13 (Patau's syndrome), Turner's syndrome and mosaicism may present as hydrops fetalis. Other chromosomal anomalies that are incompatible with life, such as polyploides and triploidies, may also present as hydrops fetalis.

Fetal chondrodysplasias

Fetal bony defects, such as thanatophoric dwarfism, osteogenesis imperfecta, achondrogenesis and hypophosphatasia, are reported with hydrops fetalis.

Twin pregnancy

Twin-to-twin transfusion syndrome can lead to hydrops fetalis. This can be managed by laser ablation of the connecting fetal vessels through amnioscopy.

An acardiac twin can also be a cause of hydrops and can be managed by fetal reduction.

Maternal

Severe maternal anaemia, hypoproteinaemia and uncontrolled diabetes mellitus can lead to hydrops fetalis.

Inborn errors of metabolism

These are rare enzyme disorders that lead to defective metabolism. The most common disorder described in the literature with recurrent fetal hydrops is mucopolysaccharidosis Type VII.[13–18] In this disorder, there is deficiency of the enzyme beta glucuronidase.

Other disorders reported infrequently are:

- infantile Gaucher's disease;
- I-cell disease;[19]
- GM1 gangliosidosis, sialidosis (neuraminidase deficiency);[20]
- mucopolysaccharidosis type IV A (Morquio's disease type A).[21]

The prognosis in all these fetuses is poor.

Idiopathic

In spite of extensive investigations after cordocentesis, in almost 15 per cent of the cases, the cause of fetal hydrops may not be diagnosed. There are case reports in the literature of recurrent fetal hydrops in the absence of any known cause. These patients are hard to counsel and treat.

Endocardial fibroelastosis has been reported on autopsy of infants with hydrops fetalis. It is postulated that thickening of the endocardium in excess of $30\,\mu m$ (normal being $5\,\mu m$) is in response to chronic prenatal myocardial stress.[22]

■ References

1. Warsof SL, Nicolaides KH, Rodeck C. Immune and non-immune hydrops *Clin Obstet Gynaecol* 1986; **29:** 533–42.

2. Levine P, Burntam L, Katzin E, Vogel P. The role of isoimmunisation in the pathogenesis of erythroblastosis fetalis. *Am J Obstet Gynecol* 1941; **42:** 925–37.

3. Allan LD, Crawford DC, Sheridan R, Chapman MG. Aetiology of non-immune hydrops. *Br J Obstet Gynaecol* 1986; **93:** 223–5.

4. Anderson MJ, Jones SE, Fisher-Hoch SP, *et al*. The human parvovirus the cause of erythema infectiosum (fifth disease). *Lancet* 1983; **i**: 1378.
5. Brown T, Anand A, Ritchie LD, Clewley JP, Reid TM. Intrauterine parvovirus infection during pregnancy. *Lancet* 1984; **ii**: 1033–4.
6. Gratocos E, Torres PJ, Vidal J, *et al*. The incidence of human parvovirus infection during pregnancy and its impact on prenatal outcome. *J Infect Dis* 1995; **171**: 1360–3.
7. Public Health Laboratory Service Working Party on Fifth Disease. Prospective study of human parvovirus B 19 infection in pregnancy. *Br Med J* 1990; **300**: 1166–70.
8. Zerbini M, Musiani M, Gentilomi G, *et al*. Comparative evaluation of virological and serological methods in prenatal diagnosis of parvovirus B 19 fetal hydrops. *J Clin Microbiol* 1996; **34**: 603–8.
9. Guidozzi F, Ballot D, Rothberg AD. Human B19 parvovirus infection in an obstetric population. *J Reprod Med* 1994; **39**: 36.
10. Joshi DD, Nickerson JH, McMannus MJ. Hydrops fetalis caused by homozygous α-thalassemia and Rh antigen alloimmunisation. *Clin Med Res* 2004; 2: 228–32.
11. Gallaher PG, Weed SA, Tse WT, *et al*. Recurrent fetal hydrops associated with a nucleotide substitution in the erythrocyte beta spectrin gene. *J Clin Invest* 1995; **95**: 1174–82.
12. Gallagher PG, Petruzzi MJ, Weed SA, *et al*. Mutation of a highly conserved residue of β1 spectrin associated with fatal and near fatal neonatal haemolytic anaemia. *J Clin Invest* 1997; 267–77.
13. Nelson J, Kenny B, O'Hara D, Harper A, Broadhead D. Foamy changes of placental cells are associated with hydrops fetalis probable beta glucuronidase deficiency. Clin Pathol 1993; **46**: 3.
14. Lowden JA, Cutz E, Conen PE, Rudd N, Doran TA. Prenatal diagnosis of GM1-gangliosidosis. *N Engl J Med* 1973; **288**: 225–8.
15. Gillan JE, Lowden JA, Gaskin K, Cutz E. Congenital ascites as a presenting sign of lysosomal storage disease. *J Pediatr* 1984; **104**: 225–31.
16. Nelson A, Peterson L, Frampton B, Sly WS. Mucopolysaccharidosis VII (8-glucuronidase deficiency) presenting as nonimmune hydrops fetalis. *J Pediatr* 1982; **101**: 574–6.
17. Irani D, Kim H-S, El-Hibri H, Dutton RV, Beaudet A, Armstrong D. Postmortem observations on β-glucuronidase deficiency presenting as hydrops fetalis. *Ann Neurol* 1983; **14**: 486–90.
18. Sheets Lee JE, Falk RE, Ng WG, Donnell GN. β Glucuronidase deficiency. A heterogenous mucopolysaccharidosis. *Am J Dis Child* 1985; **139**: 57–9.
19. Rapola J, Aula P. Morphology of the placenta in fetal I cell disease. *Clin Genet* 1977; **11**: 107–13.
20. Beck M, Bender SW, Reiter H-L, *et al*. Neuraminidase deficiency presenting as non-immune hydrops fetalis. *Eur J Pediatr* 1984; **143**: 135–9.
21. Applegarth DA, Toone JR, Wilson RD, Yong SL, Baldwin VJ. Morquio disease presenting as hydrops fetalis and enzyme analysis of chorionic villus tissue in a subsequent pregnancy. *Pediatr Pathol* 1987; **7**: 593–9.
22. Newbould MJ, Armstrong GR, Barson AJ. Endocardial fibroelastosis in infants with hydrops fetalis. *J Clin Pathol* 1991; **44**: 576–9.

INCONTINENCE, FAECAL, AND PREGNANCY

Dilip Visvanathan

Faecal incontinence may be defined as 'any involuntary loss of faeces or flatus, or urge incontinence that adversely affects the quality of life'.[1] It is an embarrassing condition and therefore goes largely under-reported. The prevalence of faecal incontinence on direct questioning of women before delivery, at 34 weeks' gestation and after delivery was found to be 0.7 per cent, 6.0 per cent and 5.5 per cent, respectively.[2] A multicentre study found that the prevalence of persistent faecal incontinence was 3.6 per cent.[3]

Faecal continence is maintained by the coordinated action of several anatomical and physiological elements. These include the internal and external anal sphincters, and the puborectalis muscle (see Fig. 2 in Birth injuries, maternal). Defecation requires anorectal sensation plus control by the cerebral cortex. Dysfunction of any of these components may lead to faecal incontinence.

The symptoms of faecal incontinence are outlined in Box 1. The severity of incontinence may be classified depending on the frequency of incontinent episodes and the contents of incontinence (Box 2).

Box 2 Faecal continence scoring scale

0	Never
1	Rarely (<1/month)
2	Sometimes (1/week to 1/month)
3	Usually (1/day to 1/week)
4	Always (>1/day)

Minor faecal incontinence is defined as the inadvertent loss of flatus or liquid stool per rectum, whereas major faecal incontinence is described as the inadvertent and frequent loss of fully formed stool per rectum and, as such, represents the most severe degree of functional impairment of the anorectum.

Box 1 Symptoms of faecal incontinence

- Passage of any flatus when socially undesirable
- Any incontinence of liquid stool
- Any need to wear a pad because of anal symptoms
- Any incontinence of solid stool
- Any faecal urgency

Box 3 Classification of the causes of faecal incontinence

Normal sphincters and pelvic floor
- Faecal impaction
- Causes of diarrhoea (e.g. infection, inflammatory bowel disease)
- Faecal fistula/colostomy

Abnormal sphincters and/or pelvic floor
Minor incontinence

Internal sphincter deficiency
- Previous surgery
- Rectal prolapse
- Third-degree haemorrhoids
- Idiopathic
- Minor denervation of external sphincter and pelvic floor

Major incontinence
Congenital anomalies of the anorectum
Trauma

- Iatrogenic
- Obstetric
- Fractures of the pelvis
- Impalement

Denervation

- Obstetric
- Rectal prolapse
- Peripheral neuropathy (e.g. diabetic mellitus)
- Cauda equina lesion (tumour or trauma)
- Tabes dorsalis (syphilis)
- Lumbar meningomyelocele (spina bifida)

Upper motor neuron lesion

- Cerebral
  - Multiple stroke
  - Metastases and other tumours
  - Trauma
  - Dementia and other degenerative disorders

Spinal

- Multiple sclerosis
- Metastases and other tumours
- Degenerative diseases (e.g. vitamin B12 deficiency)

Rectal carcinoma
Anorectal infection (e.g. lymphogranuloma)
Drug intoxication (particularly in the elderly)

Causes of faecal incontinence

There are many causes of faecal incontinence and a complete classification is given in Box 3.[4] The commonest cause in women is considered to be due to sphincter injury following childbirth.[4,5] Damage may occur during childbirth in three ways:

Direct mechanical injury

Direct external or internal anal sphincter muscle disruption can occur, as with a clinically obvious third- or fourth-degree perineal laceration, or an occult injury subsequently noted on ultrasound scan of the anus.

Neurological injury

Neuropathy of the pudendal nerve may result from forceps delivery or persistent nerve compression from the fetal head.[6] Traction neuropathy may also occur with the following:

- fetal macrosomia;
- prolonged pushing during second stage in successive pregnancies;
- prolonged stretching of the nerve owing to persistent poor tone of the pelvic floor postpartum.

Injured nerves often undergo demyelination but usually recover with time.

Combined mechanical and neurological trauma

Neuropathy more commonly accompanies mechanical damage.

Factors in childbirth contributing to faecal incontinence

These are summarized in Box 4. The most significant factors that cause sphincter damage include forceps delivery and a previous sphincter injury. A randomized control trial found clinical third-degree tears in 16 per cent of women with forceps-assisted deliveries, compared with 7 per cent of vacuum-assisted deliveries.[7]

Box 4 Factors in pregnancy and delivery associated with faecal incontinence

- Nulliparity (primigravidity)
- Instrumental delivery, overall
- Forceps-assisted delivery
- Vacuum-assisted delivery
- Midline episiotomy
- Episiotomy, mediolateral
- Prolonged second stage of labour
- Epidural analgesia
- Birth weight >4 kg
- Persistent occipitoposterior position
- Previous anal sphincter tear

■ Prevalence of anal symptoms

The prevalence of anal symptoms in women who have undergone third- and fourth-degree tear repair ranges from 25 to 57 per cent. In these studies, the type of incontinence is mainly of flatus (30 per cent), leakage of liquid stool (8 per cent), while leakage of solid stool occurred in 4 per cent. Faecal urgency occurred in 26 per cent of women.[8]

■ Prevention

Avoiding obstetrical injury to the anal sphincter is the single biggest factor in preventing faecal incontinence among women. The strategies for prevention of this problem are outlined in Box 5.[9,10] Elective Caesarean section appears to be the only preventive measure to avoid sphincter and pelvic floor damage; however, it has been reported that there was no reduction in the prevalence of persistent faecal incontinence in women following elective Caesarean section when compared to a normal vaginal delivery.

Box 5 Strategies for preventing sphincter damage at childbirth

Primary prevention
- Spontaneous over forceps-assisted vaginal delivery
- Vacuum extraction over forceps delivery
- Restrictive use of episiotomy
- Mediolateral episiotomy over medial episiotomy
- Antepartum pelvic floor exercises and antepartum perineal massage
- Consider Caesarean section

Secondary prevention
- Early detection and proper repair of perineal injury

Tertiary prevention
- Consider lower segment Caesarean section for women with childbirth injuries to the pelvic floor in future pregnancies

---

■ Repair

Repair of sphincter damage at delivery is best done immediately. Failed repairs should be diagnosed early and specialist help enlisted.

Immediate repair

It is standard practice to repair a damaged anal sphincter immediately or soon after delivery. All women having a vaginal delivery should have a systematic examination of the perineum, vagina and rectum to assess the severity of damage prior to suturing. Repair of the perineum requires good lighting and visualization, proper surgical instruments and suture material, and adequate analgesia.

Two commonly used methods of external anal sphincter repair are:

- end-to-end approximation of the cut ends;
- overlapping the cut ends and suturing through the overlapped portions.

There is no significant difference in outcomes between these methods. The preoperative, intraoperative and postoperative standards for the successful outcome of the procedure have been described in the Royal College of Obstetricians and Gynaecologists guidelines.[11]

Secondary sphincter repair

All women who have had a third- and fourth-degree tear repaired should be offered a planned follow-up at 6–12 months by a gynaecologist with an interest in anorectal dysfunction or a colorectal surgeon. If symptomatic, they should be offered endoanal ultrasonography plus anorectal manometry and referral to a colorectal surgeon for consideration of secondary sphincter repair.

■ Management in a subsequent pregnancy

Subsequent vaginal deliveries may worsen anal incontinence symptoms. These women are also at increased risk of repeat injury to the anal sphincter complex. All women who have had a third- and fourth-degree tear in their previous pregnancy should be counselled regarding the risk of developing anal incontinence or worsening symptoms with subsequent vaginal delivery. If they are symptomatic or with abnormal endoanal ultrasonography or manometry, the option of elective Caesarean section should be discussed. If asymptomatic, there is no clear evidence as to the best mode of delivery.[1,12]

■ References

1. Royal College of Obstetricians and Gynaecologists. *Management of third- and fourth-degree perineal tears following vaginal delivery.* Guideline No. 29. London: RCOG Press; 2001.

2. Chaliha C, Kalia V, Stanton SL, Monga A, Sultan AH. Antenatal prediction of post-partum urinary and fecal incontinence. *Obstet Gynecol* 1999; **94:** 689–94.

3. Macarthur C, Bick DE, Keighley MR. Faecal incontinence after childbirth. *Br J Obstet Gynaecol* 1997; **104:** 46–50.

4. Cooper ZR, Rose S. Fecal incontinence: a clinical approach. *Mt Sinai J Med* 2000; **67:** 96–105.

5. Bartolo DC. Gastroenterological options in faecal incontinence.*Ann Chir* 1991; **45:** 590–8.

6. Sultan AH, Kamm MA, Hudson CN. Pudendal nerve damage during labour: prospective study before and after childbirth. *Br J Obstet Gynaecol* 1994; **101:** 22–8.

7. Fitzpatrick M, Behan M, O'Connell PR, O'Herlihy C. Randomized clinical trial to assess anal sphincter function following forceps or vacuum assisted vaginal delivery. *Br J Obstet Gynaecol* 2003; **110:** 424–9.

8. de Leeuw JW, Vierhout ME, Struijk PC, Hop WC, Wallenburg HC. Anal sphincter damage after vaginal delivery: functional outcome and risk factors for fecal incontinence. *Acta Obstet Gynecol Scand* 2001; **80:** 830–4.

9. Power D, Fitzpatrick M, O'Herlihy C. Obstetric anal sphincter injury: How to avoid, how to repair: A literature review. *J Fam Pract* 2006; **55:** 193–200.

10. Heit M, Mudd K, Culligan P. Prevention of childbirth injuries to the pelvic floor. *Curr Womens Health Rep* 2001; **1:** 72–80.

11. Leeman L, Spearman M, Rogers R. Repair of obstetric perineal lacerations. *Am Fam Physician* 2003; **68:** 1585–90.

12. Fynes M, Donnelly V, Behan M, O'Connell PR, O'Herlihy C. Effect of second vaginal delivery on anorectal physiology and faecal continence: a prospective study. *Lancet* 1999; **354:** 983–6.

■ Useful website

www.rcog.org.uk/guidelines

INCONTINENCE, URINARY

James Green

At least a quarter of women will experience some form of incontinence in their adult life.[1] The incidence increases with age, so prevalence in the elderly is around 50 per cent.[2] The causation is multifactorial, and the aetiology can be divided into anatomical and physiological causes. The latter can then be subdivided into bladder and/or outlet dysfunction (see Table 1).

Anatomical causes include:

- congenital – ectopic ureter, spina bifida occulta; or
- acquired – fistula, which can be due to tumour, infection and childbirth, or be iatrogenic (surgical).

Physiological causes include:

- bladder dysfunction;
- urethral/outlet dysfunction;
- a mixture of both of the above.

Anatomical causes often result in continuous leakage of urine, whereas leakage tends to be episodic if the cause is dysfunction. Transient causes of urinary incontinence (UI) include urinary tract infection, restricted mobility, constipation, acute illness, confusion, dementia, diabetes mellitus or insipidus, cardiac failure, as well as some drugs, in particular, diuretics, tranquillisers and anticholinergic agents.

Table 1 Terminology and classification of urinary incontinence

Detrusor		Outlet		Classification
Normal	+	Normal	=	Continent unless 'functional or situational'
Overactive	+	Normal	=	Urge urinary incontinence (UUI)
Underactive	+	Normal	=	Retention → overflow incontinence
Normal	+	Overactive/stenosed	=	Retention → overflow incontinence
Normal	+	Underactive	=	Stress urinary incontinence (SUI)

Neurological causes of UI (e.g. multiple sclerosis) should always be considered as a differential cause. These range from continuous 'overflow' caused by an atonic bladder (see Urinary retention) to 'functional' problems, where there is an inability to perform toileting functions due to mental or mobility problems. More rarely, 'situational' causes of incontinence can occur on intercourse or giggling.

Primary evaluation of UI is directed towards categorising the type of incontinence. This is often difficult, as a mixed pattern of UI, involving a component of urge and stress is more common than either urge or stress incontinence on their own.

The second aim is to identify any treatable causes of the incontinence.

A thorough history should explore severity (pad usage) and quality of life issues. Voiding diaries should be completed for at least 3 days and urinalysis undertaken to exclude diabetes, infection and neoplasia. A measurement of post-void residual urinary volume is useful. Cystometrogram should be considered if the type of incontinence is not clearly defined. This is paramount, if any surgical intervention is planned, as the exact form of incontinence has to be clearly defined preoperatively as inappropriate surgery on a unstable bladder may aggravate the situation by making urge incontinence worse.

Table 1 describes the types of incontinence; however, mixed forms of incontinence, such as urge and stress, can often coexist in varying degrees. This classification system corresponds to whether the detrusor muscle in the wall of the bladder is functionally overactive (sometimes termed 'unstable' or 'irritative') or areflexive (underactive), and depends on whether the bladder outlet, which includes the sphincter mechanism, is dyssynergic (overactive, see Urinary retention), stenosed or incompetent (underactive).

■ Urge urinary incontinence

The definition of urge urinary incontinence (UUI) is 'the involuntary loss of urine resulting from an increase in bladder pressure secondary to a bladder contraction'. The main symptom is the loss of urine with the feeling of urgency, voiding before the ability to get to the toilet. It can be a difficult problem to treat with varying levels of success.

The treatment for UUI is given in Box 1.

Box 1 Treatment of urge urinary incontinence

Treat any underlying cause
- e.g. infection, inflammation, obstruction, calculus, neoplasm, neurological disease

Behavioural therapy
- Timed voiding (approx. every 2–3 hours) or bladder retraining for a period of at least 6 weeks

Pharmacologic therapy
- Muscarinic cholinergic antagonists
- Tricyclic antidepressants

Surgery
- Botulinum injections
- Sacral nerve stimulation
- Augmentation cystoplasty
- Other alternatives, including subtrigonal rhizolysis, autoaugmentation

■ Stress urinary incontinence (SUI)

The definition of stress urinary incontinence (SUI) is 'the involuntary loss of urine resulting from an increased intra-abdominal pressure, which overcomes the resistance of the bladder outlet in the absence of a true bladder contraction'. The main symptom is the involuntary loss of urine with activity (coughing, laughing, sneezing, lifting or straining). SUI can be caused by hypermobility of the bladder neck and proximal urethral, or loss of the posterior urethral support mechanism.

The treatment for SUI is given in Box 2.

However, if SUI occurs with a well-supported pelvic floor, then intrinsic sphincter deficiency should be considered. Treatment of this condition involves coapting the urethral mucosa at the level of the bladder neck and proximal urethra (Box 3). The success rate for surgical treatment of SUI is 75–90 per cent.

■ References

1. Elving LB, Foldspang A, Lam GW, Mommsen S. Descriptive epidemiology of urinary incontinence in 3,100 women age 30–59. *Scand J Urol Nephrol Suppl* 1989; **125:** 37–43.
2. Department of Health, Education and Welfare. *Long-term Care and Facility Improvement Study*. Washington, DC: US Government Printing Office, 1975.

Box 2 Treatment of stress urinary incontinence

Behavioural therapy:
■ Biofeedback
■ Pelvic floor exercises (Kegel) for at least 3 months' duration
■ Vaginal cones/weights

Pharmacologic therapy
■ Alpha-adrenergic agonists
■ Tricyclic antidepressants
■ Oestrogen replacement (intermittent) may help some individuals

Surgery
■ Tension-free transvaginal/obturator mid-urethral tape procedures
■ Bladder neck suspension techniques

Box 3 Treatment of intrinsic sphincter deficiency

Surgery
■ Intraurethral bulking agents
■ Tension-free transvaginal/obturator mid-urethral tape procedures
■ Artificial urinary sphincter implantation

INFERTILITY

Anne Clark

Involuntary infertility, which affects one in six couples, is defined as the lack of conception after 1 year of unprotected regular intercourse, by which time 85 per cent of couples attempting to conceive will have been successful. Intercourse should occur 2–3 times in the week prior to ovulation, as the oocyte (egg) will only be capable of fertilisation for 24 hours but the sperm will retain potency for up to 72 hours. Intercourse prior to the day of ovulation also encourages remodelling of the endometrial lining, making implantation more likely.

Primary infertility is defined as when a couple has not had a pregnancy together, although one or both might have had a pregnancy in another relationship. *Secondary infertility* is when the couple has had at least one pregnancy together, irrespective of the outcome.

Early assessment (<12 months infertility) should be considered in the following situations:

■ the woman has a history of irregular menstrual cycles (oligomenorrhoea or amenorrhoea);
■ the woman has a known or suspected history of pelvic pathology, such as tubal disease or endometriosis;
■ the man has known or suspected reproductive tract pathology, such as a history of an undescended testis;

- the couple present because they have not conceived as quickly as they had expected;
- a couple are in their 30s, as increased age affects their chance of conceiving. Therefore, if the woman is aged 35 years or older and/or the man is aged 40 years or older, then investigations are recommended to start after only 6 months of attempting to conceive.

Some of the distress associated with fertility problems can be reduced by prompt investigation and providing appropriate factual information, if a problem exists. It is important to emphasise that establishing a diagnosis or cause of the infertility does not commit the couple to any further management.

For a couple to conceive normally, the following are required:

- the woman needs to produce and release a mature, healthy egg (oocyte) on a regular basis (ovulation);
- the man needs to have a certain number of normally shaped, healthy, motile sperm in his ejaculate with a sperm DNA fragmentation rate below 20 per cent;
- the egg and sperm need to be able to get together (i.e. there is no tubal disease, sperm antibodies or sexual dysfunction);
- the embryo needs to be able to hatch out and implant without interference (i.e. there are no intrauterine adhesions, submucosal fibroids or hydrosalpinges);
- the couple have avoided lifestyle factors that may affect egg and/or sperm quality.

As fertility is a 'couple issue', it is not uncommon for more than one pathology to be affecting their likelihood of conceiving.

The causes of infertility are classified in Box 1.

■ Female factors

If a couple presents for fertility investigations, the woman should also have her rubella status checked, so if immunisation is required, it will not significantly delay any treatment, as conception is not recommended within 1 month of vaccination.

Ovulation disorders

Ovulation disorders are present in more than 25 per cent of women with fertility problems. They

---

Box 1 Classification of causes of infertility

Female factors
- Ovulation disorders
- Tubal pathology
- Uterine pathology
- Endometriosis
- Antibodies to sperm
- Age

Male factors
- Sperm-production problems
- Azoospermia (no sperm in the ejaculate)
- Sperm DNA fragmentation
- Antibodies to sperm
- Sexual problems
- Hormonal problems
- Age

Lifestyle factors
- Smoking
- Increased weight – raised body mass index (BMI)
- Increased alcohol intake
- Increased caffeine intake
- Recreational drugs (marijuana decreases sperm count) and anabolic steroids

Unexplained infertility

---

range from amenorrhoea (see Menstrual periods, absent) through oligomenorrhoea (see Menstrual periods, infrequent) to irregular cycles. The majority of these women have polycystic ovary syndrome (PCOS). The initial diagnosis is made by taking a history about the regularity of the menstrual cycle length and taking blood for a serum progesterone level in the mid-luteal phase (1 week, i.e. 7 days, prior to when menstruation is expected to commence). A serum progesterone level of >30 nmol/L is consistent with a normal ovulatory cycle. Basal body temperature charts are not helpful and should be avoided, particularly as they can increase the woman's stress, thereby exacerbating any ovulatory disorder.

Polycystic ovaries

Polycystic ovaries, which occur in one in five women, can be diagnosed by ultrasound scanning. Box 1 in Hirutism/virilism shows the 2003 consensus statement on the diagnosis of polycystic ovaries, which can be made on transvaginal ultrasound scan alone, and polycystic ovary syndrome, which occurs in one in ten women. The investigations for the assessment and management of hirsutism, which is associated with hyperandrogenic conditions causing infertility, are dealt with in Hirutism/virilism.

If the woman has a history or physical signs consistent with increased insulin levels – a family history of late-onset diabetes, body mass index (BMI) >30 or acanthosis nigricans (a grey-brown velvety discoloration of the skin found at the neck, groin, axillae and vulva) – a 2-hour glucose tolerance test should also be done.

Weight gain or loss

Weight gain or loss also results in ovulatory disorders. If a woman has polycystic ovaries and her BMI increases, she is more likely to develop or exacerbate the PCOS, although this may be reversed by a weight loss of only 5–7 kg.

A woman with a BMI of <18 will often become anovulatory (i.e. does not release oocytes).

Hyperprolactinaema

Hyperprolactinaema (prolactin >1000 IU/L) as a consequence of a pituitary adenoma, results in anovulation and is associated with galactorrhoea in 30–50 per cent of cases. It may be diagnosed clinically with changes in the visual field, but is more likely on imaging using magnetic resonance imaging or computerised tomography of the pituitary fossa. However, the prolactin levels should be repeated initially to confirm the raised concentration, as stress alone can increase levels. Moderately raised prolactin levels are present in 15 per cent of women with PCOS.

Hypothyroidism should be excluded by checking thyroid-stimulating hormone levels.

Ovarian failure

Ovarian failure needs to be considered if there is a history of anovulation for some months, particularly if there is a family history of early or premature (<40 years of age) menopause. It can be diagnosed by a raised serum level of follicle-stimulating hormone (>20 IU/L) and low serum oestrogen level on more than one occasion.

Tubal pathology

Damaged Fallopian tubes are present in 10 per cent of women with fertility problems who have never been pregnant and in 20 per cent of those who have, irrespective of the outcome of the pregnancy. It is uncommon for a woman to be aware she has had a pelvic infection unless it is related to an infection following pregnancy. Tubal disease should always be suspected in women with a history of secondary infertility, particularly if there has been a previous history of retained products of conception.

Diagnosis can be made by watching passage of fluid through the Fallopian tubes using X-ray (hysterosalpingogram; HSG) or ultrasound technology (hysterosalpingo-contrast sonography; Hy-Co-Sy), or laparoscopy and dye studies (Figs 1 and 2).

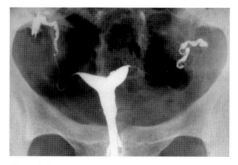

Figure 1 Normal hysterosalpingogram showing passage of contrast through the Fallopian tubes.

If a hydrosalpinx is present it can be visualised on a pelvic ultrasound. A history of an ectopic pregnancy is also suggestive of bilateral tubal damage. It is important to remember that a normal HSG or Hy-Co-Sy does not guarantee normal Fallopian tubes. They can only show tubal patency and an internal silhouette of the tubes, but will not reflect damage to the lining cilia of the tubes, which alters their function to waft the fertilised egg to the uterine cavity.

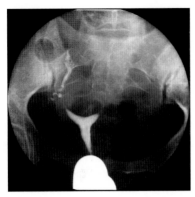

Figure 2 Hysterosalpingogram showing left tubal blockage at cornua.

Laparoscopy and dye studies are the only absolute way to assess if a woman has damage to the tubes that impairs the passage of sperm or an embryo, or external adhesions that compromise the function of the fimbrial ends as well as movement of the Fallopian tube (Fig. 3). Similarly, proximal occlusion at HSG or Hy-Co-Sy may be due to cornual spasm, which does not occur under general anaesthesia for laparoscopy. At laparoscopy, it is very important that a good cervical seal is made for the dye studies. Often a Spackman catheter is insufficient and a Leach–Wilkinson catheter is required.

If pelvic infection is suspected, *Chlamydia* testing should also be performed and the tubal investigations carried out under antibiotic cover to avoid reactivation of disease.

Laparoscopy also enables the diagnosis and treatment of unsuspected endometriosis at the same procedure.

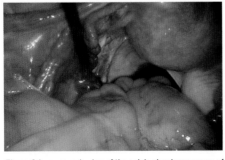

Figure 3 Laparoscopic view of the pelvis showing passage of dye through normal Fallopian tubes.

Uterine pathology

Uterine pathology should be detected at the same time as the tubal assessment and may require hysteroscopy. Types of pathology encountered include polyps, uterine fibroids, uterine septa and occasionally Asherman's syndrome (intrauterine adhesions – most likely occurring after a curettage for previous retained products of conception.)

Endometriosis

Endometriosis is found in up to 30 per cent of women with fertility problems, particularly if the woman is in her 30s. It is reported that it takes 8–11 years from the time a woman first presents to a doctor with symptoms before a diagnosis is made. However, a likely diagnosis can be made on history alone in many cases. The following factors may point to a diagnosis of endometriosis in an infertile woman:

- family history of endometriosis;
- if the woman complains of 'old blood' or brown premenstrual spotting, and/or pain with menstruation, especially if it starts several days before menstrual flow and these are symptoms that have developed over time, rather than being present since her teenage years;
- increased lifetime history of menstruation, i.e. early menarche, shorter menstrual cycles, prolonged or heavier periods, few or no pregnancies, minimal or no use of hormonal contraception;
- history of deep dyspareunia;
- if no other cause for the couple's fertility problem can be found, there is a strong likelihood that the woman has endometriosis.

It is important to remember that a third of women with endometriosis have no pain with their periods and only one in eight will have an endometrioma visible on pelvic ultrasound. Therefore, in the majority of cases, diagnosis can only be made by laparoscopy, but that does enable surgical removal to occur at the same operation, with histology confirming the diagnosis of endometrial glands in the biopsies. If there is ureteric and/or bowel involvement at laparoscopy, having made the diagnosis, referral to a laparoscopic specialist should be undertaken.

Table 1 Interpreting the results of investigation of female partners

Test	Result	Interpretation
Progesterone	<30 nmol/L	Anovulation: but check cycle length and timing correct in mid-luteal phase; complete other endocrine tests; scan for polycystic ovaries – glucose tolerance test if obese; advise weight gain or loss; may need ovulation induction; clomifene should not be started without tubal patency test
	10–30 nmol/L	Likely ovulation, but timing of test incorrect
Follicle-stimulating hormone	>10 IU/L	Reduced ovarian reserve: may respond poorly to ovulation induction
	>20 IU/L	May need egg donation
Luteinising hormone	>10 IU/L	May be polycystic ovaries: ultrasonography to confirm
	>5 nmol/L	Congenital adrenal hyperplasia: check 17-OHP and DHEAS
Testosterone	>2.5 nmol/L	May be polycystic ovaries: ultrasonography to confirm
	>5 nmol/L	Congenital adrenal hyperplasia: check 17-OHP and DHEAS
Prolactin	>1000 IU/L	May be pituitary adenoma: repeat prolactin to confirm raised concentration; exclude hypothyroidism; arrange magnetic resonance image or computerised tomography of pituitary gland; if confirmed hyperprolactinaemia, start dopamine agonist
Rubella	Non-immune	Offer immunisation and 1 month of contraception
HSG or HyCoSy	Abnormal	May be tubal factor: arrange laparoscopy and dye test to evaluate further May be intrauterine abnormality, e.g. fibroid or adhesions: evaluate further by hysteroscopy
Laparoscopy and dye	Blocked tubes	Tubal factor confirmed: possibly suitable for surgery or *in-vitro* fertilisation (decision also depends on semen quality and couple's age)
	Endometriosis	Assess severity: may benefit from surgical excision; medical suppression not helpful for fertility; may need *in-vitro* fertilisation after excision

DHEAS, dihydroepiandrosterone sulphate; HSG, hysterosalpingogram; Hy-Co-Sy, hysterosalpingo-contrast sonography; 17-OHP, 17-hydroxyprogesterone

Antibodies to sperm

Up to 6 per cent of women can develop antibodies to sperm over time, which impair sperm function and transport in the woman's reproductive tract. It is unclear, as sperm are foreign to all women, why most sexually active women avoid producing antisperm antibodies.

Age

It is important to remember that it is not just the woman's age that affects a couple's chances of conceiving. Although it is known a woman's fertility decreases with age, particularly after the age of 35 years, it is also important to remember that a woman in her late 30s is likely to be partnered with a man of a similar age or older. If a woman in her mid to late 30s is trying to conceive with a partner 5 years older than herself, she has half the chance of conceiving each month compared to a woman whose partner is the same age or younger.

A good guide to timing of reduced ovarian reserve is to ascertain the age of menopause of the woman's mother or any older sisters. An ultrasound scan to assess the number of antral follicles present (>6) at one time and absence of any reduction in ovarian size is a good indicator of normal ovarian reserve.

Table 1 covers the investigations and their interpretations for female fertility factors.

Box 2 Known causes of male infertility

Sperm production problems

- Chromosomal or genetic causes
- Undescended testes (failure of the testes to descend at birth)
- Infections
- Torsion (twisting of the testes in the scrotum)
- Heat
- Varicocoele
- Drugs and chemicals
- Radiation damage
- Unknown cause

Blockage of sperm transport (azoospermia; see Table 2)

Sperm DNA damage or fragmentation

- Male age >40 years
- Long periods of abstinence
- Lifestyle factors (e.g. smoking, alcohol, poor diet, medications)

Sperm antibodies

- Vasectomy
- Injury or infection in the epididymis
- Unknown cause

Sexual problems (erection and ejaculation problems)

- Retrograde and premature ejaculation
- Failure of ejaculation
- Infrequent intercourse
- Spinal cord injury
- Prostate surgery
- Damage to nerves
- Some medicines, such as antihypertensives

Hormonal problems

- Pituitary tumours (hyperprolactinaemia)
- Congenital lack of LH/FSH (pituitary problem from birth)
- Anabolic (androgenic) steroid abuse

Male age

- >40 years
- Lifestyle factors (e.g. smoking, alcohol, poor diet and medications) exacerbate the problem

---

FSH, follicle-stimulating hormone; LH, luteinising hormone.

Table 2 Blockage of sperm transport

Cause	Obstructive	Non-obstructive	Hypothalamic–pituitary
	Post-testicular	Testicular	
Congenital	Cystic fibrosis or cystic fibrosis carrier, Müllerian cysts	Genetic causes, cryptorchidism, anorchia, Sertoli cell only	Kallmann's syndrome, isolated FSH deficiency
Acquired	Sexually transmitted diseases (gonorrhoea, *Chlamydia*), tuberculosis, prostatitis, vasectomy	Radiotherapy, chemotherapy, orchitis, trauma, torsion	Craniopharyngioma, pituitary tumour or ablation, anabolic steroid use, hyperprolactinaemia
Testicular size	Normal	Small, atrophic	Small, prepubertal
FSH	Normal	Raised	Low
Testosterone	Normal	Low	Low

FSH, follicle-stimulating hormone.

Male factors

The known causes of male infertility are outlined in Box 2 and Table 2. A total of 40–50 per cent of couples with fertility problems will have a male factor contributing to their infertility. The most common are sperm production problems; therefore, a semen analysis is the first step in assessing a man's fertility.

Table 3 outlines a normal semen analysis. The period of abstinence prior to the sample should be no longer than 3 days, otherwise abnormal morphology and DNA fragmentation rates can rise, if the sperm have been sitting in the epididymis too long. This is in contrast to advice given only a few years ago to increase periods of abstinence in the hopes of increasing the sperm count. The number of normal, functioning sperm is now recognised as a more important indicator of a man's fertility than the total number per ejaculate. If a man has a

Table 3 A normal semen analysis[a]

Parameter	Normal	Abnormal
Volume	2–5 mL	If volume is low, check the collection was complete. The majority of sperm are in the first part of the ejaculate
Count	$20–250 \times 10^6$/mL	Repeat sample. Check no acute illness has occurred in the 2 months before the sample was taken. If total count $<5 \times 10^6$, consider testing for chromosomes and Y chromosome deletions
Motility	>25% rapidly	If reduced, check the time between ejaculation and assessing of progressive sample is <1.5 hours. Repeat the sample and check lifestyle factors
Morphology	>15% normal shape	A very important parameter. Even if there are sufficient motile sperm, if they do not have a shape that gives 'the key to the door' of the egg, the couple can have fertility problems. Repeat the sample, and check lifestyle factors and abstinence
Sperm antibodies	<50% binding	Prevalence in the general population cannot be estimated; 50–70% of men with vas deferens obstruction (surgical or congenital) are positive
DNA fragmentation	<20%	Increased fragmentation does not affect fertilisation but does result in decreased pregnancy and increased miscarriage rates. Specialised assays (TUNEL or SCSA) are required

[a]If an assay is not available, advise men >39 years, plus those that smoke, take marijuana, drink alcohol and/or caffeine heavily, or have a poor diet to take antioxidant supplements (vitamin E and C 1000 mg/day plus a good-quality multivitamin/mineral tablet).

reduced number of sperm in his ejaculate, it is called oligospermia, as opposed to a complete absence of sperm in the ejaculate, which is azoospermia.

A man's age is important to take into account in fertility assessments, as even in a *in-vitro* fertilisation (IVF) treatment setting, if a man is aged 40 years or greater, his partner's chance of conceiving can be half that compared to if the man was in his 30s.

Just because a man has fathered a pregnancy in the past does not mean he can be excluded from investigations. Men's fertility, as well as women's, changes over time, and unless DNA testing has been done, it is only an assumption that he is the father of any previous pregnancies. Studies have shown that, on average, 10 per cent of children have not been fathered by the person named on the birth certificate.

■ Lifestyle factors

Lifestyle factors play a significant part in a couple's chance of conceiving and having an ongoing healthy pregnancy.

It is estimated that smoking alone causes 13 per cent of fertility problems. For women, it reduces the chance of conceiving each month 2–3 times and doubles the risk of miscarriage. Men who smoke increase sperm DNA fragmentation rates and increase the risk of the resulting child developing cancer in childhood by four times. Studies have also shown passive smoking decreases a woman's chance of conceiving to a similar level as if she was a smoker herself.

Increased weight affects both male and female fertility. An increase of just 9 kg has been reported as significantly reducing a man's fertility. If a woman's BMI rises to just 27 she is three times more likely to have ovulatory problems. However, a loss of just 5–7 kg can reverse ovulatory and miscarriage problems (normal BMI is 18–25).

The evidence for alcohol affecting fertility is less secure. However, woman should drink a maximum of three drinks/units a week (not in the same night) and men can average ten drinks/units a week, provided there is no binge drinking.

Studies have shown that women who consume more than 100 mg of caffeine a day (one cup of percolated coffee or two instant) can halve their chance of conceiving and double their risk of miscarriage in that month. Information is less certain in relation to male fertility, so 'all things in moderation' is the best advice.

Recreational drugs, such as marijuana, have an impact on sperm, the chances of conception and sexual function, and should be avoided. Anabolic steroids can render a man azoospermic or a woman anovular. Depending on the dose and length of use, these changes are not always reversible, so once again they should be avoided or stopped.

■ Unexplained infertility

Unexplained infertility is a diagnosis of exclusion, i.e. all the above investigations or lifestyle factors are normal. It can occur in up to 25 per cent of couples. It does not mean there is no cause for the couple's infertility, only that the cause has not been found in the investigations available. For example, a woman with abnormal oocytes would only have that diagnosis made if she proceeded to an IVF treatment cycle. Similarly, if the sperm were unable to penetrate the shell of the egg (zona pellucida) and fertilisation it, this diagnosis could only be made at the time of an IVF treatment cycle.

It is important to reassure a couple that all fertility problems can potentially be solved with current fertility treatments. It is the man's sperm and the woman's Fallopian tubes that will most determine their choices. If eggs and/or sperm are absent, then a pregnancy is still possible with the use of donor gametes. If the uterus is absent, surrogacy is possible.

Finally, most couples want a family rather than one child. Therefore, the couple's age in relation to the last pregnancy should be taken into account when considering the timing of investigations and/or referral to a specialist centre.

INTRAUTERINE FETAL DEATH AND MID-TRIMESTER PREGNANCY LOSS

Nigel Bickerton

In the UK, intrauterine fetal death (IUFD) is defined as fetal death after 24 weeks' gestation. Any fetal loss before that time is classed as a miscarriage.

The Confidential Enquiry into Maternal and Child Health defines stillbirth as an *in-utero* death delivering after the 24th week of pregnancy, and defines late fetal loss as an *in-utero* death delivering between 20 weeks and 23 weeks 6 days of gestation. Using this classification, in the UK in 2003, there were 642 899 live births, 2764 late fetal losses and 3730 stillbirths, giving a stillbirth rate of 5.77 per 1000 live births and stillbirths.

In the USA, the 2003 revision of the Procedures for Coding Cause of Fetal Death under ICD-10, the National Center for Health Statistics classifies fetal death as:

- early – <20 weeks' gestation;
- intermediate – 20–27 weeks' gestation;
- late – >27 weeks' gestation.

Individual states within the USA in the past have used different interpretations of late fetal loss, making national data difficult to interpret.

The World Health Organization recommends that fetal death data should exclude fetuses weighing less than 500 g from stillbirth data. It follows that there are discrepancies when comparing the fetal loss rates between different countries.

Perinatal death (stillbirth and neonatal death) occurs in 1 per cent of pregnancies in the USA. It is estimated that 10–25 per cent of pregnancies end before 28 weeks. Fetal death before the onset of labour may be diagnosed when the mother stops feeling fetal movements or the symptoms of pregnancy subside, the former being the commonest presentation. The obstetrician or midwife is unable to hear fetal heart

tones either by stethoscope or by Doppler. However, ultrasound scanning by an experienced practitioner remains the gold standard for diagnosis, as mistakes can be made through auscultation alone (Fig. 1).

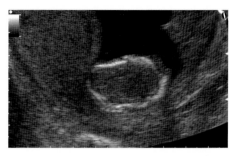

Figure 1 Ultrasound scan of Spalding's sign (overlapping of fetal skull bones), diagnostic of intrauterine fetal death.

The pregnant woman may have no other symptoms, the diagnosis being made at a routine antenatal clinic visit. On the other hand, the woman may have noted an absence of fetal activity with abdominal pain, as in placental abruption, or she may be brought in to a hospital emergency unit following a road-traffic accident or gunshot/shrapnel injury. With such different presentations, it is important that the attending clinician considers the whole clinical picture and calls upon the skills of other professionals, as the case requires.

When fetal death is suspected during labour, the diagnosis should be confirmed by ultrasound scan. A possible diagnostic pitfall is to apply a fetal scalp electrode after loss of the fetal heart tones through an abdominal recorder. Maternal cardiac electrical activity may be conducted through the dead fetus. This can lead to misdiagnosis and unnecessary Caesarean section.

General risk factors for fetal death include:

- maternal age – both teenage and over 35 years;
- single parent status;
- multiple pregnancy;
- high multiparity;
- a fetal presentation other than cephalic;
- prematurity.

■ History

A history is not always helpful in pointing to the cause of a fetal death. Emotionally, this is a very distressing time for the woman and so history-taking may be difficult, if she knows the baby is already dead. Aspects specific to the patient and/or the pregnancy may help with the diagnosis.

Aspects specific to the pregnancy include:

■ a history of pain;
■ a history of bleeding;
■ concerns from previous ultrasound scans, e.g. growth restriction;
■ possible fluid leakage (premature membrane rupture);
■ fetal number, i.e. gestational order and also multiple pregnancy.

Multiple pregnancy carries a greater risk than singleton pregnancy of IUFD. In the UK, the increased risk is 3.5-fold. Sometimes one twin dies whilst the other remains alive. The risk of the living twin dying depends on the chorionicity, being far higher in monochorionic twins.

Aspects specific to the patient include:

■ pre-existing medical conditions. including diabetes, hypertension, renal disease, thromboembolic disease and thrombophilia;
■ recent physical symptoms, including itching suggestive of cholestasis;
■ recent exposure to any infectious illnesses, e.g. malaria, toxoplasmosis and parvovirus;
■ any recent use of any prescribed or recreational drugs;
■ the possibility of trauma, including road accidents or domestic violence. The history of domestic violence may only be revealed when the woman feels comfortable with disclosing it.

■ Examination

General examination of the woman should include vital signs to exclude sepsis, shock from bleeding and to look for signs of pre-eclampsia. Urine testing for proteinuria is essential (see Proteinuria in pregnancy).

Abdominal examination may be unremarkable or may reveal the signs of placental abruption or reveal local signs of maternal injury implicating uterine injury. After excluding a major placenta praevia, vaginal examination may show signs of bleeding or septic discharge. Appropriate bacteriology swabs should be taken during examination.

In the UK, once an IUFD has been diagnosed, the majority of women opt to have active management to end the pregnancy. Of those who opt for conservative management, 80 per cent will commence spontaneous labour within 2 weeks of fetal death.

The question of investigations to find the cause of IUFD should be explored, especially around postmortem, before delivery. This includes examination of the fetus and placenta. The acceptance of full fetal autopsy by parents is variable according to geography and culture. Some will opt for a more limited external fetal examination with an X-ray, together with placental examination.

Pregnancy is arbitrarily divided into trimesters, athough it is really a continuum. It has been said that the common causes for fetal loss in the first trimester are genetic, infective in the second and placental/cord accident in the third. However, this is by no means invariable. Fetal death in the second and third trimester can be due to a single cause or a multifactorial, and may be acute, subacute or chronic in onset.

■ Causes of fetal death

In many cases, the underlying cause may not be diagnosed. Fetomaternal haemorrhage of an amount to cause fetal death has been reported in about 10 per cent of otherwise unexplained cases.

Acute

■ Placental abruption (see Bleeding in late pregnancy).
■ Umbilical cord accidents and pathology. Umbilical cord pathology has recently been recognized to play a part in a proportion of IUFDs (about 10 per cent in one study). There is an association between

hypercoiling (more than one coil of cord per 5 cm) and cord thinning, leading to constriction and mal-perfusion of the fetus. This is known as thin cord syndrome. Careful cord examination in IUFD may reduce the proportion of unexplained cases of fetal death.

■ Trauma, including road accidents, gunshot, blast or shrapnel injury – anything causing maternal shock or hypoperfusion of the uteroplacental unit. The associated cause will present with wide geographical variations.

■ Burns – these injuries bring about significant morbidity and mortality in developing countries. The risk of fetal death is linked with the total body surface area affected by burns, which in turn may be related to impaired uteroplacental circulation caused by severe and acute maternal body fluid loss.

Subacute

■ Cervical incompetence – mid-trimester pregnancy loss has been strongly linked with cervical incompetence. Cervical cerclage has been used widely throughout the world in women whose previous pregnancy loss was attributed to cervical incompetence. Recently the place of cervical cerclage has been questioned. A recent Cochrane review found no conclusive evidence about the benefit of cerclage for all women. It would appear that cerclage might benefit women at very high risk of second trimester miscarriage due to a cervical factor. The difficulty is in identifying those women who would benefit from treatment; therefore, some women may receive unnecessary treatment.

■ Infections due to *E. coli*, *Listeria monocytogenes*, Group B streptococcus, *Ureaplasma urealyticum*.

■ Parvovirus B19, cytomegalovirus (CMV), Coxsackie virus and toxoplasmosis. Swedish investigators recommend polymerase chain reaction studies of placental and fetal tissue for parvovirus B19 DNA, CMV DNA and enterovirus RNA. This is deemed important, as many women with viral infection-associated IUFD have no clinical signs of infection during pregnancy.

■ Malaria – in malaria endemic areas the diagnosis of malaria-induced fetal death will feature highly.

■ Maternal infections.

Chronic

■ Congenital malformations; as a group, this is a major determinant of perinatal mortality.

■ Premature rupture of fetal membranes and infection. In the mid-trimester, the leading cause of IUFD is amnion infection, followed by placental separation and placental insufficiency.

■ Intrauterine growth restriction.

■ Maternal diabetes.

■ Chronic maternal hypertension (see Blood pressure problems in pregnancy).

■ Pre-eclampsia (see Blood pressure problems in pregnancy).

■ Thrombophilias – third trimester IUFDs have a significant association with thrombophilias, particularly prothrombin mutation and protein S deficiency. Therefore, a full thrombophilia assessment is indicated for all women who suffer a third-trimester fetal death.

The loss of a pregnancy at any stage can be devastating to the mother and her partner, causing all the phases of the bereavement reaction. Their major concerns are around whether they could have done anything to cause or prevent the loss, and whether this will happen again in a subsequent pregnancy. In order to give the best advice to women about the cause of fetal death and the possible implications on future pregnancy, the clinician requires a test protocol that is extensive and at the same time suitable for the patient population.

■ Investigations

The investigations of IUFD will depend upon the resources available locally, but they may include the following.

For fetoplacental causes

■ Karyotype from either amniotic fluid, fetal blood sample or skin biopsy.

■ External examination of the fetus.

- X-ray of fetus.
- Magnetic resonance scan of the fetus.
- Infection screen from either fetal blood sample, fetal or placental swabs, or maternal serology including syphilis, *Toxoplasma*, parvovirus (maternal B19, IgM and IgG levels), rubella and cytomegalovirus. Some of these tests will have been undertaken early in the pregnancy and so may not need repeating. There is debate about the cost effectiveness of some of this serological screening (e.g. Herpes simplex virus) and it may need to be decided by any appropriate history.
- Fetal and placental pathological examination, both grossly and microscopically.

Maternal tests

Blood tests should include:

- full blood count;
- Kleihauer–Betke blood stain looking for fetomaternal transfusion;
- rhesus antibody status;
- clotting screen (see Bleeding disorders in pregnancy);
- lupus anticoagulant;
- anticardiolipins;
- thrombophilia screening;
- biochemistry, including urea and electrolytes, liver function tests, glucose and HbA_{1c} levels.

Despite extensive investigation, one-quarter to one-third of cases of IUFD will remain unexplained. It is wise to warn the woman of this possibility when the investigations are commenced, especially the postmortem examination. In the vast majority of cases, the risk of a similar event in a subsequent pregnancy is small. The woman should be reassured that she could try for a pregnancy when she and her partner feel emotionally ready to embark on another one. It is always worthwhile to warn the couple that the time of the expected delivery could possibly be emotionally difficult for them.

■ Useful website

www.sands.org.uk

ITCHING IN PREGNANCY (SEE ALSO Rashes in pregnancy)

Anthony Bewley

■ Itching related to pregnancy

As so often in medicine, the diagnosis, when a patient presents with itching (pruritus) during pregnancy, can frequently be made from taking a history and careful examination. Investigations are rarely required. The differential diagnosis (Table 1) is made up of causes specific to and causes unrelated to pregnancy.

Table 1 Common causes of itching in pregnancy

Itching related to pregnancy	Itching unrelated to pregnancy
Rashes in pregnancy[a]	**Rashes from skin disease**
Polymorphic eruption of pregnancy	Atopic eczema
Pemphigoid gestationalis	Eczema (other causes; e.g. contact)
Prurigo of pregnancy	Psoriasis
Pruritic folliculitis of pregnancy	Xerosis (dry skin)
	Lichen planus
	Pityriasis rosea
	Urticaria
Rashes from metabolic changes of pregnancy	**Metabolic causes**
Hyperthyroidism/ hypothyroidism[b]	Hyperthyroidism/ hypothyroidism
Cholestasis[c]	Liver disease
Renal impairment	Renal impairment
Iron deficiency	Iron deficiency
	Other causes
	Scabies and infestations
	Tinea (fungal skin disease)
	HIV-related skin disease
	Localised itching
	Vulval itch[d]

[a]See Rashes in pregnancy.
[b]See Thyroid problems in pregnancy.
[c]See Jaundice and liver disease in pregnancy.
[d]See Vulval itching.

Rashes specific to pregnancy (most of which are intensely itchy) usually follow specific patterns and are discussed in Rashes in pregnancy. Both hyperthyroidism and hypothyroidism (Thyroid problems in pregnancy) may lead to itching as a primary presenting complaint; and cholestasis (Jaundice and liver disease in pregnancy) is a common cause of itching during pregnancy. Renal impairment may be exacerbated by pregnancy and iron deficiency (from poor nutrition or multiple successive pregnancies) may also present as itching.

Itching unrelated to pregnancy

A patient's pre-existing dermatological disease may improve or deteriorate during pregnancy. Most patients with pre-existing skin disease can identify the cause of their itching, or else can identify others within their family who have similar conditions.

Atopic eczema (Fig. 1) is intensely itchy and so is characterised by excoriations (scratch marks), thickening (from rubbing the skin), pigmentation changes, oozing and scaling of, usually, flexural skin. Patients with eczema may also have hay fever, perennial conjunctivitis and asthma.

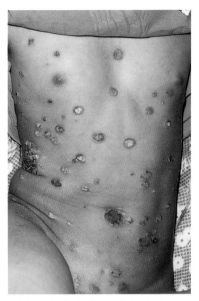

Figure 2 Psoriasis. Scaly plaques, but note that some are excoriated indicating pruritus.

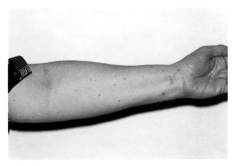

Figure 3 Lichen planus (classical); note the flat-topped, polygonal, violaceous (purple) papules affecting the flexures.

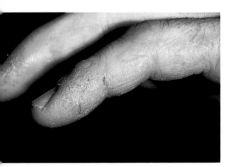

Figure 1 Atopic eczema; note fissuring and thickening (lichenification) of the skin.

Psoriasis (Fig. 2) usually presents as scaly, well-demarcated plaques affecting the extensors. Many patients with psoriasis also have nail, scalp and genital (see Vulval itching) disease.

Lichen planus (Fig. 3) is a self-limiting disease, so, unlike eczema and psoriasis, the patient

usually presents *de novo* with characteristic purplish, polygonal flat-topped papules affecting the anterior surfaces (especially the wrists). About 30 per cent of patients will have oral lichen planus.

Pityriasis rosea, appears to be more common in pregnancy. It certainly affects young adults. It is the *herald patch* (a scaly, often annular patch, usually found on the abdomen or back, usually pre-dating the main rash) that is so helpful in ascertaining the diagnosis. The smaller, scaly, ovoid macules, which form a 'Christmas tree' pattern on abdomen, chest and back, appear a few days after the herald patch. The rash of pityriasis rosea rarely extends below the knees and elbows, and rarely affects the head.

Scabies (Fig. 4) is usually sexually transmitted in adults. It is characterised by curvilinear, intensely itchy burrows. The total mite population of an infested individual is surprisingly small (often just 20 mites). Burrows often affect the hand's web spaces, the genital and periareolar skin. If scabies is suspected, take a look at the patient's partner, as similar lesions may help to make the diagnosis.

Tinea (Fig. 5) (ringworm) is characterised by an annular rash, which often has small

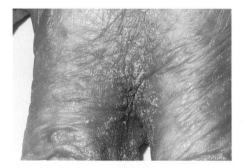

Figure 4. Scabies; note scaling adjacent to curvilinear papules affecting the hand web spaces.

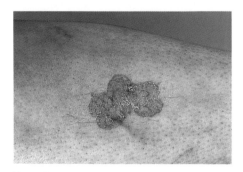

Figure 5. Tinea corporis. The scaly edge of this lesion has small studded pustules. This lesion had been mistakenly treated with steroids (tinea incognito), hence the atrophy.

pustules and scaling at the edge of individual ring-shaped lesions. Scraping of the edge may show fungal hyphae, and culture of the scrapings may identify causative organisms. Topical treatments only are safest during pregnancy.

Chickenpox (varicella) is uncommon in pregnancy but, when a patient presents with chickenpox in pregnancy, it is important to recognise the condition, as transplacental spread of the virus may lead to fetal varicella syndrome. Chickenpox presents initially as 'tear drops on a rose petal' vesicles. The often intensely itchy lesions spread centripetally and usually involve mucosal membranes.

Use of zoster immune globulin (ZIG) with in 24 hours of the infection may be used at various stages of the pregnancy according to national/local guidelines (in the UK, see www.rcog.org.uk). ZIG may be used when a non-zoster-immune pregnant woman comes into contact with chickenpox or shingles, or when a neonate is exposed around the puerperium. Aciclovir, although not licensed during pregnancy, is thought to be safe, and is frequently used to treat pregnant women who develop chickenpox or shingles during pregnancy.

Finally HIV-related skin disease is often itchy. The virus itself can lead to various, very itchy inflammatory dermatoses. Medication for HIV commonly leads to skin rashes, many of which are itchy and, of course, skin disease associated with opportunistic infections is more common in HIV-infected individuals.

◼ Management of itching in pregnancy

Management of itching in pregnancy is limited and follows a stepwise pattern (Box 1). Management of specific dermatological problems may involve specific treatments together with advice from the local dermatology department. Primarily dermatological conditions such as eczema and psoriasis (which are frequently itchy despite what the textbooks say) may require ongoing treatment with topical steroids. When advocating topical steroids, it is advisable to prescribe ointments, to keep to the lowest strength possible (no stronger than betamethasone 0.1 per cent on the body and hydrocortisone 1 per cent on the face), and to use steroids for pulses of no longer than 6 weeks. Topical steroids are treatment for inflammation (although cessation of inflammation means cessation of itch) and so should be stopped as soon as the disease improves.

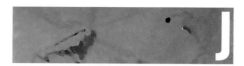

JAUNDICE AND LIVER DISEASE IN PREGNANCY

Margaret Myszor

Liver diseases in pregnancy include:

- those present at conception;
- those that occur coincidentally;
- those that occur as a result of pregnancy

Functions of the normal liver are:

- production of plasma proteins (albumin, coagulation factors, globulins);
- metabolism of amino acids, carbohydrates and lipids;
- metabolism and excretion of bilirubin and cholesterol;
- biotransformation of drugs and toxins.

A list of liver function tests (LFTs) in the non-pregnant state is shown in Table 1.

Box 1 Management of itching in pregnancy

- Emollients (into the bath or on to the skin)
- Bath additives containing lauromacrogols (e.g. Balneum Plus®or oat extract (e.g. Aveeno® may be additionally antipruritic
- Topical emollients range from very watery (e.g. aqueous cream) to very greasy (e.g. white soft paraffin). Let the patient decide which is best
- Avoidance of soaps and detergents. Use soap substitutes (e.g. aqueous cream)
- Non-sedating antihistamines (e.g. loratidine) are usually not licensed for pregnancy but are probably safe
- Sedating antihistamines (e.g. chlorpheniramine) have been used safely in pregnancy
- Topical steroid ointments (rather than creams) are probably safe (although not licensed) in pregnancy. Try to keep to the lowest strength possible for no longer than 6 weeks
- (Rarely) Phototherapy (usually narrow-band ultra-violet B)

Table 1 Liver function tests in the non-pregnant state. (NB No single test can quantify liver function as a panel of tests is needed to help) The following are serum blood tests

Serum level	Cause
AST (aspartate aminotransferase) ↑	Liver cell injury or necrosis
ALT (alanine aminotransferase) ↑	
Albumin ↓	
Prothrombin time (INR) ↑	Reduced liver synthetic function
ALP (alkaline phosphatase) ↑	Cholestasis or biliary obstruction
Bilirubin ↑	Cholestasis, biliary obstruction or haemolysis

↑, increased; ↓, decreased; INR, international normalised ratio.

◼ History

If liver disease is suspected, the most important factor is to determine the gestational age of the pregnancy, as the differential diagnoses change with the stage of the pregnancy (Table 2). However, taking a careful history that includes a drug history is vitally important. Most women minimise the use of prescribed and over-the-counter medication whilst pregnant, but there is a general increase in the use of alternative and herbal remedies, some of which can be associated with abnormal liver function. A history of intravenous drug use or alcohol abuse will make certain forms of liver disease much more likely. If there are abnormal LFTs, then it is important to determine whether this was also the case in any previous pregnancies, as both intrahepatic cholestasis and acute fatty liver of pregnancy can recur.

Table 2 Differential diagnosis of abnormal liver function tests or jaundice in pregnancy

Trimester	Differential diagnosis
First	Hyperemesis gravidarum
	Drug-induced hepatitis
	Gallstones
	Viral hepatitis
Second	Intrahepatic cholestasis of pregnancy
	Gallstones
	Viral hepatitis
	Drug-induced hepatitis
Third	Intrahepatic cholestasis of pregnancy
	Pre-eclampsia/eclampsia
	HELLP syndrome
	Acute fatty liver of pregnancy
	Hepatic rupture
	Gallstones
	Viral hepatitis
	Drug-induced hepatitis

HELLP, haemolysis, elevated liver enzymes and low platelets.

Clinical features that can be elicited from the history include pruritus (itch). In intrahepatic cholestasis of pregnancy, pruritus initially affects predominantly the hands and feet, but will eventually become more generalised. It is usually worse at night and will usually pre-date abnormal LFTs. Although the commonest cause of itch and abnormal LFTs is intrahepatic cholestasis of pregnancy, other causes should be excluded, such as a gallstone in the bile duct leading to cholestasis.

Abdominal pain, particularly in late pregnancy, may be extremely important as it can be a sign of acute fatty liver, hepatic rupture or eclampsia, or rather less worrying but more common, gallstones.

Fever and malaise may be prominent in viral hepatitis or cholecystitis, but when there are the classical clinical features of pre-eclampsia in association with abnormal LFTs, then the HELLP (haemolysis, elevated liver enzymes and low platelets) syndrome or hepatic rupture must be considered.

◼ Examination

Some of the clinical signs associated with chronic liver disease in the non-pregnant state are normal occurrences in pregnancy. For example, spider naevi and palmar erythema are common findings, and should not be overinterpreted. Jaundice is rare during pregnancy, and has no prognostic importance in terms of the severity of the liver disease. Liver tests are much more likely to be abnormal in the absence of jaundice. Excoriations with abnormal LFTs are a sign of intrahepatic cholestasis of pregnancy or other causes of cholestasis (less common).

Abdominal tenderness, particularly over the liver may indicate cholecystitis associated with gallstones or imminent hepatic rupture. It is usually constant, but if severe, and in the appropriate clinical setting, must raise the possibility of hepatic rupture or subcapsular haemorrhage.

◼ Investigations

- ◼ Ultrasound examination of the liver and biliary system is safe in pregnancy, and should be performed where there is any abnormality of liver function. If intrahepatic cholestasis of pregnancy is suspected it is important to rule out other causes of cholestasis, such as gallstones with biliary obstruction.
- ◼ Serum bile acid estimation (where available) will help in the diagnosis of intrahepatic cholestasis of pregnancy.
- ◼ Low platelets and evidence of haemolysis occur in HELLP syndrome, as can disseminated intravascular coagulation.

■ If viral hepatitis is suspected, check hepatitis A, B and C markers and, if the patient has travelled to the appropriate part of the world, check hepatitis E.

The pattern of LFTs in pregnancy-associated liver disease is shown in Table 3.

Diagnoses

Hyperemesis gravidarum

Intractable vomiting in the first trimester commonly leads to slightly abnormal LFTs. The diagnosis is usually fairly easy to make because of the clinical situation and stage of pregnancy.

Intrahepatic cholestasis of pregnancy (or obstetric cholestasis)

Characterised by intense pruritus and abnormal LFTs associated with other signs of cholestasis, such as dark urine and pale stools. It affects 0.9 per cent of pregnancies, although the incidence is higher in those from the Indian subcontinent and rare in Afro–Caribbean patients. It is also commoner in those with a family history or those who have experienced it in a previous pregnancy, and typically occurs in the third trimester. As the pruritus is particularly severe at night, it can lead to significant sleep deprivation, and has been reportedly associated with intrauterine death

(not confirmed by the most recent studies) and premature delivery. It is thought to be related to oestrogen metabolism. Jaundice occurs in a small minority of patients.

Treatment is symptomatic and sometimes unsuccessful. In recent years the bile acid ursodeoxycholic acid (15 mg/kg per day) has been widely used and is well tolerated, although there is no conclusive evidence that it works. Parenteral vitamin K should be given to those with prolonged cholestasis to minimise the effects of malabsorption of fat-soluble vitamins. There has also been a trend to deliver at 36 weeks to minimise the risk of stillbirth. Once again, there is insufficient evidence to sustain this practice and certainly early delivery should not be undertaken for abnormal LFTs alone in obstetric cholestasis. Liver function tests return to normal within 2 weeks of delivery.

Acute fatty liver of pregnancy

This is a rare pregnancy-associated liver disease most commonly presenting in the third trimester. It occurs as a result of fat accumulation in the liver. It is potentially fatal to both mother and baby, and is thought to occur as a result of an interaction between a fetus that is homozygous for long-chain 3-hydroxyacyl-coenzyme A deficiency and a

Table 3 Pattern of liver function tests in pregnancy-associated liver disease

Condition	Bilirubin	AST/ALT	ALP	Bile acids
Normal pregnancy	Normal	Normal	Slightly raised	Normal
Hyperemesis gravidarum	Normal	Slightly raised	Slightly raised	Normal
Intrahepatic cholestasis of pregnancy	Normal	Slightly to moderately raised	Slightly raised	Markedly raised
Acute fatty liver of pregnancy	Slightly raised	Slightly to moderately raised	Slightly raised	Normal
Pre-eclampsia/eclampsia	Normal	Slightly to markedly raised	Slightly raised	Normal
HELLP syndrome	Moderately raised	Slightly to markedly raised	Slightly raised	Normal
Hepatic rupture	Slightly raised	Slightly to markedly raised	Variably raised	Normal

Slightly raised: 1–2 × upper limit of normal.
Moderately raised: 3–5 × upper limit of normal.
Markedly raised: 5–100 × upper limit of normal.
ALP, alkaline phosphatase; ALT, alanine aminotransferase; AST, aspartate aminotransferase; HELLP, haemolysis, elevated liver enzymes and low platelets.

heterozygous mother. The mother is frequently symptomatic with headache, malaise, nausea, vomiting and abdominal pain, which is often located over the site of the liver. Jaundice is not common but liver failure may develop with encephalopathy, a coagulopathy and renal failure. In liver failure, a change in the international normalised ratio (INR) or prothrombin time is the most sensitive and rapid indicator of liver synthetic function, and hence liver failure.

Treatment is rapid delivery of the baby, which should lead to rapid improvement of the mother. However, fulminant hepatic failure may develop; therefore, the patient should be put under the joint care of an obstetrician and hepatologist.

Pre-eclampsia and eclampsia

Elevated transaminases are fairly common in these conditions. The incidence rises with the severity of the condition, such that almost 90 per cent of patients with eclampsia will have abnormal LFTs. Treatment is for the underlying condition and no specific treatment is necessary for the liver.

HELLP syndrome (haemolytic anaemia, low platelets and elevated LFTs)

This can complicate the course of up to 10 per cent of those with pre-eclampsia and is due to microangiopathic damage, platelet activation and vasospasm. Patients present with right upper quadrant discomfort and malaise, and typical haematological and biochemical abnormalities. There is a significant maternal mortality rate of 2 per cent with a much higher fetal mortality rate of 33 per cent; therefore, prompt delivery is vital for fetomaternal health.

Hepatic rupture

This is an exceedingly rare complication of pre-eclampsia or eclampsia, but can also be associated with acute fatty liver of pregnancy, HELLP and hepatic adenoma. It usually occurs in the last trimester, and is characterised by sudden onset of severe abdominal pain, nausea and vomiting. There is rapid abdominal distension and hypovolaemic shock, and the prognosis for both mother and baby is very poor. Prompt delivery is

mandatory with surgical or radiological intervention to stop the bleeding from the liver.

■ Pregnancy in patients with chronic liver disease

Fertility is reduced in patients with cirrhosis and chronic liver disease. If pregnancy does occur, the clinical course of the liver disease is generally not altered, in the absence of portal hypertension. Most of the drugs used for the treatment of liver disease are safe in pregnancy, i.e. ursodeoxycholic acid for primary biliary cirrhosis, prednisolone and azathioprine for autoimmune chronic active hepatitis, and penicillamine for Wilson's disease. However, treatment of chronic hepatitis B and C with interferon and ribavarin should be avoided, and patients are advised not to become pregnant for 6 months after discontinuation of treatment.

If varices are present at the time of conception, then there is an increased incidence of bleeding whilst pregnant; therefore, varices should be treated prophylactically, preferably with oesophageal variceal band ligation performed at endoscopy. Despite this, there is a reported increase in maternal mortality and stillbirth rate in these patients.

Finally, there is an increasing number of patients who have had successful pregnancies after a stable liver transplant for chronic liver disease, such as primary biliary cirrhosis, autoimmune chronic active hepatitis, Wilson's disease and primary sclerosing cholangitis, as well as those that are transplanted in childhood for biliary atresia, etc. It is recommended that there is a period of 2 years between transplantation and conception to allow the likelihood of rejection to diminish, and any initial problems with antirejection medications to be resolved.

■ Liver disease coincidental to pregnancy
Viral hepatitis

Infection with hepatitis B virus (HBV) and C (HCV) is probably the commonest cause of liver disease in pregnancy worldwide, although there is great geographical variation, even within a single country owing to ethnicity and country of birth. The clinical course is generally unaltered by the pregnancy, although treatment with interferon or ribavarin is not possible, and will have to await delivery, if clinically indicated.

Delivery of babies to mothers that are HBV or HCV positive needs special consideration. Mothers infected with HCV can deliver vaginally, if indicated, as the risk of transmission is much less than that of HBV or human immunodeficiency virus. There has been no proven transmission of HCV to a baby by breast feeding and certainly HCV-positive mothers should not be advised against breast feeding. Babies are tested for HCV at between 12 and 18 months of age, depending on the local policy.

With hepatitis B, there is a real risk of transmission of HBV to the baby at birth but the risk is minimised, if the baby receives a full course of immunisation starting shortly after birth. This policy has been shown to be 90–95 per cent effective in preventing chronic infection. The immunisation schedule should be accelerated by giving the vaccine at birth, and at 1 and 2 months. The baby should be tested at 2 months to confirm negativity. In births to mothers that are highly infectious, those with a high viral load, babies should in addition be given HBV immunoglobulin at birth.

Hepatitis E, a rare waterborne virus, found in developing countries after flooding, is associated with high maternal mortality rates. Although rare, it must be considered if the mother has travelled to an appropriate area.

Cholelithiasis in pregnancy

Gallstones can be found in as many as 6 per cent of pregnant women but are usually asymptomatic. If symptomatic, they can present with abdominal pain, fever and a raised white cell count suggestive of cholecystitis. There are usually associated changes in the LFTs with a rise in the transaminases. Surgery is sometimes indicated either during or shortly after delivery (see Epigastric pain in pregnancy).

Choledochocholelithiasis accounts for as much as 7 per cent of patients with jaundice in pregnancy and will present as an emergency,

with or without pancreatitis. Endoscopic retrograde cholangiopancreatography can be performed safely during pregnancy with adequate shielding of the fetus from radiation, and can allow safe removal of the intraduct stones, particularly important in gallstone pancreatitis.

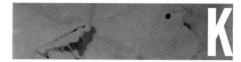

KELOIDS AND HYPERTROPHIC SCARS

Anthony Bewley

Keloids (Fig. 1) and hypertrophic scars (Fig. 2) occur where there is exaggerated fibroblastic activity and collagenous scar deposition within the dermis of the skin. The term '*keloid*' tends to refer to spontaneous scar formation (although, in fact, keloids tend to be at sites of minor skin trauma, e.g. on shoulder skin from clothing friction). The tendency to develop spontaneous keloids tends to run in families and is more common in Afro–Caribbean individuals. Keloids are also more common in the midline of the body, especially the neck and chest.

Hypertrophic scars appear the same as keloids clinically, but have a clear precipitant cause (e.g. incisions for Caesarean sections, or body piercing). Individuals who form spontaneous keloids are very likely to form hypertrophic scars as well, but a purely hypertrophic scar

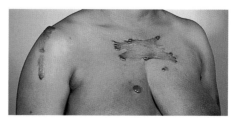

Figure 1 Keloids are more common in Afro–Caribbean patients and may occur spontaneously.

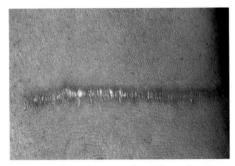

Figure 2 Hypertrophic scar on the abdomen of a woman following abdominal surgery.

(such as may develop following abdominal surgery) may have a better prognosis.

Hypertrophic scars may be very itchy and treatment of the itch may be all the patient seeks. Slow (over 5 years or more) softening of hypertrophic scars is usual. Interventional management of hypertrophic scars from obstetric and gynaecological surgery is described in Box 1.

Box 1 Management of hypertrophic scars following obstetric and gynaecological surgery

- Reassurance that the scar will soften with time (often best advice)
- Intralesional triamcinolone, 1 mL of 10 mg/mL, every 4 weeks for six doses (remember to consent as hypopigmentation and atrophy are possible, especially in Asian and Afro–Caribbean skin)
- Massage with emollient (e.g. vitamin E cream)
- Silicon gel and plasters (little evidence base)
- Very rarely; surgical repair sometimes with additional topical chemotherapy (recurrence and exacerbation of scarring is common)

Individuals who form keloids and hypertrophic scars are likely to have similar reactions following future trauma and should be advised accordingly.

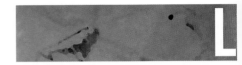

LABOUR, PRECIPITATE

Nigel Bickerton

The definition of precipitate labour varies depending on geographical location. In the UK, midwifery texts have defined precipitate labour as an interval of 1 hour or less between the onset of labour and delivery. The International Federation of Obstetrics and Gynaecology (FIGO) describes precipitate labour as 1 hour or less from 3 cm cervical dilatation to delivery for primigravid women, and half an hour or less for multiparous women. More recently, the Royal College of Obstetricians and Gynaecologists in its guidelines has adopted 2 hours as the cut-off point, in line with the definition most commonly used in the USA. Several countries in the Middle East use 3 hours or less from the start of uterine contractions until delivery as their definition. In many definitions the inclusion of the third stage is not clearly stated.

It follows that epidemiological comparisons within and between countries is, therefore, difficult. Inevitably, the diagnosis of labour is retrospective and many women are not precise about the time of onset of their labour. Some women may not be aware of uterine contractions until labour is well established and consequently may appear to have had a precipitate labour using the definitions given. A true precipitate labour is characterized by rapid dilatation of the cervix with rapid descent of the fetus through the pelvis, caused by frequent and strong uterine contractions. It was thought that precipitate labour was associated with fetal distress and hypoxia, but this is an extremely rare event.

Using the 2-hour definition, it is estimated that 2 per cent of women will experience a precipitate labour, which can occur in spontaneous or induced labour. Induction of labour in women of high parity may be associated with an increased incidence of precipitate labour, uterine rupture and postpartum haemorrhage. In a large study of outcomes of induction of labour, it was found that there was no higher incidence of fetal distress in the subgroup of babies born to women with precipitate labour.

When presented with a possible precipitate labour, the following possibilities should be considered:

- a normal labour of undetermined start time;
- a rapid labour;
- uterine hypertonus – often iatrogenic, owing to prostaglandin use;
- placental abruption.

In precipitate labour there is an adequate duration of each uterine contraction with an interval of rest between. In uterine hypertonus, there are contractions of prolonged duration with a reduced intervening relaxation phase. A common working definition is a single uterine contraction that lasts longer than 2 minutes.

A hard tender uterus that does not relax characterizes placental abruption. Tenderness may be localized or general, depending upon the severity.

Predisposing factors for precipitate labour include:

- increased parity/*grand multiparity*;
- induction of labour in women of high parity;
- placental abruption;
- some variants of Ehlers–Danlos syndrome;
- congenital hypoplasia of the cervix.

However, in the majority of cases, there is no apparent cause.

A precipitate labour may lead to delivery in an unplanned location, especially if the woman is travelling to hospital whilst in labour. The woman will often need emotional support during and after the event, as many women find this type of labour most distressing.

The chance of a similar labour in a subsequent pregnancy is significant, and appropriate timing and planning will need to be given due consideration. There is an association with postpartum atonic uterus and primary postpartum haemorrhage. Whilst it would appear a logical approach, there is no proven benefit in using tocolytic agents to 'normalize' the labour.

Assessment of fetal well-being in labour should follow normal practice. If fetal compromise is suspected, then it should be assessed and managed in the usual way, including fetal blood sampling to aid decision-making where indicated.

■ Further reading

Erkkola R, Nikkanen V. Precipitate labour. *Ann Chir Gynaecol* 1978; **67**: 150–3.

Sheiner E, Levy A, Mazor M. Precipitate labour: higher rates of maternal complications. *Eur J Obstet Gynaecol Reprod Biol* 2004; **116**: 43–7.

LABOUR, PREMATURE

Nigel Bickerton

In the UK, there are 650 000 babies born each year and, of these, 45 000 (7 per cent) are premature by being born before 37 completed weeks of pregnancy. In the USA, 490 000 premature babies are delivered per year, giving a rate of 12 per cent.[1] There is evidence that preterm delivery rates have been increasing over the past 20 years.[2]

Premature labour occurs when any process disrupts the normal physiology that maintains the pregnant uterus quiescent until parturition at term. The normal parturition cascade is usually inhibited until term. Removal of this inhibition plus an increase in myometrial receptors for prostaglandins and oxytocin, as well as raised levels of the gap junction component connexin-43, leads to activation of uterine activity. Long-duration, low-frequency contractions change to high-intensity and more frequent contractions. At the same time, there is softening, effacement and dilatation of the uterine cervix.

The common pathway in labour, activated through the different causes of premature labour, is prostaglandin synthesis. This occurs whether it is due to infection, cytokine activity or bleeding in placental abruption. The physiology of the onset of premature labour is still not fully understood and extensive research continues in this fascinating and important area.

Clinically, the importance of premature labour is to recognise it, so that the mother is in the optimal place for safe delivery, which will be determined by local models of care and rationalisation of services. Extreme prematurity carries the greatest risk to the neonate, with appropriate and immediate specialist neonatal care being vital to avoid death and to minimise morbidity. Survival of the newborn is dependent on both gestational age and weight.

There have been many comparative studies on the use of tocolytics to suppress labour. Whilst the use of tocolytics reduces the proportion of births after treatment starts, there is little available evidence about its effect on perinatal mortality or severe morbidity.

The main indications for tocolytic drugs in premature labour in the short term are:

- to allow a course of maternal steroid injections for fetal lung maturation;
- to allow transfer of the mother to a maternity unit with appropriate neonatal intensive care unit facilities for that particular gestation.

Making a correct diagnosis and then giving the patient informed treatment options is at the centre of good medical practice. The treatment for premature labour requires maternal treatment for perceived benefits to the fetus. With the exception of the benefits of short-term use in selected cases for steroid administration or patient transfer, one should remain mindful of potential maternal risks in a treatment that has limited evidence of fetal benefit.

Currently in the UK, there are four licensed tocolytic drugs:

- atosiban;
- ritodrine;
- salbutamol;
- terbutaline.

If threatened premature labour becomes established labour, there is no convincing evidence to support the use of elective forceps for delivery, or for the routine use of episiotomy. Both practices used to be common in the UK during the last century, before the matter was carefully reviewed.

Babies born prematurely are at risk of respiratory/ventilation problems, and this is a major cause of mortality and morbidity. Respiratory distress syndrome (RDS) will occur in 40–50 per cent of babies born before 32 weeks' gestation. Antenatal steroid treatment causes a significant reduction in the severity of RDS, intraventricular haemorrhage and neonatal death. In addition, steroid treatment reduces the cost and duration of neonatal intensive care. Steroid treatment is contraindicated if the mother is suffering from systemic infection, including active tuberculosis.

Other problems for the neonate from prematurity include hypothermia, hypoglycaemia, jaundice, infection, feeding difficulties, hypocalcaemia, hypomagnesaemia, as well as intraventricular haemorrhage and necrotising enterocolitis, especially in the very premature baby.

As in many areas of obstetrics, the diagnosis of premature labour is not a precise art: two-thirds of those considered in preterm labour will remain undelivered 48 hours later, and one-third will continue the pregnancy to term. It should not be forgotten that, in Western Europe, approximately one-third of all premature labours are iatrogenic. A woman with a history of spontaneous premature labour has a 15 per cent chance of premature labour in a subsequent pregnancy.

The diagnosis is made by abdominal palpation and by using a uterine tocograph, if one is available. The strength, frequency and the patient's response to the uterine contractions are recorded. Vaginal examination using a speculum may reveal some effacement or even dilatation of the cervix. Any amniotic fluid leakage through the cervical os should be noted. Digital examination should be avoided, as it may increase the chance of ascending infection. During the examination, high vaginal bacteriology swabs are taken and a urine sample is taken for bacterial culture.

The general and clinical risk factors for premature labour are listed in Boxes 1 and 2.

Box 1 General risk factors for premature labour

Maternal age

- <20 years
- >35 years

Weight

- Low body mass index

Obstetric history

- Relative subfertility
- Previous miscarriage 16–24 weeks
- Previous premature labour

Social

- Lower social class
- Single parent

Lifestyle activities

- Smoking
- High caffeine intake
- Recreational drugs (cannabis, cocaine, ecstasy)

Box 2 Clinical risk factors for premature labour/delivery

Congenital

- Uterine and cervical anomalies

Maternal disease

- Pre-eclampsia
- Diabetes
- Obstetric cholestasis
- Renal disease
- Systemic lupus erythematosus
- Antiphospholipid syndrome (Hughes' syndrome)
- Ehlers–Danlos syndrome

Cervical surgery

- Previous termination of pregnancy, especially late dilatation and evacuation procedure
- Cone biopsy
- Large loop excision of the transformation zone (LLETZ);

Infections

- Genital tract
- Bacterial vaginosis
- *Chlamydia*
- Gonorrhoea
- Group B Streptococcus
- Trichomoniasis
- Other infections
- Severe urinary tract infection
- Appendicitis
- Diverticular abscess
- Pelvic abscess

Fetoplacental unit

- Multiple pregnancy
- Polyhydramnios
- Fetal growth restriction
- Placental abruption

Maternal trauma

- Domestic violence
- Deceleration injuries – road traffic accident
- Civil unrest – blast injuries

■ References

1. *Premature Birth Rate in U.S. Reaches Historic High; Now Up 29 Percent since 1981.* www.marchofdimes.com/aboutus/10651_10763.asp (accessed 30 August 2006).
2. Danielian P, Hall M. The epidemiology of preterm labour and delivery. In: Norman J, Greer I, eds. *Preterm Labour: Managing Risk in Clinical Practice.* Cambridge: Cambridge University Press, 2005.

LABOUR, PROLONGED

Nigel Bickerton

A successful labour requires uterine contractions of adequate strength to dilate the uterine cervix and then to expel the fetus.

Labour is subdivided into the following phases/stages.

- *A latent phase of the first stage:* the softening and thinning of the cervix (effacement). This is a slow process until the cervix is 3–4 cm dilated.
- *An active phase of the first stage:* regular uterine contractions cause the cervix of the primigravid woman to dilate at approximately 1 cm per hour until the cervix is fully dilated (no cervix palpable around the fetal head).
- *A second stage,* which involves descent of the fetal presenting part through the pelvis leading to birth of the baby. This part of the labour will take about 1 hour in primigravid women. In multiparous women the time is usually less.
- *A third stage,* involving the delivery of the placenta and membranes.

The process of a woman's labour is recorded on a partogram chart. These differ in their layout between countries and between units in the same country. The majority are rectangular, although in some countries a circular partogram is used (developed by the National University Hospital of Ouagadougou). The partogram is used to record the progress of a woman's labour. It can be used to alert the carer to poor progress that may warrant intervention (Fig. 1).

The World Health Organization's definition of prolonged labour is when a woman has experienced labour pains for 12 hours or more without delivery. It is often difficult to pinpoint the time of onset of labour. It is defined as the time when uterine contractions become regular and cause cervical effacement and dilatation.

Many studies have shown that the mean times for the duration of labour differ for primigravid and multiparous women. In Europe, the mean labour time for primigravid women is 10 hours, compared with a mean time of 5.5 hours for multiparous women, but the normal range either side of these figures is wide. As a general rule, the cervix should dilate at the rate of at least 1 cm per hour once the active phase of labour has been reached.

This fact should be remembered in clinical practice. A multiparous woman whose progress in labour is slow requires particular caution in assessment. An unduly large baby or a malposition needs to be excluded. Augmentation of labour using oxytocin should proceed with caution and regular assessment of progress is required.

Prolongation of labour can be considered accordingly:

- false labour or the misdiagnosis of labour;
- a prolonged latent phase of labour;
- a prolonged active phase of labour;
- a prolonged expulsive phase of labour.

False labour may be suspected when abdominal palpation reveals no palpable uterine contractions or the occasional infrequent contraction only, together with a vaginal examination that shows no cervical effacement or dilatation. A *prolonged latent phase of labour* has to be made retrospectively. When uterine contractions become regular and cervical dilatation progresses beyond 3–4 cm, a woman is said to have been in the latent phase of labour. It is important to recognise false labour and a prolonged latent phase of labour. This will help to avoid unnecessary intervention, which may diminish patient satisfaction and carry an increased risk of operative delivery.

Prolonged labour in the active phase is more common in the primigravid woman, and is usually due to:

- ineffective uterine contractions;
- occipitoposterior position of the fetal head;
- cephalopelvic disproportion.

The assessment of the quality of uterine contractions is notoriously difficult and inaccurate by abdominal palpation. The printout on the cardiotocograph is a representation of the frequency of uterine contractions and cannot be used to infer or quantify the strength of the contractions. The use of intrauterine pressure-transducer catheters to measure the strength of a contraction and the work done per contraction is rarely performed in the UK nowadays.

Serial examination of the cervix, preferably by the same examiner, which shows progressive dilatation, is reassuring of adequate uterine contractions and progress in labour, especially if an appropriate partogram path of progress is achieved. If the uterine contractions are not dilating the cervix, then, save for the rare case of cervical dystocia, it is most likely that the uterine activity is inadequate. It is important that cephalopelvic disproportion and obstructed labour are excluded before coming to this conclusion.

The management of inadequate uterine activity is amniotomy, if the fetal membranes are intact, followed by augmentation with an oxytocin infusion. It is important that the oxytocin infusion is given at the adequate dose to cause regular and strong contractions with relaxation in between. If the woman becomes dehydrated and develops ketones in her urine, then fluid replacement can very often positively affect the efficiency of her contractions. Progress should be assessed by abdominal and vaginal examination after regular, strong, uterine contractions are established.

The routine use of enemas during early labour is very much an outdated practice; however, on occasion, it can be extremely useful in facilitating descent of the presenting part if the woman has become very constipated during her pregnancy. Likewise, a full urinary bladder can affect the descent of the presenting part and catheterisation may be necessary, particularly in women with an epidural catheter *in situ*.

The occipitoposterior (OP) position of the fetal head is a relatively common event, occurring in approximately 10 per cent of labours, with the fetal occiput lying in the posterior part of the maternal pelvis. It can be a particular problem in women with a raised body mass index, where excess adipose tissue in the ischiorectal fossae results in poor descent of the fetal head into the pelvis. In the OP position, the fetal head presents a larger diameter to the maternal pelvis and it may be deflexed (Fig. 2).

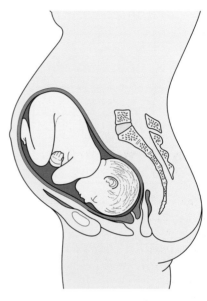

Figure 2 Diagram of the occipitoposterior position.

The diagnosis may have been made antenatally by inspection and palpation. The fetal head tends to be readily palpable in an unengaged state. In Europe, this position of the fetus is the commonest cause of a high fetal head at term. During labour, the mother may complain of a gnawing and persistent backache, worsened during uterine contractions. There is an association with incoordinate uterine contractions that may require an oxytocin infusion to improve them.

Women who labour with an OP fetal position tend to experience the urge to bear down before completion of the first stage of labour. This in part is due to the fetal occiput pressing on the maternal rectum. Premature bearing down may cause cervical oedema together with the development of fetal caput and skull moulding (Fig. 3). This can be a trap for the inexperienced

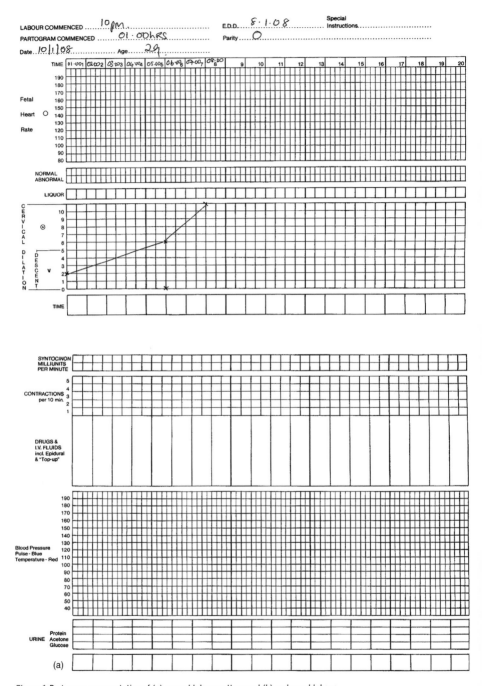

Figure 1 Partogram representation of (a) normal labour pattern and (b) prolonged labour.

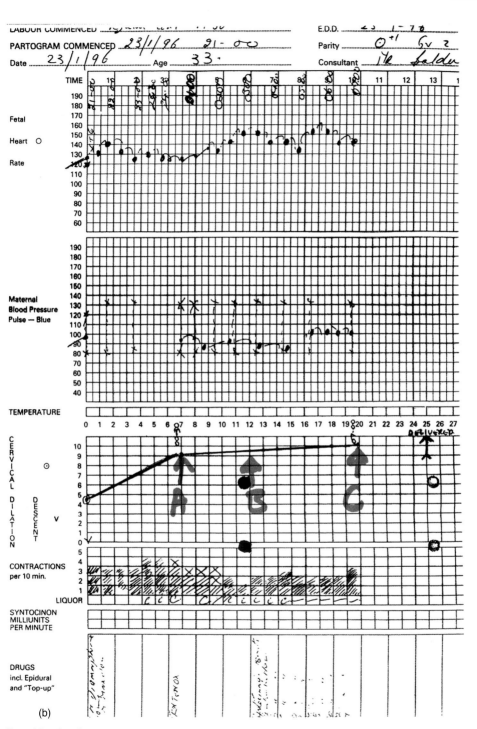

(b)

Figure 1 (continued)

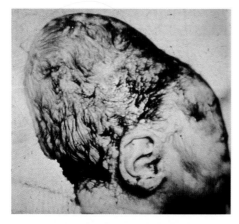

Figure 3 Caput and moulding of a baby's head.

attendant, as the elongated fetal scalp often comes into view before the cervix is fully dilated. Enthusiasm in encouraging the patient to bear down at this stage can seriously demoralise the woman when subsequent examination reveals the true state of cervical dilatation.

Occipitoposterior positions are associated with:

- the need for syntocinon infusion owing to inadequate contractions in the second stage of labour;
- a prolonged second stage of labour;
- an increased need for operative delivery;
- an increased risk of failed operative vaginal delivery and second stage Caesarean section.

Obstructed labour is diagnosed when there is no progressive descent of the fetal presenting part despite strong uterine contractions. Often, in primigravid women, this is associated with an eventual fall off of uterine activity.

Absolute cephalopelvic disproportion is a disparity between the fetal size and the maternal pelvis to a degree that vaginal birth is not possible. The problem of a contracted pelvis is an uncommon finding in a well-nourished population, but may be more problematic in the developing world or in young girls who find themselves pregnant before their full growth

potential has been achieved. Delivery by Caesarean section is required in such cases.

Relative cephalopelvic disproportion occurs when the presenting fetal head is not optimally aligned, through malposition. Management of such cases requires an experienced clinician. Following a period of satisfactory uterine contractions, re-examination will reveal either progress, or it will reveal increasing scalp oedema (caput) and moulding of the fetal skull bones with no further fetal descent at re-examination. The management for the latter is Caesarean section.

Another cause for prolonged labour is deep transverse arrest – at the level of the ischial spines following incomplete rotation from an OP position. The fetal occipitofrontal diameter becomes fixed. The sagittal suture lies in the transverse plane and usually both fontanelles are palpable. Management involves operative delivery. According to local practice, this will be by manual rotation, ventouse or Keilland's (rotational) forceps. In all cases, the fetal head is brought on to the occipitoanterior position before delivery. Adequate analgesia is required, usually through epidural anaesthesia.

It is wise to consider the possibility of other fetal presentations in cases of prolonged labour. A brow presentation or even more rarely a shoulder presentation may be diagnosed late in the day. A shoulder presentation cannot deliver vaginally and must be delivered by Caesarean section. A brow presentation rarely delivers vaginally unless there is spontaneous flexion to a vertex or extension to a face presentation (mentoanterior; Fig. 4).

Rare causes have become even rarer, as nowadays most women receive antenatal ultrasound scans. They include hydrocephalus and conjoined twins. Abnormalities of the uterus and adnexa that may obstruct labour are usually discovered before labour, and include large or multiple fibroids in the lower segment of the uterus and large ovarian masses impacted in the pelvis. Ovarian cysts are not usually an impediment to vaginal birth, as the majority lie at the

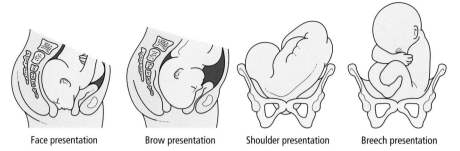

Face presentation   Brow presentation   Shoulder presentation   Breech presentation

Figure 4 Diagrams of malpresentations.

side of or above the pregnant uterus, so that they do not obstruct.

LEG PAIN IN PREGNANCY (DEEP VENOUS THROMBOSIS)

Naim Akhtar

Deep venous thrombosis (DVT) and venous thromboembolic disease remains the leading cause of illness and death in pregnancy in the Western world. In the UK, pulmonary embolism (PE) remains the leading cause of maternal death, and obviously DVT is the underlying cause.

Leg pain and swelling in pregnancy is, however, fairly common (Box 1), and may not have a sinister cause. Leg oedema from venous insufficiency is not dangerous, with symptoms of pain, heaviness, night cramps and paraesthesiae, but requires further investigation. Leg pain may also result from infected varicose veins and superficial thrombophlebitis. Prolonged standing and sitting (long-haul flights, car journeys) are fairly common benign causes for leg pain and swelling.

Leg pain and swelling in pregnancy may also be a sign of pre-eclampsia when associated with raised blood pressure and proteinuria. However, oedema can be found in almost all pregnant women as they get closer to term.

The physiological changes associated with pregnancy result in the haemostatic balance

Box 1 Causes of leg pain and swelling in pregnancy

- Pregnancy with increasing gestation
- Prolonged standing or sitting
- Venous insufficiency
- Pre-eclampsia (associated with hypertension, proteinuria)
- Infection (superficial thrombophlebitis)
- Ruptured Baker's cyst (popliteal bursa)
- Lymphatic obstruction (lymphadenopathy)
- Previous deep venous thrombosis (DVT)
- Previous abdominal/pelvic surgery
- Previous trauma
- Age, obesity
- Co-morbidities (heart failure, liver/renal disease)
- Drugs (e.g. calcium-channel blockers, antidepressants)
- DVT/venous thromboembolism (new onset)

favouring procoagulation and thrombosis (Box 2). As a consequence, Virchow's triad of coagulation, vessel wall damage and blood flow are affected in pregnancy, making venous thromboembolic disease a serious and potentially life-threatening complication. Therefore, the pregnant woman with leg pain/swelling or chest pain/breathlessness

Box 2 Physiological procoagulant changes in pregnancy

- Prohaemostatic changes – shortened clotting times
  - increased fibrinogen concentration
  - increased Factor VIII and some other coagulation factors
- Reduced systemic fibrinolysis – slower dissolution of clot
  - increased plasminogen activator inhibitor
- Reduced protein S concentration – variable effects
- Increased protein C concentration – variable effects

should be suspected and investigated appropriately for a diagnosis of DVT or venous thromboembolism (VTE). There appears to be reluctance to investigate pregnant women with suspected VTE thoroughly.

The clinical diagnosis and differential diagnoses are based on:

- clinical history (including family history, additional risk factors);
- physical examination;
- initial screening tests;
- confirmatory investigations.

■ Clinical history

The history will exclude other likely causes of leg pain and swelling, such as venous insufficiency or pre-eclampsia. VTE occurs in 1:1000 pregnancies, which is a fivefold increase from the non-pregnant state. Although the risk is carried throughout pregnancy, it is substantially higher in the last trimester and delivery, and even higher in the postpartum period.

The risk assessment for a patient is based on several factors (Table 1). A previous history of

VTE, in addition to obesity and multiparous state are major contributing risks for DVT and VTE.

Table 1 Thrombotic risk assessment in pregnancy

Risk factor	Risk
Pregnancy	5-fold increase (1:1000 risk)
Previous VTE	3.5-fold increase
Inherited thrombophilia	3–15-fold increase
Prothrombin variant	Estimated risk 1:200
Factor V Leiden	Estimated risk 1:400
Protein C + S deficiency	Estimated risk 1:100
Antithrombin III deficiency	Estimated risk 1:40
Obesity (BMI > 30)	siginificant risk factors identified in multivariate analysis but remain ill defined in terms of absolute risk
Parity (multiparous > 4)	
Co-morbidities: heart failure, sickle cell disease, malignancy, myeloproliferative disorders, paraplegia, inflammatory disorders, gross varicose veins	
Antiphospholipid syndromes	
Lupus anticoagulant (strongly positive and persistent)	
Anticardiolipin antibodies (moderate levels > 20 units)	
Age (risk increases with age > 35)	
Additional risk factors	
Trauma	
Major surgery	
Central venous catheters/lines	
Hyperemesis	
Dehydration	
Immobilisation (including long-distance travel)	

BMI, body mass index; VTE, venous thromboembolism.

The antiphospholipid syndrome poses significant risk (threefold increase) for arterial, venous and small vessel thromboses, in addition to the well-recognised association with pregnancy losses (Box 3).

Left-leg DVT predominates (90 per cent) in pregnancy owing to the anatomical circulation of the left iliofemoral veins and the compressive effect of the gravid uterus. The postphlebitic syndrome is also fairly common. A total of

Box 3 Antiphospholipid syndromes (APS) and pregnancy

APS

- Increased risk of venous thromboembolism (arterial, venous, small vessel thrombosis)
- Pregnancy losses (early, late), fetal growth retardation
- Pre-eclampsia, abruption (poor placental perfusion)

Diagnosis

- Lupus anticoagulant (two or more times, 6 weeks apart)
- Anticardiolipin immunoglobulin G (IgG) or IgM at moderate levels (> 20 u)

Therapy

- Thromboprophylaxis – low-molecular-weight heparin (LMWH) + low-dose aspirin
- Thrombosis – therapeutic anticoagulation (LMWH) + postpartum heparin or warfarin for 6 weeks

Box 4 Clinical risk for deep vein thrombosis (DVT) and pulmonary embolism (PE)

DVT	PE
Paralysis/paresis	Signs of DVT
Recent confinement to bed > 3 days	Alternative diagnosis less likely
Major surgery within 12 weeks	Heart rate > 100
Localised deep vein tenderness	Immobilisation or surgery within previous 4 weeks
Swelling of entire leg	Previous DVT or PE
Calf circumference difference > 3 cm	Haemoptysis
Pitting oedema	Cancer
Collateral flow	
Previous DVT	

70 per cent of VTEs in pregnancy are not associated with any inherited thrombophilias, and in 25 per cent there are no obvious risk factors other than pregnancy.

■ Physical examination

A full physical examination is mandatory, to exclude other potential conditions and establish co-morbid risk factors. Pain and tenderness over the deep veins is common. Leg swelling may be significant and no other signs may be apparent. Pain on dorsiflexion of the foot (Homan's sign) has not been found to be particularly discriminatory. A clinical risk and probability score can be based on the absence or presence of significant findings on physical examination (Box 4) and is the basis of pre-test probability (PTP) scores.

Objective measurements include circumferential measurements of the leg at fixed points in comparison with the normal leg, or presence of spreading cellulitis are useful baseline recordings. The presence of varicose veins and synovial joint swellings should also be detected and recorded. The presence of a haematoma and ecchymosis should alert the clinician to consider a bleeding diathesis as a potential cause.

■ Screening tests

These include the following routine tests.

- *Full blood count and erythrocyte sedimentation rate (ESR)* to exclude potential secondary causes, including myeloproliferative disorders, malignancy and infection. A normal platelet count and subsequent drop with the introduction of heparin raises the clinical suspicion for heparin-induced thrombocytopenia (HIT).
- *Coagulation profile* to establish a baseline, and exclude possibilities of a coagulopathy associated with lupus anticoagulant, consumptive thrombocytopenia in disseminated intravascular coagulopathy,

or haemolysis associated with elevated liver enzymes and low platelets (HELLP syndrome).

- *D-Dimers* are useful when negative to exclude a diagnosis of DVT or VTE. If elevated, D-dimers may support a diagnosis for VTE and hence further definitive investigations. Raised D-dimers, however, may result from many other causes, including inflammation and malignancy. There are some models to use D-dimers as part of a risk assessment score, which essentially raises the clinical suspicion of VTE. However, the clinical suspicion of DVT and VTE in pregnancy is high, irrespective of the D-dimer level.

The investigation of inherited thrombophilia factors is not encouraged in the acute setting. The levels of many of these factors are likely to be erroneous as a result of the dynamic situation of production and consumption in VTE. Secondly, the immediate management is not altered by the absence or presence of these factors. Pregnancy, in addition, will in any case alter the steady levels of these factors.

■ Definitive investigations

The diagnosis of DVT and VTE may be problematical in pregnancy. Historic venography is no longer the investigation of choice for suspected DVT and leg swelling. Venography has, therefore, been phased out in all patients owing to clinical risks associated with an invasive investigation and the complications associated with a radioactive tracer. The current imaging modalities are listed in Box 5.

In pregnant women with suspected PE or with a suspected DVT and PE, a limited ventilation/perfusion (V/Q) scan may be diagnostic. The use of a spiral computerised tomography pulmonary angiography (CT-PA) scan is now considered to be a good alternative, but both investigations are associated with modest radiation doses and inherent risks in pregnancy.

For suspected leg DVT, duplex ultrasound scan is the main diagnostic tool and is in widespread routine use (see Fig. 1 in Leg swelling in pregnancy). These later scans are useful for detecting

Box 5 Current imaging modalities for suspected venous thromboembolism

Venography (for DVT)

- Historic gold standard for DVT
- Significant risks (invasive, allergy, post-phlebographic DVT)

Ultrasonography (for DVT)

- Compression with transducer
- Non-compression
- Colour duplex
- Pelvic veins not accessible
- Higher sensitivity for proximal DVT

Ventilation/perfusion scan (for PE)

- ^{99}Tc-labelled albumin
- Limited perfusion scan suitable for pregnant patient

Spiral computerised tomography pulmonary angiography (for PE)

- Radiation dose to lactating breasts of concern

Invasive pulmonary angiography (for PE)

- Investigation of last resort in an emergency setting in consideration of thrombolysis

---

DVT, deep vein thrombosis; PE, pulmonary embolism.

proximal DVTs, but may miss the less clinically significant distal leg DVTs. Negative duplex scans should be repeated within a few days if the clinical suspicion remains high, and the patient treated for a DVT or VTE in the interim.

It is important to note that CT-PA, V/Q scanning and limited venography have modest radiation doses, and pose negligible risks to the fetus.

Risks in subsequent pregnancies

There is substantial risk of recurrence in subsequent pregnancies for a variety of reasons, including age, parity and damaged veins due to previous VTE. Some of these risks are quantified in Table 1. Thromboprophylaxis is mandatory in subsequent pregnancies.

Management of obstetric thromboprophylaxis

Both warfarin and unfractionated heparin (UH) have side effects limiting their use in pregnancy. Warfarin is contraindicated in early pregnancy and the first trimester, as it can cross the placenta and disrupt normal bone and cartilage development (warfarin embryopathy).

Unfractionated heparin has no direct teratogenic effects, but risks to the mother include allergic skin reactions, heparin-induced thrombocytopenia and, with long-term use, significant risk of osteoporosis. Most patients are comfortable with self-injection with a longer-acting, low-molecular-weight heparin (LMWH), and the avoidance of monitoring required with both UH and warfarin.

Assessment of thrombotic risk factors (Table 1) should be made in all women in early pregnancy as part of the booking procedure. High-risk women should be managed jointly with a haematologist in a thrombophilia clinic. All women should have their body mass index calculated based on early pregnancy weight. Risk reassessment should occur during pregnancy, if intercurrent problems arise.

Consider prophylaxis with LMWH (enoxaparin 40 mg daily subcutaneously) if three or more of the risk factors (Table 1) are present. For specific recommendations based on risk categories, please see Box 6a–c.

Treatment of VTE in pregnancy

Low-molecular-weight heparin is recommended for treatment of suspected or proven VTE in pregnancy. A twice daily dose is recommended in view of the rapid clearance in pregnancy (Table 2). The guidance is based on enoxaparin,

---

Box 6 Obstetric thromboprophylaxis

(a) High risk

- Antiphospholipid syndrome (previous VTE or fetal loss)
- Recurrent VTE
- Antithrombin deficiency

Recommendations

- Antenatal: enoxaparin 0.75–1 mg/kg twice a day SC + aspirin 75 mg daily
- Intrapartum: enoxaparin 40 mg/day SC
- Postpartum: enoxaparin 0.75–1 mg/kg twice a day SC until 6 weeks postpartum

(b) Intermediate risk

- Personal history VTE (spontaneous or precipitated)
- Thrombophilia
- Family history of VTE (first-degree relatives)

Recommendations

- Antenatal: enoxaparin 40–80 mg/day SC from 10 to 16 weeks
- Intrapartum: enoxaparin 40 mg/day SC
- Postpartum: enoxaparin 40–80 mg/day SC until 6 weeks postpartum

(c) Low risk

- No personal history VTE but with thrombophilia
- Previous VTE, precipitated now resolved
- Family history

Recommendations

- Antenatal: aspirin 75 mg daily
- Intrapartum: enoxaparin 40 mg/day SC
- Postpartum: enoxaparin 40 mg/day SC until 6 weeks postpartum

---

SC, subcutaneously; VTE, venous thromboembolism.

but would be equally applicable to other low molecular weight heparins.

Monitoring is required using anti-Xa levels (target 1 IU/dL 3 hours post dose). Continue treatment throughout pregnancy and the puerperium, with a minimum of 3 months anticoagulation following VTE in pregnancy. Women may breast feed with both LMWH and warfarin.

Table 2 Treatment of venous thrombosis in pregnancy

Early pregnancy weight (kg)	Initial enoxaparin dose
<50	40 mg SC twice daily
50–69	60 mg SC twice daily
70–89	80 mg SC twice daily
>90	100 mg SC twice daily
Target anti-Xa levels	1 IU/dL

SC, subcutaneously.

LEG SWELLING IN PREGNANCY

Nigel Bickerton

Leg swelling is very common in pregnancy. By term, over 60 per cent of women will have noticed it to some degree. The clinical issue with leg swelling is to differentiate between the physiological and the pathological in order to decide whether treatment is necessary and its degree of urgency.

Leg swelling is most often due to oedema, but enlargement of any of the tissues of the leg may give the clinical impression of swelling. Box 1 gives a broad summary of the causes of leg swelling, both acute and chronic, which may occur irrespective of pregnancy. A brief summary of the physiology of peripheral fluid homeostasis may be helpful.

■ Physiology

Tissue capillaries are porous rather than watertight. In the normal state, there is tissue fluid exchange from the capillary into the interstitial space. This is a filtration of liquid and the hydraulic pressure in the capillaries determines

Box 1 Causes of leg swelling

Acute leg swelling

Oedema

- 'Physiological of pregnancy'
- Pre-eclampsia

Thrombotic

- Thrombophlebitis
- Deep vein thrombosis (DVT)

Infective/inflammatory

- Cellulitis
- Dermatitis
- Necrotising fasciitis

Traumatic

- Fracture
- Dislocation
- Disrupted joint – effusion or haemarthrosis
- Ligamentous tear
- Torn leg muscles
- Ruptured Achilles' tendon
- Ruptured popliteal fossa cyst – Baker's
- Sunburn
- Insect bite

Chronic leg swelling

Congenital lymphoedemas

- Hereditary lymphoedema Type I
  - Milroy's disease
  - presents after birth
  - may initially be unilateral
  - the one everyone knows; it accounts for about 2–5 per cent of cases
- Hereditary lymphoedema Type II
  - Meige's lymphoedema – familial lymphoedema praecox
  - presents at puberty
  - accounts for 80 per cent of cases
- Hereditary lymphoedema Type III
  - hereditary lymphoedema tarda
  - presents at 35+ years
  - accounts for 10–15 per cent of cases

Acquired

- Traumatic
  - post lymphatic dissection
  - post radiotherapy
- Venous
  - chronic insufficiency
  - venous obstruction
  - post DVT syndrome
  - pelvic tumour obstructing venous return
- Cardiac
- Congestive heart failure
- Pericardial effusion
  - valvular disease
  - tricuspid valve regurgitation/stenosis
  - pulmonary stenosis

Low serum albumin

- Production
  - malnutrition
  - cirrhosis
  - enteropathy
  - malabsorption
- Loss
  - nephrotic syndrome

Drugs

- Calcium-channel blockers
  - amlodipine
  - diltiazem
  - felodipine
  - nifedipine
- Steroids
- Monoamine oxidase inhibitors
  - phenelzine
- Tricyclics
  - amitriptyline
  - desipramine
  - nortriptyline

the rate of flow. There are different forces at work during this process and an imbalance will lead to oedema.

Hydraulic pressure moves fluid through the capillary wall in the direction of the interstitial tissues. The hydraulic force in the capillary is countered by the pressure in the interstitial fluid and by the osmotic suction in the capillary fluid. Under normal circumstances, the direction of fluid flow is towards the interstitial tissues.

Older physiology texts describe a significant distal capillary reabsorption of water. However, in most tissues, the majority of fluid is returned to the body's circulation by way of the lymphatic system.

The lymphatic drainage of fluid away from the tissue starts at the cellular level and then the lymph fluid flows towards small collecting tubules that in turn convey the lymph into the main trunks. These trunks mirror the layout of the major arteries. Lymph movement at this level is by muscular contraction in the lymph trunks and one-way flow is ensured through a series of valves. In the pregnant woman, up to 10 L of lymph is transported daily. The lymph returns to the circulation through two routes, the lymph nodes and the thoracic duct.

Understanding the process will help in appreciation of ways that the steady state may be altered. An increase in capillary hydrostatic pressure, a fall in plasma osmotic pressure or a fall in lymph drainage rate will all lead to oedema formation. Most cases of clinical oedema occur after the capillary filtration rate exceeds the handling capacity of the lymphatic system, even though this has some degree of biological reserve.

■ Assessment

Assessment of the pregnant woman with leg swelling starts with taking a history of events. Some useful questions are listed below.

- Did the swelling start suddenly?
- Was it there before pregnancy, but is now worse?
- Is it unilateral or bilateral?
- Is there any associated swelling of the face and hands?
- Is there any history of injury? Most people will recall the episode, with pain commencing immediately or soon afterwards.
- Is there any localized pain?
- What drugs are being taken?

Specific questions should focus around the three causes of oedema mentioned above. For example, questions about increased hydrostatic pressure would include an enquiry about varicose veins, any history suggestive of deep vein thrombosis (DVT) or recent, large-volume, fluid infusion. Diminished plasma osmotic pressure as a cause may be suggested by any disease that lessens plasma protein production or by loss of protein through the kidneys or skin.

■ Examination

Examination should be carried out in good light and with both of the patient's legs at the same level. Ideally, the patient should be lying down to allow examination of the abdomen and groin. The urine should be tested for proteinuria and the blood pressure checked. The examiner should look for any asymmetry of swelling and for the degree of oedema. Testing for pitting oedema should involve gentle and prolonged pressure over the area, preferably against a bony area, e.g. 2 cm above the medial malleolus. Leg circumference measurement should be standardized. One approach is to measure the circumference at 10 cm below the tibial tuberosity. A girth increase of more than 3 cm is clinically significant. In DVT, there may be marked pain induced by palpation over the deep venous system. However, the classical features of increased skin warmth and increased venous collateral circulation may not be present.

Acute unilateral leg swelling, with or without pain, and in the absence of any local cause, such as cellulitis, should be regarded as due to DVT until the diagnosis can be confidently excluded. In pregnancy, the use of the D-dimer test for the diagnosis of DVT is clinically unreliable and its continued use by maternity units as a screening test before applying more reliable imaging studies should be discouraged. Ultrasound scanning of the lower limbs with duplex Doppler studies (Fig. 1) or venography with adequate maternal abdominal shielding from X-rays are the tests of choice. Despite this, one potential catch is to have

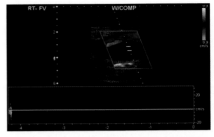

Figure 1 A sagittal scan through the femoral vein (FV) showing lack of compressibility and absence of Doppler signal. A tributary vessel shows marginal flow around the recent sonolucent clot. Reproduced by kind permission of Dr Carl Wright FRCR, Department of Radiology, Ysbyty Glan Clwyd, Bodelwyddan, North Wales.

negative Doppler studies after early presentation. In such cases, if all other causes for unilateral leg swelling have been excluded, then a request for a further scan should be made 2 to 3 days later.

The oedema of pregnancy or of pre-eclampsia is rarely unilateral, with the exception that, in its early stages, it may appear so in women who have undergone unilateral lymphatic disruption, as this leads to less biological reserve on the affected side.

■ Pitfalls in diagnosis

In pregnancy, the significant diagnoses that should not be missed are leg swelling due to pre-eclampsia for a bilateral swelling and DVT for a unilateral swelling. Bilateral swelling in pregnancy may antecede the hypertension and proteinuria of pre-eclampsia, and caution requires that women with significant oedema should be reviewed at an interval for blood pressure checking and urinalysis.

With the exception of oedema due to pre-eclampsia, unilateral leg swelling is more significant in its possible clinical urgency. Approximately one in four women with untreated DVT will develop a pulmonary embolus and, of those who do, one in seven will die as a direct result.

Leg swelling postpartum must be considered with a similar degree of suspicion because only one-half of pregnancy-related DVTs happen antenatally. Pregnancy comes with a fivefold increase in the risk of DVT in part due to the physiological adaptation that leads to a hyper-coagulable state. The DVT risk is further increased by operative delivery, either by the vaginal or abdominal route. Both will reflect a change in the factors of Virchow's triad and increase the risk of DVT. (Virchow's triad refers to the vessel wall, stasis of blood flow and the change in vessel contents' coagulability.) Box 2 lists the additional factors that increase this risk of DVT during pregnancy.

Box 2 Additional factors increasing the risk of deep vein thrombosis (DVT) during pregnancy

---

- History of DVT
- Family history of DVT
- Thrombophilia
- Maternal age > 40 years
- High parity
- Obesity
- Varicose veins
- Immobility
- Heart failure
- Sepsis
- Dehydration
- Long distance air/train travel
- Sickle cell disease
- History of smoking

Four-fifths of DVTs are left sided and 7/10ths are ileofemoral in pregnancy. This is a remarkably high proportion compared with the non-pregnant rate.

Unfortunately, clinical diagnosis alone is not reliable for DVT in pregnancy. Up to one in two suspected cases will prove negative. Once diagnosed, management with anticoagulants should follow local guidance.

LOSS OF LIBIDO

Cynthia Farquhar

Libido is the desire to cause one to be receptive to or to initiate sexual activity. Both men and women experience a range of sexual desire from low to high. For women, the emotional aspect and quality of the relationship are important factors affecting the satisfaction gained from a physical sexual relationship. From a purely physiological viewpoint, libido requires circulating androgens derived from the adrenal glands and ovaries in women. This is controlled in turn by the hypothalamic–pituitary axis. There is a steady decline in the concentration of available circulating androgens in both men and women with increasing age, commencing in the third decade of life. This, together with a number of psychosocial issues, may lead to a decrease in sexual interest.

Whilst not a medical condition *per se*, the menopause is a time of end-organ failure (namely the ovaries) and may compound the situation. Box 1 lists medical conditions that can affect libido, whilst Box 2 gives a list of medications that

---

Box 1 Medical conditions affecting libido

- Hypothyroidism
- Addison's disease
- Parkinson's disease
- Hyperprolactinaemia
- Chronic renal failure
- Severe chronic obstructive pulmonary disease/congestive heart failure
- Alcoholism
- Liver disease
- Depression
- Chronic fatigue
- Fibromyalgia
- Post mastectomy

Box 2 Drugs associated with loss of libido

- Anti-androgens GnRH analogues
- Anti-arrhythmics
- Anticancer drugs
- Cholesterol lowering drugs
- Anticholinergics
- Antihistamines
- Antihypertensives including atenolol and methyldopa
- Antivirals
- Corticosteroids
- Diuretics – spironolactone
- Neuroleptics
- Recreational drugs
- Opiates
- Psychotropics – phenothiazines, haloperidol
- Sedatives – hypnotics

Box 3 Key features in the sexual history

The patient should be asked the following:

- To describe the problem
- When she first noticed the problem and the course of the problem
- What she believes to be the cause of the problem
- What she has tried to help resolve the problem
- What are her expectations and goals

affect desire. A history of painful intercourse may also lead to a reduced desire for physical activity (see Pain during intercourse).

The categories of desire problems are as follows.

- *Primary low libido*: some women never experience sexual desire. This is a difficult challenge and no therapies have been shown to be useful.
- *Secondary inhibited sexual desire*: a number of factors have been found to inhibit desire including recent childbirth, painful conditions, relationship problems and depression. Reviewing the role of these factors may be useful in finding strategies to overcome them.
- *Desire discrepancy*: women frequently report that they do not want sex as often as their male partner. Differing levels of sexual interest are inevitable in long-term relationships and counselling may be helpful.

In establishing a differential diagnosis in a woman presenting with loss of libido, a full medical history (being mindful of conditions in the two attached tables) plus a sexual problem history should be taken (Box 3). Direct questioning about symptoms related to the conditions listed in Box 1 may be useful. Investigations are usually not indicated unless trying to exclude an underlying medical cause as listed.

Management of this problem may prove difficult. If there is an underlying medical condition, then appropriate treatment may improve the condition. Likewise, changing medication that has been linked with loss of libido would seem a sensible option. Lifestyle changes may be helpful including decreasing alcohol consumption, weight loss, exercise, smoking cessation and stress management. Pharmacological agents may include vaginal lubricants and the use of androgenic progestogens (levonorgestrel, norgestrel, desogestrel) as appropriate. Pubococcygeal exercises can increase blood flow to the perineum and can improve the sensation of arousal. If these measures are ineffective. then the help of a psychosexual counsellor should be recommended.

■ Further reading

Nusbaum MRH. *Sexual Health*, Monograph 267, Home Study Self-Assessment Program. Leawood, Kan: American Academy of Family Physicians, 2001.

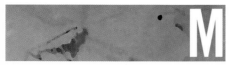

MENSTRUAL PERIODS, ABSENT (AMENORRHOEA)

Tony Hollingworth

Amenorrhoea can be defined as the absence of menstruation, which can be either temporary or permanent. It may occur as a normal physiological event before puberty, as a result of pregnancy and subsequent lactation, or the onset of the menopause. It may be a symptom of a non-physiological problem, which may be systemic or gynaecological in origin.

Primary amenorrhoea is the failure to menstruate by the age of 16 years, when the girl has developed normal secondary sexual characteristics, *or* failure to menstruate at the age of 14 years in the absence of any secondary sexual characteristics. This definition aids the diagnostic differentiation of causes, which include reproductive tract anomalies, gonadal quiescence or gonadal failure. Primary amenorrhoea may result from congenital abnormalities in the development of the ovaries, genital tract or external genitalia, or disturbance of the normal endocrinological events at the time of puberty. Some of these structural abnormalities may lead to cryptomenorrhoea, where menstruation is taking place but the menstrual flow is unable to escape owing to some closure of part of the genital tract (see Puberty, delayed).

Most causes of secondary amenorrhoea can cause amenorrhoea, if the problem occurs before puberty. Delay in the onset of puberty is often constitutional. It is important to exclude the possibility of primary ovarian failure or dysfunction of the hypothalamic–pituitary axis. As a general rule, 40 per cent of cases of primary amenorrhoea are due to endocrine disorders and the remainder (60 per cent) are due to developmental abnormalities.

The definition of *secondary amenorrhoea* has usually been taken to be the cessation of menstruation for six consecutive months in a woman who has had regular periods, although recently it has been suggested that cessation of periods for 3–4 months may be considered pathological and warrant investigation.

Irrespective of the type of amenorrhoea, a thorough history and examination should be undertaken. Examination needs to include the stature and body form of the individual; the height and weight should be measured and converted into a body mass index [BMI = weight, in kilograms/(height, in metres)^2]. Inspection should concentrate on the presence or absence of secondary sexual characteristics and the appearance of the external genitalia. It is essential that this be undertaken before requesting any investigations. Most cases of secondary amenorrhoea by definition would exclude congenital anomalies unless the individual had been using the oral contraceptive pill, which would induce a withdrawal bleed each month. Vaginal examination may be inappropriate in someone under the age of 16 years or who had not been sexually active. Abdominal ultrasound scanning is very useful to define the anatomy. It is *always* important to exclude pregnancy. Serum investigations should include prolactin, gonadotrophins [follicle-stimulating hormone FSH and luteinising hormone (LH)] and thyroid function tests.

Raised serum prolactin levels (>1500 IU/L) may indicate the need for a computerised tomography (CT) or magnetic resonance imaging (MRI) scan of the pituitary fossa to exclude a hypothalamic tumour. Serum FSH levels >40 IU/L usually suggest irreversible ovarian failure. Raised serum FSH and LH levels usually suggest ovarian failure, but raised LH levels alone may indicate polycystic ovarian syndrome (PCOS), which can be confirmed by ultrasound scan of the ovaries. Amenorrhoea in PCOS is secondary to acylical ovarian activity and continuous oestrogen production. Abnormally low serum levels of FSH and LH suggests failure at the level of the hypothalamus and pituitary giving hypogonadotrophic hypogonadism. Kallmann's syndrome is associated with hypogonadotrophic hypogonadism, and these patients have hyposmia and/or colour blindness. Hormonal patterns in amenorrhoea with their associated diagnoses are shown in Table 1.

Table 1 Hormonal patterns in amenorrhoea with their associated diagnoses

Condition	Serum biochemistry
Ovarian failure	Raised FSH and LH
Polycystic ovarian syndrome	Raised LH, raised free androgen index
Hypogonadotrophic/hypogonadism	Low FSH and LH

FSH, follicle-stimulating hormone; LH, luteinising hormone.

The free androgen index is the relationship or ratio of the total testosterone concentration (slightly raised) to the sex hormone-binding globulin concentration, which is lowered in PCOS. This is on a molar/molar basis and may be rescaled by a factor of 10, 100 or 1000. It is often raised in severe acne, male androgenic alopecia, and hirsutism, as well as PCOS, for which it can be a sensitive and specific indicator if elevated in the early follicular phase.

Chromosomal abnormalities (e.g. Turner's syndrome 45XO) can be diagnosed by karyotyping. Autoantibody screens should be undertaken in women with a premature menopause. Premature menopause can be associated with an increase risk of heart disease and, consequently, it may be useful to check serum cholesterol levels in these patients. Women with PCOS and prolonged amenorrhoea have an increased risk of endometrial hyperplasia and carcinoma; endometrial sampling may be useful if any abnormal bleeding occurs.

■ Primary amenorrhoea

Chromosomal

Turner's syndrome (gonadal dysgenesis), in which there is also dwarfism, web neck, cubitus valgus and an XO sex-chromosome pattern (Fig. 1) is the commonest form of gonadal dysgenesis. These women may develop spontaneous menstruation; however, premature ovarian failure is common. The gonadotrophin levels may be

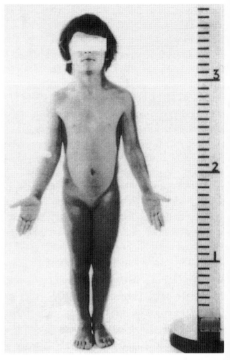

Figure 1 Turner's syndrome. (Courtesy of Professor Paul Polani.)

raised and they may require hormone replacement therapy (HRT). Although spontaneous conceptions have been reported, some form of assisted conception is likely to be required, if they were to want a pregnancy.

Testicular feminization (which is, in reality, androgen insensitivity) in which the form is female with well-developed breasts, but with absent or sparse pubic and axillary hair, and the gonad, which may be found in the groin or in the abdomen, is a testicle. The gonadal tissue should be removed because of the increased risk of malignancy.

In *ovarian dysgenesis*, there are streak ovaries, an infantile uterus and absent secondary sexual characteristics (Figs. A.11–A.14). In these cases, a buccal smear for sex chromatin and a chromosome analysis on a sample of peripheral blood are indicated.

In ovarian dysgenesis, there is a chromatin-negative smear but only 45 chromosomes – a single X chromosome (XO). In testicular feminization, the smear is also chromatin negative but there are 46 chromosomes (XY). Gonadal biopsy is also helpful in diagnosis

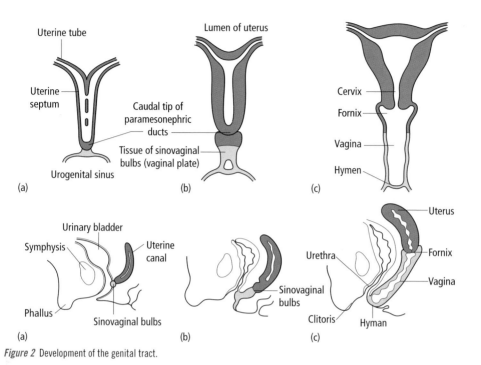

Uterine tube

Uterine septum

Caudal tip of paramesonephric ducts

Tissue of sinovaginal bulbs (vaginal plate)

Urogenital sinus

(a)

Lumen of uterus

(b)

Cervix

Fornix

Vagina

Hymen

(c)

Urinary bladder

Symphysis

Uterine canal

Phallus

Sinovaginal bulbs

(a)

(b)

Sinovaginal bulbs

Urethra

Clitoris

Hymen

Uterus

Fornix

Vagina

(c)

Figure 2 Development of the genital tract.

■ Müllerian duct abnormalities

The Wolffian ducts regress in the embryo after the sixth week, if there is no Y chromosome present. The Müllerian ducts will develop into the tubes and uterus, and fuse caudally with the urogenital sinus to produce the vagina (Fig. 2). Abnormalities may occur in the process of fusion and these may be medial or vertical, and give rise to primary amenorrhoea. Complete or partial Müllerian agenesis may occur. In these cases, the genotype is 46XX with normal secondary sexual characteristics and normal ovarian tissue, but the vagina is short and may require surgery. There may also be associated urinary tract abnormalities.

The commonest form of abnormality is that of an imperforate hymen, which leads to primary amenorrhoea or cryptomenorrhoea (hidden menses). The secondary sexual characteristics are normal, but the individual may complain of cyclical lower abdominal pain and abdominal distension. It is not unusual for theses cases to present with retention of urine and, on inspection, have a bulging hymen (Fig. 3). A cruciate incision releases the menses and that is all that is necessary.

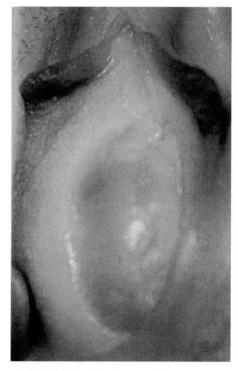

Figure 3 Imperforate hymen.

■ Secondary amenorrhoea

Genital tract abnormalities

There is a potential for scarring anywhere within the genital outflow tract. Ashermann's syndrome is a condition where intrauterine adhesions develop, which prevent normal endometrial growth. It is an uncommon condition, and usually occurs following vigorous curettage at the time of an evacuation of the uterus or suction termination of pregnancy.

Cervical stenosis can cause cryptomenorrhoea with development of a haematometra, and may occur due to repeated treatment of the cervix for precancerous lesions. Radiotherapy may have an effect on the cervix and uterus, if used for advanced cancer of the cervix, and may cause vaginal stenosis. In these cases, the amenorrhoea is more likely to be related to the radiotherapy effect on the ovaries than outflow obstruction.

Systemic disorders

Chronic disease may cause menstrual disorders as a consequence of the general disease state, weight loss or effects on the hypothalamic–pituitary axis. Certain disorders will affect gonadal function directly. Chronic renal disease will act by increasing the serum LH level and also prolactin levels, possibly due to reduced renal clearance. Other causes would include systemic conditions in the form of tuberculosis or sarcoid.

Weight-related amenorrhoea

Body weight/BMI can have a significant effect on the regulation and release of serum gonadotrophins. Menstruation will not occur regularly if the BMI falls below 19, and it is estimated that the 22 per cent of female body weight should be fat to ensure ovulatory cycles. Fat in the form of adipose tissue is a source of oestrogen by the aromatization of androgens to oestrogen. This ensures the appropriate feedback mechanism of the hypothalamic–pituitary–ovarian axis. The weight loss may be due to illness, exercise or dieting. Potential sequelae of a low BMI include the long-term effects on bone mineralisation.

Stress in itself is unlikely to give amenorrhoea lasting longer than 2 months unless associated with debilitation. Exercise, particularly in the endurance events, is a common cause of amenorrhoea and this is also usually related to the BMI and body fat content as described above.

Hypothalamic causes

These causes are uncommon and include craniopharyngioma, gliomas and dermoid cysts. The mechanism of action may be to destroy local tissue or disrupt dopamine production resulting in hyperprolactinaemia. Treatment is usually surgical and possibly radiotherapy. HRT may be necessary together with other hormonal supplementation depending on the extent of the local damage in the pituitary. Head injury or irradiation may have a similar effect.

Pituitary causes

The commonest pituitary cause of amenorrhoea is hyperprolactinaemia, which may be physiological due to lactation, iatrogenic or pathological. A non-functioning tumour or pituitary adenoma may affect dopamine secretion levels, as may prothiazines and metoclopramide. The consequence is a raise in the serum prolactin level. Galactorrhoea may occur in up to a third of patients and, very occasionally, there may be visual field impairment.

Unless the serum prolactin is markedly raised, it is unlikely to show any effect on the sella turcica on a lateral skull X-ray. CT or MRI scanning may be more appropriate investigations.

Box 1 Drugs associated with secondary amenorrhoea

- Amoxapine
- Carbenoxolone
- Cyclophosphamide
- Danazol
- Domperidone
- Fluvoxamine
- Glucocorticoid
- Imipramine
- Isoniazid
- Leuprorelin
- Methyldopa
- Neuroleptic agents
- Procainamide
- Tamoxifen

Box 2 Classification of amenorrhoea

Physiological
- Before puberty
- After the menopause
- During pregnancy
- During lactation

Hypothalamic
- Primary hypothalamic–pituitary failure
- Following oral contraceptives (post-pill)
- Anterior pituitary failure (Sheehan's disease)

Pituitary

Ovarian
- Congenital absence of ovaries (rare)
- Ovarian agenesis
- Gonadal dysgenesis (Turner's syndrome)
- Destruction of both ovaries by double ovarian growths
- Polycystic ovarian disease
- Resistant ovarian syndrome
- Certain rate functioning tumours of the ovary: arrhenoblastoma, granulosa-cell tumour

Genital outflow (uterine, cervix, vagina and vulva)
- Imperforate vagina
- Imperforate hymen
- Absence of the vagina
- Imperforate cervix
- Double uterus with retention
- Congenital absence of uterus
- Uterine hypoplasia of infantile type
- Uterine hypoplasia of adult type
- Haematocolpos
- Haematometra
- Haematosalpinx

Acquired
- Ashermann's syndrome
- Pelvic inflammation
- Closure of the vagina:
  - due to specific fevers
  - due to injury
- Closure of the cervix
  - due to injury
  - following operations, e.g. loop cone biopsy

Endocrine
- Myxoedema
- Addison's disease
- Thyrotoxicosis
- Adrenal hyperplasia
- Adrenal cortical tumours
- Acromegaly

Iatrogenic
- Pelvic irradiation
- Hysterectomy
- Depo-Provera
- Progesterone-only contraception
- Mirena coil
- Drugs mentioned earlier (see Box 1)

General
- Anaemia
- Leukaemia
- Hodgkin's disease
- Malignant growths
- Tuberculosis
- Prolonged suppuration
- Diabetes
- Late stages of nephritis
- Late stage of some forms of heart disease
- Late stage of cirrhosis of the liver
- Dietetic deficiencies, the result of attempts to lose weight
- Toxic
- During and after specific fevers
- Chronic poisoning by lead, mercury, morphine, alcohol
- Anorexia nervosa or loss of weight
- Obesity
- Dystrophia adipose-genitalis (Frohlich's syndrome)
- Cretinism
- Stress

Treatment involves the use of a dopamine antagonist, usually bromocriptine or a related drug. This should be discontinued if the patient becomes pregnant: a quarter of adenomas will increase in size during pregnancy.

Profound hypotension following delivery can cause Sheehan's syndrome, which can affect the pituitary causing necrosis, as it has an end artery with no collateral supply to protect it in these circumstances. Appropriate induction agents will be needed to induce ovulation.

Treatment needs to be given to correct the amenorrhoea and oestrogen deficiency, improve libido and effect tumour shrinkage in cases with hyperprolactinaemia. It is safe to use the combined oral contraceptive pill in these women, if they require contraception.

Ovarian causes

Premature ovarian failure may occur and is defined as the cessation of periods before the age of 40 years. This may be due to chromosomal abnormalities, which have already been discussed and also chromosomal mosaicisms. The most common causes include autoimmune disease, as well as infection, previous surgery, chemotherapy or radiotherapy.

Tumours are an unusual cause of amenorrhoea, but arrhenoblastomas can cause virilism as well as amenorrhoea, atrophy of the breasts and hirsutism.

Iatrogenic causes

The obvious causes include radiotherapy and chemotherapy for malignant disease. Others that may need to be considered are forms of contraception, including Depo-Provera, the progesterone-only pill, the Mirena coil, post-pill amenorrhoea as well as gonadotrophin-releasing hormone analogues. A list of drugs that have also been associated with secondary amenorrhoea is shown in Box 1.

■ Classification of amenorrhoea

Although the basic classification is primary and secondary, amenorrhoea can also be classified as shown in Box 2.

MENSTRUAL PERIODS, HEAVY AND/OR IRREGULAR (MENORRHAGIA/ METRORRHAGIA)

Cynthia Farquhar

Heavy menstrual bleeding (HMB) refers to excessive menstrual flow and is also known as menorrhagia. The patient is free from bleeding during the intermenstrual period. The term irregular uterine bleeding or intermenstrual bleeding is used for bleeding that occurs between the periods and is sometimes known as metrorrhagia. HMB is an important symptom of many well-defined conditions, which may or may not be associated with irregular cycles. As a rule, delayed menstruation is often associated with an increase in the menstrual blood flow. These terms are limited to patients who menstruate and must not be used for bleeding after the menopause.

Heavy menstrual bleeding is a subjective symptom, and menstrual loss consists not only of blood but also tissue and other secretions. Objectively, periods are considered to be heavy if there is more than 80 mL blood loss per month, which will result in iron-deficiency anaemia. The diagnosis of heavy menstrual bleeding is of necessity a self-diagnosis, although even mild anaemia (haemoglobin <12 g) is a good indication of the severity. Sleep disturbance, clots and flooding all provide some indication that menstruation is excessive. Heavy bleeding is the second most common cause for hospital referrals, and up to one-third of women may consult their primary care physician about this symptom.

An excess of menstrual loss in women without evidence of pathology is sometimes called dysfunctional menorrhagia or dysfunctional uterine bleeding, or unexplained HMB. Acute endometritis of gonococcal or pyogenic origin tends to cure itself, owing to the shedding of the endometrium during menstruation. Tuberculous endometritis, a rare cause of infertility in the UK, is due to spread from the Fallopian tubes and is, therefore, associated with menorrhagia

---

Box 1 Causes of heavy menstrual bleeding (HMB)

Unexplained or dysfunctional HMB	Underlying pathology
Anovulatory	**Fibroids**
■ At puberty	Chronic pelvic infection
■ At maturity without obvious lesions	Endometriosis
■ In relation to the menopause, and in the years preceding	Adenomyosis
Ovulatory HMB	Intrauterine contraceptive devices
	Bleeding disorders
	Thyroid disorders
	Tuberculous endometritis

---

owing to the tuberculous salpingo-oophoritis. If a tuberculous infection is suspected, the uterine curettings should be examined for the typical tubercles and the organism isolated by culture. Adenomyosis may also cause HMB. The causes of heavy menstrual bleeding are given in Box 1.

■ Heavy menstrual bleeding with irregular cycles

During puberty, HMB can occur as a result of hypofunction of the anterior pituitary body, with consequent failure of ovulation and therefore no corpus luteum is formed. The ovaries contain unruptured Graafian follicles; there is increased oestrogen production and a lack of the luteal hormone progesterone. Once the pituitary gradually assumes its normal cyclic activity, then the cycles often occur spontaneously. These are anovulatory cycles and are usually painless.

Perimenopausal women may experience heavy menstrual bleeding secondary to cessation of regular ovulatory cycles. When there is a complete absence of progesterone in the second half of the menstrual cycle, the cycle is referred to as anovular, drawing attention to failure of ovulation and formation of a corpus luteum. The endometrium may undergo polypoidal thickening with a characteristic microscopic appearance known as 'Swiss cheese' endometrium or 'complex hyperplasia'. Episodes of amenorrhoea of some weeks may be followed by prolonged irregular and heavy bleeding.

■ Heavy menstrual bleeding with pathology

Heavy menstrual bleeding can be associated with fibroids (benign leiomyomas), adenomyosis, pelvic infection, endometrial polyps, endometriosis and the presence of an intrauterine contraceptive device. Of all the causes of pure HMB, leiomyoma (fibroids) of the uterus stands out as the only important growth associated with this symptom and a simple bimanual examination, as a rule, suffices to show that such a tumour exists. The size and shape of the uterus is dependent on the number and size of the fibroids, as there may be more than one tumour in the uterus, whose shape may be exceedingly irregular. The uterus feels firm and, in most cases, is mobile.

The only difficulty in diagnosis, as a rule, lies in distinguishing a fibroid of the uterus from an ovarian cyst. This is sometimes difficult, for it is not always possible to say that a given tumour is actually the enlarged uterus. Ultrasound scanning is helpful in the diagnosis of fibroids by establishing whether a pelvic swelling is both uterine and solid. Fibroids may be submucous, intramural, subserosal or pedunculated. Distortion of the uterine cavity with an increase in the surface area from which menstruation occurs will lead to menorrhagia (Fig. 1).

Chronic pelvic infection (in the form of a pyosalpinx, a hydrosalpinx, a tubo-ovarian abscess or chronic interstitial salpingitis) and ovarian endometriosis both give rise to HMB

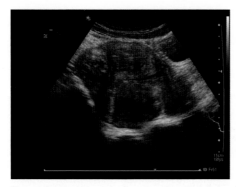 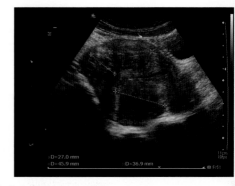

Figure 1 Ultrasound scan showing enlarged and distorted cavity due to fibroids.

due to inflammation, but dysmenorrhoea, pelvic pain, dyspareunia and backache are usually more prominent symptoms. In either case, a firm tender swelling in the pouch of Douglas is felt on bimanual palpation. Intermenstrual or irregular bleeding is also common in these cases.

Adenomyosis is a condition that can present with HMB and pain at the time of menstruation; on examination the uterus may be tender. The diagnosis can only be confirmed histologically, as endometrial tissue is found invading the myometrium (Fig. 2). The condition is more common in parous women and, in essence, there has been bleeding in the myometrium that gives rise to the pain and tenderness.

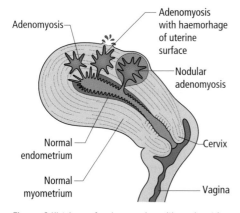

Figure 2 Histology of adenomyosis, with endometrium extending into the myometrium.

There is almost always some increase of the menstrual blood loss with the use of intrauterine contraceptive devices (IUCDs; copper devices) and, in some cases, the loss amounts to HMB. This results from the inflammatory reaction the coil sets up in the myometrium to prevent implantation of the fertilised egg. Changing the IUCD to a progestogen-releasing IUCD usually improves the situation.

■ Clotting defects

There are certain haemorrhagic disorders that can cause excessive menstrual loss. These include thrombocytopenic purpura, von Willebrand's disease and Christmas disease. These women may suffer excessive menstrual loss and may require surgical intervention. In thrombocytopenia, the blood loss relates to the platelet level and, in some cases, splenectomy for the underlying cause has improved the menstrual symptoms.

Anticoagulation in women who are on long-term anticoagulants for prosthetic heart valves, previous pulmonary embolism or, in some cases, antiphospholipid syndrome may develop significant period problems depending on the international normalised ratio level.

Thrombocytopenia can sometimes complicated by HMB. As soon as the platelet level is back to normal, the blood loss usually becomes normal.

Medical disorders

The function of the thyroid and adrenal glands can influence the menstrual loss, although the mechanism is unknown. HMB tends to be more common in hypothyroidism than thyrotoxicosis, and is not uncommon with Cushing's disease.

Intermenstrual uterine bleeding

Intermenstrual uterine bleeding means loss of blood vaginally between the menstrual periods, and the term should be applied strictly only to irregular haemorrhages during the reproductive age range, i.e. from puberty to the menopause. It may be used for losses of actual blood or for blood-stained discharges in which mucus is mixed with blood. For the purposes of discussion, irregular vaginal bleeding will be considered here under three headings:

- irregular bleeding during menstrual life;
- irregular bleeding before puberty and after the menopause;
- irregular bleeding during pregnancy.

It is important to emphasise that, if a woman has had regular periods and then starts to get irregular bleeding for no apparent reason, one must exclude pregnancy and where that pregnancy is located, i.e. an ectopic pregnancy, as this is still a major cause of maternal death in the UK.

Irregular bleeding during menstrual life

The causes of irregular bleeding during menstrual life are given in Box 2.

Malignancy
Carcinoma of the cervix
Cervical cancer is an uncommon disease with an incidence that is reducing as a result of the cervical screening programme. It is estimated that a general practitioner in the UK will see one case of cervical cancer every 7–9 years. The cervix is replaced with a friable mass, which causes irregular bleeding as well as postcoital bleeding. The lesion can be diagnosed macroscopically,

---

Box 2 Causes of irregular bleeding during menstrual life

Generative system

- Malignant growths
- Carcinoma of the cervix

- Carcinoma of the uterus
- Sarcoma
- Chorionic carcinoma
- Carcinoma of the Fallopian tube
- Carcinoma of the ovary

Benign growths
- Submucous fibroids
- Endometrial and endocervical polyps

Other
- Endometriosis
- Ectropion of the cervix
- Tuberculosis of the uterus

Endocrine

Anovulatory heavy menstrual bleeding
- Breakthrough bleeding on the oral contraceptive pill and hormone therapy

although many of these women will be seen in the colposcopy clinic so that a directed biopsy can be undertaken (see Cervical swellings).

Carcinoma of the uterine body

Endometrial carcinoma does occur during the reproductive age group but it is much more common in postmenopausal women. It is the second most common genital tract tumour and presents with irregular bleeding. Risk factors include obesity (raised BMI), nulliparity and history of polycystic ovarian disease. It is unusual to diagnose this condition before the age of 40 years, hence the Royal College of Obstetricians and Gynaecologists recommendations suggesting that women with menstrual irregularities before the age of 40 years should receive treatment for 3 months. If the irregularity persists, then a hysteroscopy and endometrial sampling should be undertaken. If the woman is over the age of 40 years, then this would be a first-line investigation (see Uterine swellings).

Sarcoma of the uterus

This is a very uncommon tumour and occurs in fibroids. It may present with irregular bleeding, but many of these women will be postmenopausal and present with a rapidly expanding pelvic mass. The risk of a fibroid becoming malignant is estimated at about 1 in 1000. This tumour may occur in an existing fibroid or appear *de novo*. The difficulty with this condition is the highly aggressive nature of the disease, which does not respond well to radiotherapy or chemotherapy as a rule (see Uterine swellings).

Chorionic carcinoma

This condition is *fortunately* very rare, and follows hydatidiform mole in about 5 per cent of recorded cases, and it always follows pregnancy, never having been seen in the uterus where pregnancy could be excluded, although the pregnancy may have occurred some years earlier. It is associated with profuse bleeding and the rapid development of a fetid discharge due to decomposition of blood and necrosing tissues *in utero*. Secondary deposits of chorionic carcinoma

appear as small plum-coloured ulcerating nodules in the vagina and secondaries in the lungs cause haemoptysis. The patient rapidly becomes ill with pyrexia and profound anaemia. A raised level of chorionic gonadotrophin is found in the urine. The diagnosis depends upon the finding of masses of trophoblastic cells in uterine curettings without any evidence of villous formation (see Bleeding in early pregnancy).

Other malignancies

Carcinoma of the Fallopian tube is a rare tumour and tends to present in the postmenopausal woman, but may present with irregular bleeding. Ovarian cancer is unlikely to cause bleeding unless it has invaded the uterus. Clear-cell carcinoma of the vagina is also rare and has been reported in teenage girls exposed to stilboestrol *in utero*.

Benign lesions that may cause irregular bleeding

Fibroids

Leiomyomas may cause a mixture of HMB and intermenstrual spotting. The irregular bleeding tends to occur when they are submucous. They may be in the process of extrusion when they may become infected and sloughing occurs. The reason for this is that, in these conditions, the tumours are partly strangulated by uterine contractions and consequently congested with venous blood. This results in bleeding, which is unpredictable in timing and amount.

Polyps

Polyps can occur within the cervix and endometrium. Cervical polyps are usually identified at the time of taking a routine cervical smear test but, if the tip becomes inflamed, then it can give rise to vaginal bleeding or postcoital bleeding. Polyps within the endometrial cavity, whether fibroid or mucous, are common causes of intermenstrual bleeding, and are usually quite definitive growths. The mucous polyp is soft strawberry-red in colour, pedunculated and contains cystic spaces filled with glairy mucus. It rarely gives rise to a malignant growth. The fibroid poly is hard and shows the glistening whorled appearance so well known in fibromyomas on section. These growths are liable to infection and sloughing, and are then apt to be mistaken for carcinoma or sarcoma macroscopically.

Endometriosis

This condition is defined as the finding of tissue outside the uterus that is histologically similar to that of endometrium, and is not strictly an inflammatory lesion. However, it is one of the commonest benign gynaecological conditions and may present with a myriad of symptoms, including painful bleeding and dyspareunia.

Ectropion of the cervix

This is a physiological condition in which there is eversion of the columnar epithelium from the endocervical canal towards the vagina. The columnar epithelium appears reddened because it is one-cell thick and consequently translucent, allowing the blood supply below to be seen. The term erosion should be avoided. as it suggests something pathological. The epithelium can become inflamed and gives rise to discharge, which sometimes results in contact bleeding, although intermenstrual bleeding is unusual. The columnar epithelium may undergo metaplastic change to squamous epithelium owing to pH changes within the vagina. This area is known as the transformation zone. It is in this area that pre-cancerous changes may occur. Pre-cancerous changes within the cervix are asymptomatic and usually only diagnosed by cytology and at time of colposcopy.

Tuberculosis

Tuberculosis (TB) may affect the genital tract and give rise to irregular bleeding and infertility. It is an uncommon problem within the UK but is much more common in the developing world. Histology of the endometrial curettings may give the diagnosis, although a strong suspicion of TB suggests the need to involve a physician in the care of the woman.

Heavy menstrual bleeding without obvious pathology

Heavy menstrual bleeding without obvious pathology is also sometimes known as dysfunctional bleeding. It may occur at any age between puberty and the menopause, but 50 per cent occurs between the ages of 40 and 50 years, about 10 per cent at puberty, and the remainder between these ages. When it occurs in association with longer menstrual cycles, it is most likely the results of anovulation and for this reason is more likely seen in adolescents, at the time of the perimenopause and in women with polycystic ovarian syndrome. When the bleeding is usually preceded by amenorrhoea for some weeks then the length of bleeding may be prolonged.

The histology of any curettings may prove to be essentially normal, although in women with a increased body mass index, polycystic ovarian syndrome or a perimenopausal woman, then endometrial hyperplasia may be present. Endometrial hyperplasia (Fig. 3) can occur as a

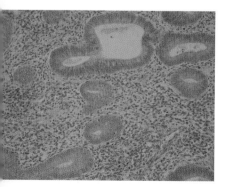
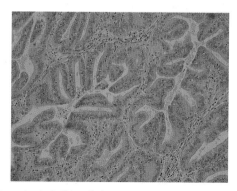

igure 3 Histology of simple hyperplasia of the endometrium and complex atypical hyperplasia.

result of excess oestrogen production. It is a premalignant condition that is rarely a cause of heavy menstrual bleeding but should be excluded in women who are overweight or are perimenopausal. These conditions are histological diagnoses and how the woman is treated will depend on her age and fertility status. Women with complex hyperplasia with atypia are at risk of developing endometrial cancer and hysterectomy is usually recommended.

Contraception and heavy menstrual bleeding

There are three main areas that can give rise to HMB as listed below.

- The copper-containing IUCDs can give rise to HMB and, in some cases, the low-grade inflammatory response of the endometrium to the coil can result in irregular shedding. The treatment would be to remove the coil in the first instance.
- Progesterone contraception, whether as the progesterone only-pill, the Mirena IUCD or Depo-Provera, will usually result in the woman being amenorrhoeic. There are a number of women who develop irregular bleeding, which may be completely unpredictable, although it is usually not particularly heavy.
- The combined oral contraceptive pill usually gives good cycle control. However, breakthrough bleeding can occur owing to gastrointestinal upset, absorption and metabolism problems due to other medications (e.g. antibiotics and antiepileptic drugs), diet affecting the enterohepatic circulation and a dosage too low for the individual.

Bleeding associated with ovulation

It is not uncommon for women to bleed very slightly about midway between the periods at the time of ovulation. When this is accompanied by lower abdominal pain (Mittelschmerz), the diagnosis is straightforward.

Bleeding due to granulosa-cell tumour

When irregular bleeding occurs in the presence of an ovarian swelling, the possibility of a granulosa-cell tumour arises. Removal of the tumour and histology reveal its nature. The presence of an intrauterine lesion and a non-secreting ovarian tumour must not be overlooked.

■ Irregular bleeding before puberty and after the menopause

The bleeding that occurs from the vagina occasionally in newborn infants is usually due to a high concentration of oestrogen in the fetal circulation. It is usually trivial but a fatal case has been reported. Bleeding later in childhood may be due to sexual precocity, when secondary sexual characteristics will be in evidence, or due to a new growth, such as an embryonal rhabdomyosarcoma (sarcoma botryoides). Vaginoscopy under anaesthesia (and biopsy, if a lesion is found) is essential.

After the menopause, the differentiation of malignant growths, polyps and senile endometritis can only be established by uterine curettage (see Bleeding, post menopausal) Carcinoma of the body of the uterus (endometrial adenocarcinoma) is the commonest malignant growth after the menopause. In any doubtful case, routine dilatation and curettage of the uterus must never be omitted. Senile (atrophic) vaginitis must not be overlooked as a possible cause: the vaginal walls at the fornice become inflamed and may bleed if the surface rub together; the surfaces may be partly adherent, and the separation brought about by the examining finger may cause bleeding. Pyometra or distension of the uterus with pus, may cause haemorrhage, with a foul discharge. Although this is almost always due to malignant growth, it may be only the result of infection. The only growth of the ovary that produces uterine haemorrhage, is the granulosa-cell tumour and may occur at almost any age (see Ovarian swellings)

In women with postmenopausal bleeding ultrasound scanning to measure the endometrial thickness may be a useful way to triage these patients. If the endometrial thickness is 5 mm or less in thickness, then no further action is needed unless the bleeding continues

Otherwise hysteroscopy and endometrial sampling is recommended.

MENSTRUAL PERIODS, INFREQUENT (OLIGOMENORRHOEA)

Tony Hollingworth

Oligomenorrhoea is a term that defines menstrual periods that occur repeatedly at intervals between 6 weeks and 6 months. It is an arbitrary definition and may be misleading. It is considered that the normal menstrual cycle has an upper limit of 35 days. The proliferative phase, that is, the time during which the follicle (the egg) develops, is the variable part of the cycle. The secretory or luteal phase is the time from ovulation to menstruation, which is usually constant at 14 days. Cycles of 6 weeks duration seem to show no difference from normal-length cycles from the point of follicular and hormone development.

There are several conditions that lead to oligomenorrhoea, and these range from normal (for that woman) to the same causes as amenorrhoea (see Menstrual periods, absent). Some common causes are listed below.

■ *Polycystic ovarian syndrome* accounts for about 90 per cent of cases of oligomenorrhoea compared with only 33 per cent of amenorrhoea. In this situation, the menstrual periods are usually light and the woman may not ovulate (anovulation).

■ A *prolonged proliferative phase* is associated with ovulatory oligomenorrhoea. It often occurs in adolescent girls or at the time of menarche, and in older women in the perimenopausal phase.

■ *Prolonged corpus luteum* activity may also lead to oligomenorrhoea and a prolonged cycle, but is usually associated with prolonged menstruation.

Clinically, oligomenorrhoea should be considered in the same way as amenorrhoea for the purpose of investigations and further management.

MENSTRUAL PERIODS, PAINFUL (DYSMENORRHOEA)

Cynthia Farquhar

Painful periods are also known as dysmenorrhoea, which comes from the Greek meaning 'difficult monthly flow'; however, it is taken to mean 'painful menstruation'. It is a symptom complex, which includes cramping lower abdominal pain radiating to the back and legs, and is often associated with gastrointestinal upset, malaise and headaches. This chapter should be read in conjunction with Menstrual periods, heavy and/or irregular. The problem can be divided into primary and secondary dysmenorrhoea.

Primary dysmenorrhoea occurs when the periods are painful, and no organic or psychological cause can be found. It usually occurs at the beginning of reproductive life when the girl starts ovulating. The pain starts with the onset of menstruation and is generally associated with ovulatory cycles. There is an abnormally high production of endometrial prostaglandins, which causes excessive uterine contractions. Examination findings are usually normal and further investigation may only be necessary if treatment fails to alleviate the symptoms. The options for treatment include the combined oral contraceptive pill to inhibit ovulation, or non-steroidal anti-inflammatory agents, which act as prostaglandin synthetase inhibitors to decrease the concentration of local prostaglandins, and thereby reduce pain and also menstrual loss.

Secondary dysmenorrhoea occurs when the woman experiences painful periods where an organic or psychosexual cause can be found. The differential diagnosis includes:

■ pelvic inflammatory disease;
■ endometriosis or adenomyosis;
■ fibroids;
■ intrauterine contraceptive device;
■ cervical stenosis following treatment for pre-cancer;
■ ovarian tumour;
■ previous pelvic or abdominal surgery;

- pelvic congestion syndrome;
- previous history of sexual abuse or other psychological problems.

Taking a detailed history is important in order to guide diagnostic tests. Pelvic examination should be performed and swabs taken, if indicated. A tender uterus may indicate the possibility of adenomyosis; restricted mobility or a fixed retroverted uterus may suggest the presence of adhesions secondary to endometriosis, pelvic inflammatory disease or previous surgery. A previous history of cone biopsy or other excision procedures for cervical intraepithelial neoplasia might suggest the possibility of cervical stenosis, which can require dilatation of the cervix.

Investigations will depend upon the history. An ultrasound scan may be a useful, especially if vaginal examination is difficult or painful. In many cases, laparoscopy may be indicated to exclude a particular pathology, especially endometriosis. If the findings are normal, then often reassurance in itself may be sufficient.

MISCARRIAGE, RECURRENT

Mala Arora

Recurrent miscarriage is a term coined by Malpas from Liverpool to define women who had three or more consecutive miscarriages. *Miscarriage* is defined as the loss of a pregnancy less than 20 weeks' gestation or losing a fetus that weighs less than 500 g. This is so defined because fetuses below this weight and gestation will not survive.

Sporadic miscarriages occur in up to 25 per cent of pregnancies. A woman may have three sporadic miscarriages during her obstetric career, but these are interspersed with viable births and are not classified as recurrent miscarriages.

Primary aborters are women who have no previous issue and *secondary aborters* are women who have one or more pregnancies that have proceeded beyond 20 weeks' gestation.

The incidence of recurrent miscarriage is 1–2 per cent and the incidence of sporadic miscarriage is 10–11 per cent. By simple statistical extrapolation, the chance of a woman having three sporadic miscarriages in a row is 0.35 per cent. However, since the incidence of recurrent miscarriages is 1–2 per cent (i.e. 3–6 times higher), it points to the fact that a definitive pathology exists in these patients with recurrent miscarriages.

The causes of recurrent miscarriage are listed in Box 1.[1] More than one factor may operate in

---

Box 1 Causes of recurrent miscarriage

Immunological
- Primary antiphospholipid syndrome
- Secondary antiphospholipid syndrome

Genetic
- Fetal trisomy, polyploidy, monosomy
- Parental balanced translocations, inversions, deletions, duplications

Hormonal
- Polycystic ovarian syndrome
- Luteal phase defects
- Hyperandrogenism
- Uncontrolled diabetes mellitus
- Hypothyroidism/hyperthyroidism
- Hyperprolactinaemia
- Premature ovarian failure
- Adrenal hyperplasia/Addison's disease

Anatomical
- Müllerian abnormalities, septate uterus
- Fibroids – submucous, intramural
- Uterine synechiae
- T-shaped uterus
- Cervical incompetence

Inherited thrombophilia
- Antithrombin III deficiency
- Deficiency of protein C and protein S
- Factor V Leiden mutation
- Methyl tetrahydrofolate gene homozygosity (hyperhomocysteinaemia)
- Prothrombin gene mutation

Infections
- Genital bacterial vaginosis, tuberculosis
- Systemic syphilis, Lyme's disease, toxoplasmosis, brucellosis

Systemic conditions
- Hypertension
- Chronic renal disease
- Chronic pulmonary disease
- Heart disease
- Severe rhesus sensitisation

Miscellaneous
- Smoking, alcohol, drugs
- Exposure to irradiation
- Exposure to environmental toxins, pesticides
- Exposure to anaesthetic gases

Idiopathic
- Cytokine abnormalities
- Increased uterine natural killer cells
- Lack of pinopode formation

successive pregnancies, e.g. early miscarriages due to any cause may be coupled with a late miscarriage due to cervical incompetence. On the other hand, early miscarriages may be coupled with a late fetal demise in patients with either congenital or acquired thrombophilia.

■ Immunological causes

Antiphospholipid antibody syndrome (APS) is the commonest immunological cause of recurrent miscarriage. Antibodies are directed against negatively charged phospholipids, which are the major constituents of trophoblast. These antibodies can cause placental thrombosis, infarction, impaired trophoblastic function and abnormal placentation, and thus may lead to pregnancy-induced hypertension, intrauterine growth retardation (IUGR), intrauterine fetal death and recurrent miscarriage.[2,3] Pregnancy loss usually occurs in the mid-trimester between 14 and 18 weeks; however, both early first-trimester losses

and late third-trimester losses can occur. There is an ultrasound confirmation of a viable pregnancy prior to the pregnancy loss in most first trimester losses.

Diagnosis of APS

The diagnosis of APS is made by the presence of *one clinical criterion and one laboratory criterion, which must be positive on two occasions 3 months apart.*

Clinical criteria include the following:[4]

- one or more unexplained deaths of a morphologically normal fetus of more than 10 weeks' gestation documented by ultrasonography or direct examination;
- one or more preterm births at or before 34 weeks' gestation due to severe pre-eclampsia or placental insufficiency with evidence of IUGR;
- three or more consecutive abortions before 10 weeks' gestation with no maternal hormonal, or anatomic abnormalities, normal maternal and paternal chromosomes and other causes of recurrent losses being ruled out.

Laboratory criteria include detection of either lupus anticoagulant or anticardiolipin antibody or both.

Autoimmune disorders, such as systemic lupus erythematosus, systemic sclerosis, and autoimmune thrombocytopenia are associated with recurrent miscarriage, and are often classified as secondary antiphospholipid syndrome (or SAPS). The mechanism of loss and the treatment are the same as those for APS.

■ Genetic causes

Genetic abnormalities in karyotypically normal parents

Various studies demonstrate that at least 50 per cent of clinically recognised pregnancy loss results from a cytogenetic abnormality,[5–8] of which 51 per cent show autosomal trisomies, 22 per cent show polyploidy, 19 per cent show monosomy, 4 per cent shows translocations, and the rest are unclassified genetic defects. The autosomal trisomies commonly encountered are those of chromosomes 3, 4, 9, 13–16, 19, 21 and 22.[9]

Genetic abnormalities in karyotypically abnormal parents

Women may have structural chromosomal abnormality in the following forms.

■ Deletions and duplications produce large chromosomal defects, which may cause severe phenotypic anomalies, thus individuals with these anomalies rarely reproduce.
■ Dicentric and ring chromosomes are mitotically unstable, so the chances of offspring acquiring these anomalies are very small.
■ In balanced translocations in men, the reproductive fitness is only slightly diminished.[10] In spite of their good reproductive performance, these individuals show a significant decrease in live births, and a significant increase in both fetal death and interval infertility; hence they will present with recurrent miscarriage.
■ In unbalanced translocations in men, not only is the reproductive fitness greatly decreased but the risk of abnormal offspring also increased.[10]

■ Hormonal disorders

A multitude of endocrinal disorders can cause recurrent miscarriage. *Polycystic ovarian syndrome* is one of the commonest endocrinal abnormalities affecting female reproductive performance. Besides infertility, it presents higher risks of first- and second-trimester abortions.[11,12]

Factors associated with a high miscarriage rate are *hyperandrogenism*, *hyperinsulinaemia* and/or *ovulatory dysfunction* that accompanies high levels of luteinising hormone and low levels of progesterone.

Women with poorly controlled *type 1 (insulin-dependent) diabetes mellitus* with glycosylated haemoglobin levels greater than four standard deviations above the mean had a higher pregnancy loss rate.[13–15] Well-controlled diabetics had pregnancy loss rates similar to those of non-diabetics.[16] Apart from frank diabetes, syndrome X,[13] which comprises impaired glucose tolerance test (GTT), hypertension, hypertriglyceridaemia and a procoagulant state with increased coronary heart disease, could also potentially cause recurrent pregnancy loss.

Abnormal maternal thyroid functions have been implicated as a cause of recurrent miscarriage.[17] However, mild or subclinical thyroid dysfunction is not associated with recurrent miscarriage, as it more often leads to infertility, but increased levels of thyroid antibodies have been associated with recurrent miscarriage.[18]

Hyperprolactinaemia usually causes infertility due to luteolysis; however, in partially treated cases, the picture may change to pregnancy losses.

Although rare, the patient with an untreated *adrenal hyperplasia* may have an increased chance of recurrent miscarriage owing to hyperandrogenism. On the other hand, incipient *Addison's disease* will also cause recurrent miscarriages; the patient often has low blood pressure and hyperpigmentation.

Premature ovarian failure remains an important factor responsible for recurrent miscarriage, owing to declining ovarian function and poor-quality oocytes. Women with follicle-stimulating hormone levels that are fluctuate between 10 and 40 mIU/mL, not only experience difficulty in conceiving but also have a higher rate of pregnancy loss.

■ Anatomic abnormalities

Anatomic abnormalities of the uterus and cervix are amenable to surgery. An estimated 15 per cent of couples (one in six) with recurrent miscarriage have an anatomic abnormality of the uterus as the primary cause. These abnormalities include the following.

■ Defects of Müllerian fusion, which include septate uterus, unicornuate uterus and bicornuate uterus with unequal uterine horns.
■ Acquired anatomical defects, such as, submucous or intramural fibroids, endometrial polyps and Ashermann's syndrome.
■ Small tubular uterine cavity: this may be secondary to diethyl stilboestrol exposure *in utero* or genital tuberculosis.
■ Cervical incompetence, which is diagnosed by shortening of the cervix on ultrasound scan.[19] It may be a congenital weakness or secondary to repeated cervical dilatation. It is also associated with unicornuate or bicornuate uteri.

■ Thrombophilias

These are rare inherited disorders that predispose an individual to venous and arterial thrombosis. They cause inadequate placental circulation owing to thrombosis in the placental vasculature, and lead to adverse pregnancy outcomes like recurrent miscarriage, fetal death and placental abruption.[20]

Congenital thrombophilias include the following.

- Activated protein C resistance (APCR)[21] due to Factor V Leiden mutation: a single missense mutation of the Factor V gene can cause 90 per cent cases of APCR and is present in 5 per cent of the UK population.
- Deficiency of antithrombin III: this occurs in 32–51 per cent patients with thrombophilia.[22]
- Deficiency of protein C and protein S: in patients with thrombophilia, 22–26 per cent have protein C deficiency, while 12–17 per cent have protein S deficiency.[22]
- Prothrombin gene mutation G 20210A leads to elevated levels of prothrombin and is present in 2 per cent of the UK population.[22]
- Homozygosity for the thermolabile mutation of methylene tetrahydrofolate reductase causing hyperhomocysteinaemia.

The most common acquired thrombophilia is the antiphospholipid antibody syndrome.

■ Systemic conditions

Severe maternal illness, such as, essential hypertension, cardiac disease, chronic pulmonary disease and chronic nephritis, are important causes of recurrent miscarriages. Pregnancy in a rhesus-sensitised woman with a high titre of anti-D antibodies will also result in recurrent pregnancy losses.

Systemic infections like syphilis were an important cause of recurrent miscarriage in the past. Currently, Lyme disease and toxoplasmosis can result in repetitive losses. Bacterial infections like *Brucella abortus* also cause recurrent miscarriage.

■ Genital infections

Genitourinary tuberculosis is classically associated with infertility but can also cause recurrent ectopic pregnancy as well as recurrent miscarriages. Bacterial vaginosis is now implicated in recurrent miscarriages, and recurrent preterm labour and preterm premature rupture of membranes.

■ Miscellaneous causes

Hyperhomocysteinaemia is associated with thrombosis and can be genetic or dietary in origin. Administration of folic acid and vitamin B6 and B12 will help in decreasing homocysteine levels. Excessive smoking, alcohol intake and the use of recreational drugs will cause recurrent miscarriage. Other factors include prolonged exposure to irradiation and anaesthetic gases, pesticides and other environmental toxins.

■ Idiopathic

In many cases, the cause of recurrent miscarriages is not clearly elucidated at present. Implantation is a complex process that involves synchronization of endometrial maturity with fertilization, expression of *HOX A 10* genes in the endometrium, formation of pinopodes, as well as the presence of cytokines of the anti-inflammatory kind, such as interleukins 4, 6 and 10, leukaemia inhibiting factor (LIF) and transforming growth factor beta (TGF-β). A disturbance in any of the above processes will lead to early pregnancy losses. Absence of the cytokine leukaemia inhibiting factor in the endometrium is associated with recurrent miscarriages in the knockout mouse model but its exact role in humans is yet to be elucidated. Other cytokine abnormalities in the endometrium are the subject of current research in recurrent miscarriages.

Hence recurrent miscarriages may occur due to a variety of causes, some well understood and others less so. Some are treatable, such as thrombophilia and those with an immunological, hormonal or anatomical cause. Genetic causes are best investigated and treated through *in-vitro* fertilisation and pre-implantation genetic diagnosis. An abnormal cytokine environment may be responsible for some of the hitherto unexplained recurrent miscarriages.

■ References

1. Arora M and Konje J, eds. *Recurrent Pregnancy Loss*. Second International edition. New Delhi: Jaypee, 2007.
2. Gharavi AE, Pierangli SS, Levy RA, Harris N. Mechanisms of pregnancy loss in antiphospholipid syndrome. *Clin Obstet Gynaecol* 2001; **44**: 11–19.
3. Hughes GR. The antiphospholipid syndrome: ten years on. *Lancet* 1993; **342**: 341–44.
4. Geis W, Branch DW. Obstetric implications of antiphospholipid antibodies: pregnancy loss and other complications. *Clin Obstet Gynaecol* 2001; **44**: 2–10.
5. Boui J, Boui A, Lazar P. Retrospective and prospective epidemiological studies of 1500 karyotyped spontaneous human abortions. *Teratology* 1975; **12**: 11.
6. Hassold T. A cytogenetic study of repeated spontaneous abortions. *Am J Hum Genet* 1980; **32**: 723.
7. Hassold T, Chiu D, Yamane JA. Parental origin of autosomal trisomies. *Ann Hum Genet* 1984, **48**: 129–44.
8. Simpson JL, Bombard AT. Chromosomal abnormalities in spontaneous abortions: frequency, pathology and genetic counselling. In: Edmonds K, Bennett MJ, eds. *Spontaneous Abortions*. London: Blackwell, 1987: 51.
9. Papa Dopoulos G, Templeton AA, Fisk N, *et al.* The frequency of chromosomal anomalies in human preimplantation embryos after in vitro fertilization. *Hum Reprod* 1987; **4**: 91.
10. Jacobs PA. Structural rearrangements of chromosomes in men. In: Hook EB, Porter IM, eds. *Population Cytogenetics*. New York: Academic Press, 1977: 81–97.
11. Regan L, Owen EJ, Jacobs HS. Hypersecretion of luteinizing hormone, infertility and miscarriage. *Lancet* 1990; **336**: 1141–4.
12. Homberg R. Influence of serum LH concentrations on ovulation, conception and early pregnancy loss in PCOD. *BMJ* 1988; **297**: 1024–6.
13. Zaveroni I, Bonini L, Fantuzzi M, *et al.* Hyperinsulinemia, obesity and Syndrome X. *J Intern Med* 1994; **235**: 51–6.
14. Miodovnik M, Mimouni F, Tsang RL, *et al.* Glycemic control and spontaneous abortions in insulin dependent diabetic women. *Obstet Gynecol* 1986; **68**: 366.
15. Mills JL, Simpson JI, Driscoll SE, *et al.* Incidence of abortion among normal women and insulin dependent diabetic women whose pregnancies were identified within 21 days of conception. *N Engl J Med* 1988; **391**: 1617–23.
16. Dicker D, Feldberg D, Samuel N. Spontaneous abortions in patients with insulin dependent diabetes mellitus: the effect of preconceptional diabetic control. *Am J Obstet Gynecol* 1988; **158**: 1161.
17. Gilnoer D, Soto MF, Bourdoux P, *et al.* Pregnancy in patients with mild thyroid abnormalities: maternal and neonatal repercussion. *J Clin Endocrinol Metab* 1991; **73**: 421–7.
18. Bussen S, Steck T. Thyroid antibodies in euthyroid non pregnant women with recurrent spontaneous abortions. *Hum Reprod* 1995; **10**: 2938.
19. Gomez R. Ultrasonographic examination of uterine cervix is better than cervical digital examination as a predictor of the likelihood of premature delivery in patients with preterm labor and intact membranes. *Am J Obstet Gynecol* 1994; **171**: 956–64.
20. Desai P. Thrombophilia in pregnancy. *Obstet Gynaecol Today* 1999; **3**: 21.
21. Younis JS, Brenner B, Ohel G, *et al.* Activated protein C resistance and factor V Leiden mutation can be associated with first as well as second trimester RPL. *Am J Reprod Immunol* 2000; 43: 31–5.
22. Nelson Piercy C. Thromboembolic disease. In: *Obstetric Medicine*, Vol. 1. London: Martin Dunitz, 2002: 42–4.

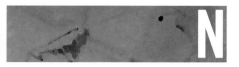

NOSEBLEEDS (EPISTAXIS) IN PREGNANCY

Mike Papesch and Eva Lunderskov Papesch

A nosebleed, or epistaxis (from the Greek *epi* meaning 'on' and *stazo* meaning 'to let fall in drops') is blood loss commonly from the front of the nose. Nosebleeds most frequently come from the front of the nasal septum called 'Little's area', which was first described by James L. Little (1836–1885), Professor of Surgery at the University of Vermont, USA.

■ Epidemiology

Nosebleeds are common in children, nearly always anterior in location and are usually brief. In older patients, bleeding from the nose can be more severe, especially if the bleeding is from the back of the nose. They occur in about 15 per cent of the population, and peak in childhood and late adult life. They can also occur in pregnancy in association with increased blood pressure and the hypervascular state.

■ Anatomy

Anterior nosebleeds occur from Little's area, a watershed of arteries in front of the nasal septum. This is a confluence of blood vessels originating from both the internal and external carotid arteries (Fig. 1). Posterior nosebleeds are less common but much more severe, and originate from the sphenopalatine artery.

■ Aetiology of epistaxis

The aetiology of epistaxis is given in Box 1.

■ Pregnancy-related nosebleeds[10]

Pregnancy hormones affect the nasal mucosa, nasal cycle and mucociliary nasal transport

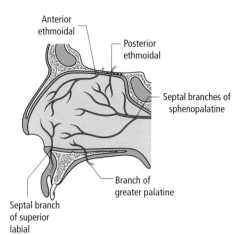

Figure 1 Arterial blood supply to the nose.

Labels:
Anterior ethmoidal
Posterior ethmoidal
Septal branches of sphenopalatine
Branch of greater palatine
Septal branch of superior labial

Box 1 Aetiology of epistaxis

- Trauma: nose picking, nasal spray, cocaine, surgery, foreign bodies, nasal septal perforation
- Nasal airflow/dry air: drying effect of septal deviation, airline travel
- Infective/inflammatory: rhinitis, sinusitis, fungal infection, Wegener's granulomatosis
- Pregnancy related: pyogenic granuloma gravidarum (nasal haemangioma of pregnancy), hypertension of pregnancy[1]
- Autoimmune: atrophic rhinitis
- Vascular malformations: haemangiomas, hereditary haemorrhagic telangiectasia[2]
- Neoplastic: inverted papilloma, adenocarcinoma
- Drugs: anticoagulants (warfarin, aspirin,[3] clopidogrel), non-steroidal anti-inflammatory drugs[4]
- Haemopoietic/coagulopathies: blood dyscrasia, idiopathic thrombocytopenia purpura, haemophilia, etc.
- Cardiac: hypertension,[5] increased venous pressure[6]
- Metabolic: renal or liver disease, vitamin C and K deficiency, folic acid deficiency (and thrombocytopenia)[7]
- Vicarious menstruation and metastasis of endometrial tissue[8,9]

time, producing rhinorrhoea and nasal obstruction.[11,12] The increased vascularity of the nasal mucosa owing to the effects of oestrogen makes bleeding secondary to minor trauma much more likely.

Pyogenic granuloma gravidarum (a form of lobular capillary haemangioma) occurs as oral (gingivitis gravidarum) or nasal lesions in less than 1 per cent of pregnant women.[13] These lesions range from a few millimetres to a centimetre in diameter, and present as an elevated red or purple mass with a smooth, lobulated, ulcerative surface and bleed easily with minimal trauma. Microscopically, the nodule consists of highly vascular granulation tissue displaying acute and chronic inflammation. They are hormone dependent, as they appear characteristically in the early months of pregnancy and, if not excised, usually regress following delivery.[14] They present with varying degrees of bleeding and nasal obstruction, and can occasionally be very large and cause massive bleeding. Treatment is by excision.[15,16] If incompletely excised, they can recur and also develop satellite lesions.

The ulcerated surface of pyogenic granulomas often contains staphylococci or streptococci. One hypothesis has been that these organisms cause an overgrowth of granulation tissue because of a retardation of re-epithelialisation of a wound. Circulating angiogenic factors also play a role, particularly in pregnancy.[17]

Hypertension of pregnancy may also contribute to serious nosebleeds that may prove difficult to control.

◼ Clinical features

It is important to be aware that women with nosebleeds may present with antepartum fetal distress, even in the absence of maternal hypotension.

Anterior bleeds are usually unilateral, occur following minimal trauma and are often brief. More severe anterior nosebleeds can occur, often from a prominent blood vessel further back on the nasal septum.

Posterior nosebleeds are often severe. They present with bilateral nasal bleeding, often with spitting up of blood. Severe nosebleeds[18] present as any acute blood loss episode with features of hypovolaemic shock[19] which includes tachycardia, hypotension, pallor and diaphoresis.

◼ Management of small nosebleeds

The side and frequency of nosebleeds is important. Examination of the nose with a headlight and mirror may reveal a prominent anterior nasal septum vessel, with associated dry crusted blood.

◼ Management of severe nosebleeds

History

On arrival, make sure you are wearing appropriate protective clothing, including gloves, glasses and a mask. Post nasal bleeding leads to significant coughing and vomiting of blood, with resultant blood spray! Take note of the side of bleeding, the length and severity of the nosebleed, and any precipitating or exacerbating factors. Usually it will be obvious if a nosebleed is minor or severe. Control of severe nosebleeds can require volume replacement and resuscitation (the Airways, Breathing and Circulation response), as well as addressing the underlying cause. Drug history is important. Coexisting coagulopathies need to be considered, as well as ruling out specific underlying systemic illnesses, such as hereditary haemorrhagic telangiectasia.

Examination

Assessment of the haemodynamic state is paramount. Once the patient is stable, with an intravenous line *in situ* and appropriate investigations and fluid replacement have been achieved, the cause of the bleed should be addressed. A good headlight, nasal speculum and suction make examination easier. The best position for examining the patient is on a bed with the head elevated about 70 degrees. Up to 90 per cent of nosebleeds can be seen originating from the anterior nasal septum (Little's area). Severe nosebleeds may be associated with bleeding from the mouth and haematemesis.

Removal of clot from the front of the nose (blowing of the nose or use of suction) allows a better view of the bleeding point, and removes the fibrinolytic factors released in clot that may prolong bleeding. A nasal speculum allows better inspection of the anterior nose. Ribbon gauze, soaked with adrenaline and lignocaine allows vasoconstriction of the mucosa and bleeding blood vessel. This provides a better view, may stop the bleeding and provides anaesthesia to allow cautery of particular blood vessels.

Bleeding not seen with this approach is further posterior. Rigid nasendoscopes allow a more detailed view of the nasal cavity, including the postnasal space.

Investigations

Full blood count, clotting profile, bleeding time and cross-match may be necessary. Other tests are directed at potential or underling pathologies.

Minor anterior nosebleeds are managed with direct pressure over the soft part of the nose, for 5 minutes (by the clock; Fig. 2). The head is in the neutral position. Cotton wool and tissues, etc. should be avoided as these lead to rebleeding when they are removed from the nose. Vaseline or other ointments (Naseptin – exclude peanut allergy as this contains arachis oil) are applied to the nose after the bleeding has stopped in order to aid healing, and prevent scabbing and drying of the anterior nose. Ice is used to reduce nasal temperature and promote vasoconstriction of the nasal vessels. It is probably of more benefit to suck ice rather that apply ice to the forehead.[20–22] Bleeds from small blood vessels in Little's area require cautery (commonly silver nitrate) if ongoing.

More severe nosebleeds are treated as for any acute blood loss. Coinciding with haemodynamic resuscitation, a full blood count, coagulation profile and cross-match may need to be done. Local control measures as above are important, but packing of the nose with adrenaline gauze (with constriction of the nasal mucosa) and suction may allow identification of the nosebleed, followed by cautery. More severe nosebleeds will require packing, occasionally in theatre. If bilateral nasal packs are used, monitoring of pO_2 is mandatory.[23] Prophylactic antibiotics are used to prevent toxic shock syndrome. Endoscopic ligation of the sphenopalatine artery at the back of the nose may be required, along with tying off the anterior ethmoid artery. Arteriography and embolisation is an effective and safe technique, and should be considered, particularly if the epistaxis is severe and has been resistant to treatment as above. A distinct advantage is that it is performed under local anaesthesia. It has been shown to be effective and safe in pregnancy.[24] Less commonly used these days is transantral maxillary artery ligation. Extreme cases will require ligation of the external carotid artery (with little morbidity).[18]

Control of hypertension and any other underlying systemic condition is very important. Caesarean section or delivery may be required to allow control of hypertension and the arrest of bleeding.[18] Bed rest is important in severe nosebleeds, with appropriate deep venous thrombosis prophylaxis.

Tranexamic acid (an inhibitor of fibrinolysis) is sometimes used also to assist control of bleeding in pregnancy. It stabilises preformed clots and prolongs their dissolution. There is no increased risk of thromboembolism with this drug in this high-risk group of women.[25–27]

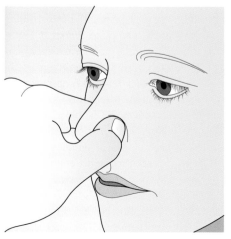

Figure 2 Treatment of minor nosebleeds.

■ Prevention

Vaseline applied to the anterior nose is useful to prevent drying of the nose, and cracking/bleeding of blood vessels. Saline nasal sprays, such as Sterimar, can also be useful.

■ Conclusion

Nosebleeds are common and occur in pregnancy. They are often trivial and anterior in situation. Simple measures, such as appropriate pressure and cautery, with use of nasal creams usually treat most bleeds. Pyogenic granulomas can occur in pregnancy and often require excision to control bleeding. Posterior nasal bleeds tend to be more severe and usually require packing. Endoscopic ligation of the sphenopalatine artery, and ligation of the anterior and posterior ethmoid arteries is often required to control these bleeds. Underlying systemic causes of bleeding must also be excluded.

■ References

1. Green LK, Green RS, Harris RE. Life-threatening epistaxis associated with pregnancy. *Am J Obstet Gynecol* 1974; **120:** 1113–4.
2. Begbie ME, Wallace GM, Shovlin CL. Hereditary haemorrhagic telangiectasia (Osler–Weber–Rendu syndrome): a view from the 21st century. *Postgrad Med J* 2003; **79:** 18–24.
3. Tay HL, Evans JM, McMahon AD, MacDonald TM. Aspirin, nonsteroidal anti-inflammatory drugs, and epistaxis. A regional record linkage case control study. *Ann Otol Rhinol Laryngol* 1998; **107:** 671–4.
4. Livesey JR, Watson MG, Kelly PJ, Kesteven PJ. Do patients with epistaxis have drug-induced platelet dysfunction? *Clin Otolaryngol Allied Sci* 1995; **20:** 407–10.
5. Jackson KR, Jackson RT. Factors associated with active, refractory epistaxis. *Arch Otolaryngol Head Neck Surg* 1988; **114:** 862–5.
6. Braithwaite JM, Economides DL. Severe recurrent epistaxis causing antepartum fetal distress. *Int J Gynaecol Obstet* 1995; **50:** 197–8.
7. Poelman AM, Aarnoudse JG. A pregnant woman with severe epistaxis – a rare manifestation of folic acid deficiency. *Eur J Obstet Gynecol Reprod Biol* 1986; **23:** 249–54.
8. Laghzaoui O, Laghzaoui M. [Nasal endometriosis: apropos of 1 case] (in French). *J Gynecol Obstet Biol Reprod* 2001; **30:** 786–8.
9. Dunn JM. Vicarious menstruation. *Am J Obstet Gynecol* 1972; **114:** 568–9.
10. Hansen L, Sobol SM, Abelson TI. Otolaryngologic manifestations of pregnancy. *J Fam Pract* 1986; **23:** 151–5.
11. Armengot M, Marco J, Ruiz M, Baixauli A. Hormones and the nasal mucosa. A bibliographic review (in Spanish). *An Otorrinolaringol Ibero Am* 1990; **17:** 317–28.
12. Hellin MD, Ruiz CV, Ruiz FM. The influence of pregnancy on mucociliary nasal transport (in Spanish). *An Otorrinolaringol Ibero Am* 1994; **21:** 595–601.
13. Kent DL, Fitzwater JE. Nasal haemangioma of pregnancy. *Ann Otol Rhinol Laryngol* 1979; **88:** 331–3.
14. Scott PMJ, van Hasselt A. Case report of a bleeding nasal polyp during pregnancy. *Ear Nose Throat J* 1999; **78:** 592.
15. Choudhary S, MacKinnon CA, Morrissey GP, Tan ST. A case of giant nasal pyogenic granuloma gravidarum. *J Craniofac Surg* 2005; **16:** 319–21.
16. Tantinikorn W, Uiprasertkul M, Assanasen P. Nasal granuloma gravidarum presenting with recurrent massive epistaxis. *J Med Assoc Thailand* 2003; **86:** 473–6.
17. McNutt NS, Smoller BR, Contreras F. Skin. In: Damjanov I, Linder J, eds.

Anderson's Pathology, 10th edn, Vol. 2. St Louis, MO: Mosby-Year Book Inc., 1996: 2465–6.

18. Howard DJ. Life-threatening epistaxis in pregnancy. *J Laryngol Otol* 1985; **99:** 95–6.

19. Cooley Sharon M, Geary M, O'Connell MP, Keane DP. Hypovolaemic shock secondary to epistaxis in pregnancy. *J Obstet Gynaecol* 2002; **22:** 229–30.

20. Teymoortash A, Sesterhenn A, Kress R, Sapundzhiev N, Werner JA. Efficacy of ice packs in the management of epistaxis. Clin Otolaryngol Allied Sci 2003; **28:** 545–7.

21. Dost P, Polyzoidis T. [Benefit of the ice pack in the treatment of nosebleed]. (in German). HNO 1992; **40:** 25–7.

22. Porter MJ. A comparison between the effect of ice packs on the forehead and ice cubes in the mouth on nasal submucosal temperature. *Rhinology* 1991; **29:** 11–5.

23. Lin Y, Orkin, LR. Arterial hypoxemia in patients with anterior and posterior nasal packing. *Laryngoscope* 1979; **89:** 140–4.

24. Elahi MM, Parnes LS, Fox AJ, Pelz DM, Lee DH. Therapeutic embolization in the treatment of intractable epistaxis. Arch Otolaryngol Head Neck Surg 1995; **121:** 65–9.

25. Lindoff C, Rybo G, Astedt B. Treatment with tranexamic acid during pregnancy, and the risk of thrombo-embolic complications. *Thromb Haemostas* 1993; **70:** 238–40.

26. Dunn CJ, Goa KL. Tranexamic acid: a review of its use in surgery and other indications. *Drugs* 1999; **57:** 1005–32.

27. Storm O, Weber J. Prolonged treatment with tranexamic acid (Cyclocapron) during pregnancy (in Danish). *Ugeskrift for Laeger* 1976; **138:** 1781–2.

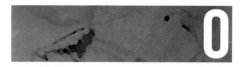

OVARIAN SWELLINGS

Karina Reynolds and Nicola Fattizzi

The ovary is essentially made up of three types of cell:

- those that produce the eggs and are, therefore, totipotential;
- those that produce the hormones;
- those that wrap it all up together.

Swellings can occur involving any of these cells.

Overall, ovarian swellings still represent one of the most difficult diagnostic problems for a gynaecologist owing to the lack of specific symptoms. Most ovarian masses cause no specific symptoms or signs because the abdomen represents a very large cavity that can cope with bulky masses without symptomatology until they become large (Figs 1 and 2). A small number of patients present with acute symptoms, if there is either severe pelvic infection, or torsion or rupture of an ovarian cyst, but for many the onset of symptoms is very gradual. Indeed, in a significant proportion of cases, large masses are an incidental finding at a routine gynaecological examination or a pelvic ultrasound scan for other reasons. The symptoms can include:

- generalised abdominal discomfort;
- dull pelvic pain and dyspareunia;
- increasing abdominal girth;
- pressure symptoms;
- urinary symptoms, frequency and urgency;
- weight loss and general debility;
- flatulence and dyspepsia.

The management of a patient presenting with an ovarian lump depends on a combination

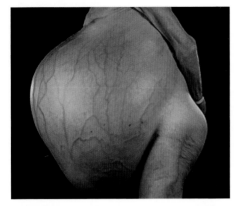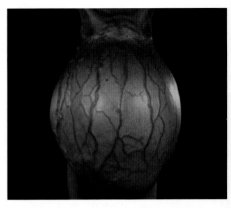

Figure 1 Woman presenting with gradually increasing abdominal girth.

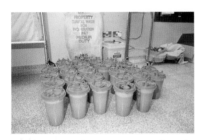

Figure 2 Fluid removed from the same woman's ovarian cyst.

of several predictive factors, which include the following.

- *Age*: one of the most important predictive characteristics for an ovarian mass.
- *Menopausal status*: in the pre-pubertal and post-menopausal age groups, an ovarian swelling must be considered to be abnormal. Consequently, further investigations are indicated and a surgical approach to treatment may be required. In the reproductive age group, the differential diagnosis of an ovarian mass may be more complex and surgery is indicated after careful evaluation.
- *Size of the mass*: an adnexal mass >5 cm in diameter that persists longer than 6–8 weeks is an indication for surgery. Functional ovarian cysts generally measure less than 7 cm and disappear within 4–6 weeks. In postmenopausal women, cysts >5 cm in diameter are more likely to be malignant, whereas the smaller unilocular cysts are almost invariably benign.

- *Ultrasound features*: including shape, size, capsular characteristics, internal septae, vegetations and solid components, and the appearance of the fluid (Figs 3 and 4). This investigation may be combined with an assessment of blood flow by means of colour/power Doppler. In fact, irregular masses with uneven capsules adherent to adjacent structures, irregular and thickened septae, vegetations, solid areas and low-resistance blood flow are all in keeping with a likely diagnosis of malignancy. Further imaging, if needed, would be by computerised tomography scanning.
- *Bilaterality*: bilaterality of an ovarian swelling, the presence of ascites and rapid growth are highly suspicious of malignancy.
- *Symptoms*: the only specific symptomatology is that secondary to the nature of the mass. These are: endocrinological, if the lump is

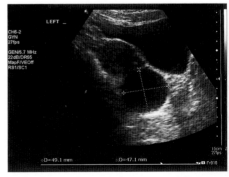

Figure 3 Ultrasound scan appearance of a simple ovarian cyst.

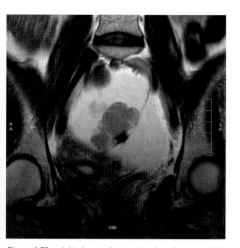

Figure 4 T2-weighted coronal scans showing a large predominantly cystic mass in the pelvis containing septations and solid components typical of an ovarian carcinoma. The uterus and cervix can be seen inferior to the mass and are separate from it.

hormone-secreting or chronic anovulation-dependant; pain in the case of endometriotic cysts; and septic in the event of acute or subacute pelvic inflammation.

■ *Tumour markers serum levels* (CA125, carcinoembryonic antigen (CEA), CA19-9, β-human chorionic gonadotrophin and AFP): CA125 can be of some help in differentiating benign and malignant tumours given that, in the majority of epithelial ovarian cancers, CA125 levels are raised (usually over 100 UI/mL). However, 50 per cent of stage 1 epithelial ovarian cancers present with normal CA125 levels. Furthermore, this is not a specific test, and levels may be elevated with endometriosis, uterine fibroids, dermoid cysts or anything that causes peritoneal irritation (see Appendix).

It is recommended that a 'risk of malignancy index' (RMI) should be used for postmenopausal women presenting with an ovarian mass to select out those women requiring surgery in a Cancer Centre (i.e. those at >75 per cent risk of having an ovarian cancer). The Royal College of Obstetricians and Gynaecologists have produced a guideline outlining the use and interpretation of the RMI

$$RMI = U \times M \times \text{CA125 level}$$

where U is ultrasound findings (0 = no features, 1 = one feature, 3 = 2–5 features), i.e.

■ multilocular cyst
■ evidence of solid areas
■ evidence of metastases
■ presence of ascites
■ bilateral lesions;

and M is menopausal status (premenopausal = 1, postmenopausal = 3). Values <25 indicate low risk, 25–250 moderate risk and >250 high risk of malignancy.

In general terms, ovarian swellings can be divided into three main groups: functional, non-neoplastic and neoplastic.

■ Functional

Epidemiologically, during the reproductive age, functional ovarian masses (follicular and corpus luteal cysts) are the most common, followed by endometriotic cysts and dermoid cysts.

A corpus luteum is formed following the release of the ovum (egg) and this will maintain a pregnancy up to 63 days' gestation (on a 28-day cycle). In most cases, the size of this 'cyst' will reach 20–25 mm in diameter. In general, most ovarian cysts of 5 cm diameter or less will regress without any need to intervene, although it may be useful to repeat an ultrasound scan after 2–3 cycles. Clinically, it may be difficult to palpate an ovarian cyst until it is greater than 5 cm. If the cyst is larger, then it may require removal to avoid the complications of torsion, rupture and haemorrhage.

In postmenopausal patients, the functional genesis of the ovarian lump is less probable since it may occur within 2 years of the last menstrual period. Functional cysts, related to the absence of the ovulation, are filled with fluid, and can be up to 5–6 cm in diameter. They can be found occasionally in healthy women and in patients with endocrine diseases. They usually regress spontaneously within a couple of weeks, when the subsequent menstrual period occurs. If they do not disappear, either a follicular or corpus luteal cyst can be formed.

The presenting symptoms may be acute due to torsion, rupture or haemorrhage, or they may present with a spectrum of menstrual problems as in endometriotic cysts. They may also be an incidental finding on pelvic ultrasound scan.

■ Non-neoplastic

Non-neoplastic benign ovarian cysts include the following.

- *Theca lutein cyst*: the formation of a theca lutein cyst is due to a process of luteinisation of an unruptured follicle and is secondary to an abnormal ovarian exposure to exogenous (ovarian hyperstimulation syndrome) or endogenous (gestational trophoblastic tumours) hormones. It may be associated with hyperemesis, pressure symptoms and can lead to pre-eclampsia-type symptoms later in pregnancy.
- *Corpus luteal cyst associated with pregnancy*: this solid, quite often voluminous, non-neoplastic, pregnancy-related mass may be an incidental finding during Caesarean section and usually regresses spontaneously after pregnancy.
- *Haemorrhagic corpus luteal cyst*: this can arise after ovulation owing to heavy bleeding from the shallow follicular microvessels. It may result in haematoma within the corpus luteum (vague or no symptoms) or can present with haemoperitoneum if the cyst ruptures (pain leading to an acute abdomen with peritoneal signs). The differential diagnosis in this situation would also include ectopic pregnancy and acute appendicitis (if on the right side).

Follicular, corpus luteal and theca lutein cysts should not be treated surgically unless complications (rupture with haemoperitoneum,

twisted cyst) occur that require such intervention.

- *Endometriotic cysts*: these often contain brown or altered blood (chocolate cysts) and can range from a few millimetres to 10 cm in diameter. They may be bilateral and may be difficult to distinguish from other benign ovarian masses. The definitive diagnosis is confirmed histologically. However, a patient's history (acute pelvic pain during the second phase of the menses, pain on intercourse or persistent pelvic pain, mainly if drug-resistant, along with the finding of some nodularity involving uterosacral ligaments and cul-de-sac) may be helpful in anticipating the diagnosis.
- *Simple cysts in postmenopausal women*: these often found on imaging and do not require intervention unless >5 cm and symptomatic. Most are small (<1 cm) and are thought to represent inclusion cysts that are the remnants of ovulation during the reproductive era.
- *Tubo-ovarian abscess* is a common cause of adnexal swelling. These usually occur bilaterally and are sequelae of acute salpingitis/pelvic inflammatory disease. Frequently, they can be palpated on bimanual examination as very firm, exquisitely tender, bilateral fixed masses, possibly located in the pelvic cul-de-sac. The symptoms and signs are similar to those of acute salpingitis, although pain and fever have often been present for longer. A ruptured tubo-ovarian abscess is a life-threatening surgical emergency, as septic shock may develop rapidly.

■ Neoplastic/malignant

In the UK, ovarian malignancy kills more women than all other genital tract cancers taken together. However, it is an uncommon disease and it is estimated that a general practitioner will see one case of ovarian cancer every 5 years. According to a simplified World Health Organisation classification, ovarian tumours can be classified as follows.

- *Epithelial*: benign (cystadenoma; Fig. 5), borderline and malignant (Fig. 6). Most epithelial ovarian

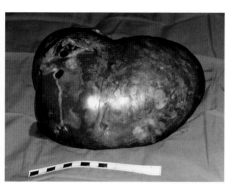

Figure 5 Cystadenoma of the ovary.

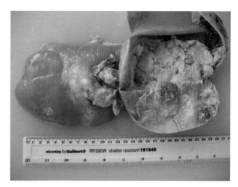

Figure 7 Dermoid cyst showing hair and sebaceous material.

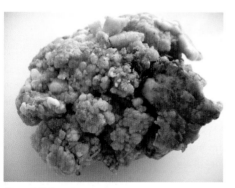

Figure 6 Malignant ovary.

cancers present late when the disease has already spread beyond the ovary. In these cases, the ovarian mass is usually associated with clear evidence of extraovarian disease, ascites and possibly pleural effusions.

■ *Germ cell*: the dermoid cyst represents a very particular benign type of germ cell tumour (Fig. 7). These cysts contain sebaceous material, hair and sometimes teeth owing to the totipotential nature of the cells. These cysts do have a markedly high risk of torsion, perhaps because of the high fat content of most dermoid cysts, allowing them to float within the abdominal and pelvic cavity. Torsion causes severe constant pain that radiates down the medial aspect of the leg and is often associated with vomiting. If the torsion is partial, the pain may be intermittent.

■ *Sex-cord stromal*: hormonal production from granulosa and thecal cell tumours can lead to precocious puberty in a child, menstrual problems during the reproductive age, and postmenopausal bleeding in the older woman owing to endometrial hyperplasia. The androgen-secreting tumours (Sertoli–Leydig tumours) are likely to cause hirsutism, acne, alopecia and behavioural alterations. Struma ovarii may present with hyperthyroidism.

■ *Uncommon*: including lymphomas, melanomas, sarcomas. A very interesting association of symptoms can be found in Meigs' syndrome, classically characterized by a fibroma associated with ascites and a right pleural effusion. Removal of the tumour cures the effusion and ascites.

■ *Metastatic*: up to 10 per cent of ovarian masses are secondary to metastases from some other organ and, in many cases, the ovarian metastases are detected before the primary tumour. The most common metastatic cancers are those arising from the colon, stomach, breast and, of course, the female genital tract. Bilaterally enlarged ovaries, which contain signet-ring cells on microscopic assessment, have been named after Krukenberg who described these ovarian tumours in patients with metastatic gastric or (less commonly) colonic cancer.

■ Reference

1. *Ovarian Cysts in Postmenopausal Women*. Green Top Guideline, no. 34 (www.rcog.org.uk).

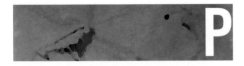

PAIN DURING INTERCOURSE

Cynthia Farquhar

Painful intercourse is also known as dyspareunia and is probably the most common sexual difficulty that presents to the gynaecologist. This pain may be classified as:

- superficial, when the pain arises at the vaginal introitus; and
- deep, when the pain is felt within the pelvis.

The pain may be continuous or intermittent in nature, and continue after intercourse is finished. The main question that needs to be asked is whether it prevents intercourse occurring. These symptoms can be further divided as follows.

- Primary dyspareunia, when intercourse has always been painful, often has a psychological background and may need expert counselling.
- Secondary dyspareunia, when the symptoms occur after a period of painless sex, may be secondary to underlying pathology, such as endometriosis.

Dyspareunia may lead to vaginismus, which is involuntary spasm of pubococcygeus muscle, such that penetration is difficult or impossible. It may occur after one episode of pain but a pattern of dyspareunia may become established. Anticipation of the pain leads to contraction of the muscles and, in addition, lubrication is reduced as pain is anticipated, also making sexual activity more painful.

■ Superficial dyspareunia

Superficial dyspareunia can be classified according to the local anatomical factors as follows.

Vulval causes

- *Infective vulvitis*, which can occur with herpes or candidal infections; relevant swabs and antibiotics or antiviral agents are needed.

- *Atrophic changes*, particularly in postmenopausal women, would respond to hormone replacement therapy or topical oestrogens. If oestrogen is contraindicated, then lubrication with KY gel may be of value, as may local moisturising preparations (Replens).
- *Bartholinitis* may be due to local infection of the Bartholin's gland but can be a site for gonorrhoea. Marsupialisation is the standard treatment to drain the cyst and create a new duct for the gland.
- *Skin conditions affecting the vulva*, including lichen sclerosus (see Vulval itching), may cause pain as a result of the development of cracks and fissures in the skin.
- *Neoplasms*, either malignant or premalignant, may cause these symptoms and would need appropriate diagnosis and treatment.

Urethral causes

These are very much anatomical problems and are not seen very often in a general gynaecological clinic.

- *Urethritis and cystitis* may require local swabs or a mid-stream urine specimen for culture and sensitivity.
- *Caruncle* should be clearly seen on inspection, usually occurs in postmenopausal women and may become inflamed and tender.
- *Diverticulum of the urethra* is an uncommon condition to present to the gynaecologist.

Vaginal causes

- *Vaginismus*, as previously described.
- *Poor lubrication* secondary to psychosexual causes, including poor sexual technique.
- *Atrophic vaginitis*, treatment is as above for the atrophic vulva.
- *Infective vaginitis* with *Candida*, *Trichomonas*, herpes and gonorrhoea. Routine local swabs need to be undertaken and appropriate treatment instituted.
- *Anatomical problems* may come to light in the form of vaginal atresia or imperforate hymen, which may require ultrasound scanning to assess any other associated anatomical problems within the pelvis,

and an examination under anaesthesia to determine the extent of the problem.

- *Contractures post surgery*, especially for episiotomy or perineal tear repairs, which can lead to narrowing of the entrance to the vagina. The introitus may be very tight and require further surgery to relieve the local tightness from the original repair.
- *Post radiotherapy* – this can be prevented to a great extent by the use of vaginal dilators around the time of initial treatment.

Disproportion in size is rarely in itself of importance, as the vagina is very distensile but if, in addition, there is any local lesion, the pain will be accentuated. Anal fissure, and thrombosed and inflamed piles are recognized by careful examination of the anus and rectum by the finger or speculum. Arthritis of the hips or lumbar spine may cause dyspareunia, although it may not be so well localised.

Deep dyspareunia

Deep dyspareunia is due to deep stretching at the time of coitus of the involved pelvic tissues, which include a fixed retroverted uterus, the uterosacral ligaments or rectovaginal septum, or pressure on enlarged ovaries. There may be no pain on penetration and no difficulty, but coitus with deep penetration gives acute pain at the time or leads to dull aching in the pelvis after intercourse. Clinically the symptoms can be mimicked with vaginal examination. The following are the usual causes.

- *Pelvic inflammatory disease* (Fig. 1), where the pelvic organs may be inflamed and adhesions may fix the tissues in place. If this is an acute episode, then antibiotics can be used and it is important to ensure that the partner is also treated. If this is a chronic picture, then pelvic clearance of the genital organs may be a final stage option.
- *Endometriosis* (Fig. 2) is a common cause of deep dyspareunia, especially when the uterosacral ligaments are involved. The degree of endometriosis

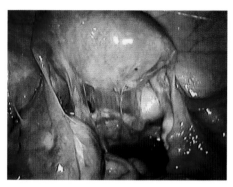

Figure 1 Laparoscopic view of pelvic inflammatory disease.

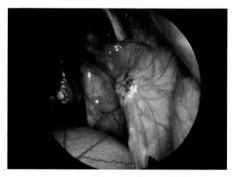

Figure 2 Laparoscopic view of endometriosis affecting the uterosacral ligaments.

does not always mirror the symptoms, the diagnosis being confirmed by diagnostic laparoscopy. Treatment options will depend on the degree of endometriosis and may involve surgery.

- *Ectopic pregnancy* may cause peritoneal irritation, which in turn causes dyspareunia. It is not a common presentation for ectopic pregnancy.
- *Chronic pelvic pain syndrome* with prominent vasculature of the pelvis (Fig. 3) may be diagnosed at laparoscopy and can be treated with progestogens.
- *Ovarian neoplasm* is an unusual cause of dyspareunia.
- *Any pelvic pathology* that causes peritoneal irritation.

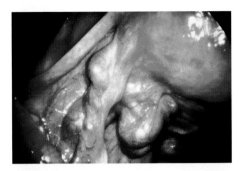

Figure 3 Laparoscopic view of prominent vasculature of the pelvis.

Despite these problems, severe constipation can cause dyspareunia in a number of women and this may be noted at the time of vaginal examination. Diagnostic laparoscopy is used to determine an obvious gynaecological cause. However, if the laparoscopy is negative, it can serve to reassure the woman that there is no pathology, and break the cycle of expecting pain and experiencing it.

PALPITATIONS IN PREGNANCY

Alamgir Kabir and Sandy Gupta

■ Introduction

Palpitation is an unpleasant awareness of an abnormal beating of the heart. The symptoms may be brought about by a number of cardiac disorders, including cardiomyopathy, valvular heart disease and coronary heart disease, or as a consequence of congenital heart disease. However, the most common cause is primary cardiac arrhythmia, where there is no underlying pathology.[1] Other non-cardiac disorders such as thyroid disease may also have an effect on the cardiac rhythm. The normal state of pregnancy can affect cardiac rhythm with or without underlying structural heart disease.

This section examines some of the issues regarding assessment and management of palpitations in pregnancy.

■ The gender difference

There are a number of predisposing factors in women for arrhythmia that may well be exacerbated during pregnancy. Women in general have a longer QT interval and also a higher incidence of atrioventricular nodal re-entrant tachycardias. Intrinsically women have higher heart rates and sinus nodal recovery times are reduced. Women have a lower incidence of atrial fibrillation (AF); however, once in AF, they have a higher mortality. It may be that sex hormones affect myocardial repolarisation and this is the mechanism that explains the sex difference.[2] Perhaps by reducing the repolarisation time of the sinus node they reduce the incidence of abnormal atrial activity triggering AF.

There are a number of factors that occur specifically in pregnancy that predispose to arrhythmogenesis. Fig. 1 demonstrates some of these factors.

The increase in cardiac output in pregnancy causes an increase in myocardial stretch, leading

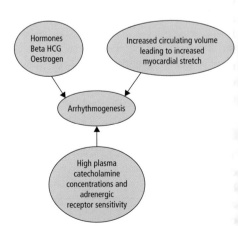

Figure 1 Factors in pregnancy that predispose to arrhythmogenesis. Beta HCG, beta human chorionic gonadotrophin.

to arrhythmias. Hormonal factors such as the increase in oestrogen and beta human chorionic gonadotrophin also predispose to the development of arrhythmias (arrhythmogenesis). Finally, increases in sympathetic tone and adrenergic receptor sensitivity related to high plasma catecholamine levels, which occur in pregnancy, affect the tendency for arrhythmia.[3]

Investigation of palpitations

There have been a number of studies assessing the incidence of arrhythmia in normal pregnancy with some interesting findings. In one study, there was no clear relationship between symptoms, such as dizziness, palpitations or syncope, and the incidence of arrhythmia on 24-hour Holter electrocardiogram (ECG) monitoring.[4] However, the same study did show an overall increase in simple and multifocal ventricular premature complexes in symptomatic patients.

The investigation of palpitations in pregnancy is similar to non-pregnant patients, and includes baseline ECGs, echocardiogram to ensure a structurally normal heart and 24-hour Holter monitoring. Caution is advised with exercise treadmill testing, as peak exercise can be associated with fetal bradycardia, so fetal monitoring and a low workload protocol are advised.

Generally, benign arrhythmias can be treated with avoidance of stimulants (e.g. caffeine or alcohol) and reassurance for the patient. However, more serious arrhythmias may need further treatment. The choice of agent used is related primarily to established safety in pregnancy. The following section will address these issues.

Supraventricular tachycardias

The data regarding supraventricular tachycardia (SVT) in pregnancy are conflicting. There have been studies showing that the incidence and exacerbation of SVT is increased in pregnancy.[5] The incidence of paroxysmal SVT is related to the menstrual cycle and they are more likely to occur in a low oestrogen state, such as pregnancy.[6] Pregnancy also appears to increase the likelihood of arrhythmia in those patients with accessory pathways as compared with AV nodal re-entrant tachycardias.[7] However, another group examining over 200 pregnant women[8] found a much lower incidence of SVT than Tawam et al.,[5] 3.9 per cent vs. 34 per cent risk of new-onset SVT. It has to be mentioned that both groups did not find any increase in exacerbation of SVT.

In terms of management of AV nodal re-entrant tachycardias, the initial protocol is the same as for a non-pregnant women. If vagal manoeuvres such as carotid massage or breath-holding fail, then adenosine may be used. The American College of Cardiology/European Society of Cardiology guidelines state that the use of adenosine in SVT for pregnant women is recommended,[9] as it has a very short half-life of less than 10 seconds. A retrospective study has shown adenosine to be safe in the second and third trimester; however, there was not enough data to validate safety in the first trimester.[10] As a second line, intravenous beta-blockade, such as propranolol or metoprolol, can be used. There are reservations about using verapamil because of the risk of prolonged hypotension.[9] Electrical cardioversion is indicated if chemical cardioversion fails or the mother becomes unstable. There is evidence to show that DC defibrillation is safe in all stages of pregnancy,[11] the amount of current reaching the fetus being insignificant.

An underlying cause, such as thyroid disease, should be excluded. There are certain indications for considering curative ablation therapy, such as drug-refractory SVT, poorly tolerated SVT and when pregnancy is planned in a woman known to have troublesome SVT. If ablation has to be carried out during pregnancy, then this should ideally wait till the second trimester. Abdominal lead shields can be used to minimise the radiation risk to the fetus.[9]

Atrial fibrillation and atrial flutter

Atrial fibrillation and flutter in pregnancy may indicate underlying structural heart disease, such as congenital heart disease/rheumatic valvular disease or endocrine dysfunction, such as thyroid disease. Patients presenting with atrial fibrillation for the first time should have an ECG, echocardiogram and routine blood tests, including thyroid function tests performed regardless of pregnancy status.

Beta-blockade or digoxin may be used to control ventricular rate. The first episode may revert spontaneously; however, if this does not occur, electrical cardioversion should be considered in the first 48 hours to reduce the need for anticoagulation for stroke prevention in AF. Maintenance of sinus rhythm with medication should be reserved for those with recurrent haemodynamically significant episodes of AF.

Anticoagulation is a difficult subject in pregnancy[12] but is necessary in patients with chronic atrial fibrillation considered high risk for embolic events. Heparin is generally considered safe, as is does not cross the placenta and is the drug of choice for anticoagulation. Warfarin should definitely not be used in the first trimester because of its teratogenic effects.

The management of atrial fibrillation and atrial flutter is essentially the same. There is increasingly successful use of catheter ablation for atrial flutter and, more recently, for atrial fibrillation. In a planned pregnancy, ablation prior to pregnancy may be considered.[13]

■ Ventricular tachycardias

Inherited long QT syndrome is a recognised cause of ventricular arrhythmia. A retrospective analysis of the over 400 pregnancies with QT abnormalities[14] suggests the postpartum period of pregnancy is associated with the highest risk of serious cardiac events, resulting in death, aborted cardiac arrest or syncope. Beta-blockade seems to reduce this risk; therefore, in terms of risk and benefit to baby and mother, continued therapy during and after pregnancy is recommended. There are many common medications that cause the QT interval on ECG to become prolonged, such as amiodarone, sotalol, cisapride, clarithromycin and chloroquine. Prolongation of the QT interval on ECG

can lead to a particular type of ventricular tachycardia (VT) with a characteristic oscillating baseline called 'torsade de pointes'. Obviously those agents that prolong the QT interval of ECG and lead to torsade de pointes should be stopped during pregnancy.

Idiopathic ventricular tachycardia may arise from the right ventricular outflow tract or the inferior left-sided ventricular septum.[15] Adenosine, verapamil or beta-blockade may be used to terminate idiopathic ventricular tachycardias.[16] Radiofrequency ablation may be an option prior to a planned pregnancy. It should be noted that right ventricular outflow tract (RVOT) tachyarrhythmia is generally benign and can occur in people with structurally normal hearts. If there is no structural abnormality detected and the ventricular tachycardia is monomorphic with left bundle branch block and an inferior axis, RVOT tachycardia is the most likely diagnosis. (Monomorphic VT has the same morphology of the QRS complex on ECG, implying a single focus in the ventricle.) If there is structural heart disease, this puts the mother at increased risk of sudden death, antiarrhythmics should be given and an implantable cardioverter defibrillator considered.

Other VTs may be terminated with lignocaine and beta-blockade may be used to avoid recurrence. Procainamide may be used as a second line to terminate tachyarrhythmia. Quinidine has also been used for termination and prophylaxis. Sotalol has been used for prophylaxis. Amiodarone should be avoided because of the range of side effects to both mother and fetus.[13] As always, haemodynamically compromising ventricular arrhythmia should be treated with electrical cardioversion.

■ Implantable cardioverter defibrillators and pacemakers

Implantable cardioverter defibrillators (ICDs) are increasing in use as indications broaden. There have been studies which demonstrate that ICDs are safe in pregnancy.[17] This study showed that three-quarters experienced no shocks, of the remainder, less than 10 per cent were multiple and 98 per cent had no major complication to the fetus.

An ICD should not deter women from pregnancy and the underlying structural heart disease is a more important factor. During delivery, the ICD should be activated. The only circumstance where the ICD may be inactivated is when Caesarean section and electrocautery may be considered, to avoid inappropriate shocks.[18]

The indications for a pacemaker are the same as for non-pregnant women. Generally the pacemaker is implanted under X-ray guidance with a radiation shield, although there have been some experiences with echo-guided lead placement.[19]

Congenital heart disease

Congenital heart disease and repair of complex abnormalities has led to an increase in the number of female patients with congenital heart disease reaching childbearing age and having successful pregnancies.[20] SVT and VT as well as high-grade atrioventricular block can lead to significant comprise during pregnancy in these patients.[21] Factors that appear to predict arrhythmia in this group are:

- poor cardiac functional status;
- polysplenia;
- residual atrioventricular regurgitation;
- specific anatomy and haemodynamic scars from surgery may cause arrhythmogenic focus, which may be uncovered by the increased preload of pregnancy.

Fetal risk

There has been an attempt to classify a system of fetal risk by the US Food and Drug Administration. Table 1 summarises the recommendations.

Table 1 US Food and Drug Administration (FDA) risk class

FDA risk class	Description		
Class A	Controlled studies show no risk		
Class B	No evidence of risk in pregnant women, but either animal studies do show risk, or no adequate human studies have been conducted		
Class C	Studies in pregnant women are lacking, and animal studies are positive for fetal risk, or lacking		
Class D	Positive evidence of risk – can be used if potential benefit outweighs risk		
Class X	Contraindicated – do not use, regardless of potential benefit		

Drug class	Drug	FDA risk class	Fetal side effects
IA	Quinidine	C	Thrombocytopenia, 8th nerve toxicity
IA	Procainamide	C	None known
IA	Disopyramide	C	Uterine contractions
IB	Lignocaine	B	Central nervous system depression at toxic levels
IB	Mexiletine	C	Little data available
IC	Flecainide	C	None known
IC	Propafenone	C	None known
II	Propranolol	C	Intrauterine growth retardation
II	Metoprolol	C	Intrauterine growth retardation
II	Atenolol	D	Intrauterine growth retardation, preterm delivery
III	Sotalol	B	None known
III	Amiodarone	D	Congenital malformations, thyroid toxicity
III	Ibutilide	C	No data available
III	Dofetilide	C	No data available
IV	Verapamil	C	Hypotension with intravenous use
IV	Diltiazem	C	Little data available
	Digoxin	C	Monitor for digoxin toxicity
	Adenosine	A	None known

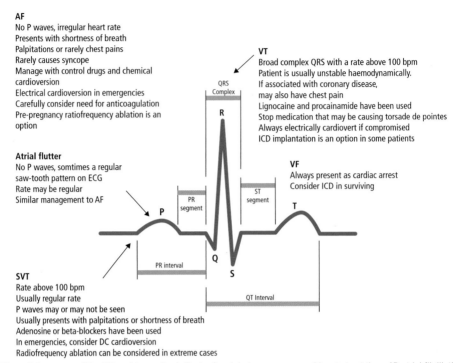

AF
No P waves, irregular heart rate
Presents with shortness of breath
Palpitations or rarely chest pains
Rarely causes syncope
Manage with control drugs and chemical cardioversion
Electrical cardioversion in emergencies
Carefully consider need for anticoagulation
Pre-pregnancy ratiofrequency ablation is an option

Atrial flutter
No P waves, somtimes a regular saw-tooth pattern on ECG
Rate may be regular
Similar management to AF

SVT
Rate above 100 bpm
Usually regular rate
P waves may or may not be seen
Usually presents with palpitations or shortness of breath
Adenosine or beta-blockers have been used
In emergencies, consider DC cardioversion
Radiofrequency ablation can be considered in extreme cases

VT
Broad complex QRS with a rate above 100 bpm
Patient is usually unstable haemodynamically.
If associated with coronary disease, may also have chest pain
Lignocaine and procainamide have been used
Stop medication that may be causing torsade de pointes
Always electrically cardiovert if compromised
ICD implantation is an option in some patients

VF
Always present as cardiac arrest
Consider ICD in surviving

Figure 2 A summary of the different types of arrhythmias found during pregnancy and how to treat them. AF, atrial fibrillation; bpm, beats per minute; DC, direct current; ECG, electrocardiogram; ICD, implantable cardioverter defibrillator; VF, ventricular fibrillation; VT, ventricular tachycardia.

Generally, it can be surmised that, for SVTs, digoxin and beta-blockers should be considered.[9] Digoxin has a long track record of safety in pregnancy. Beta-blockers should be considered after the first trimester, if possible. Atenolol should be avoided. Sotalol could be considered as second line along with flecainide (in the absence of structural heart disease).

Ventricular tachycardia may be treated with beta-blockers including sotalol. Amiodarone should be avoided if at all possible because of the risk to the mother and fetus.

During pregnancy renal blood flow increases, as does hepatic metabolism, so doses may need to be adjusted. Combination therapy at low dose may be preferable to high-dose single agents.

Women with troublesome dysrrhythmia may chose to consider radiofrequency ablation prior to conception.

■ Summary

Pregnancy may promote arrhythmogensis by virtue of hormonal and haemodynamic changes to the body. In the structurally normal heart, SVTs are more common than AF and VT. Congenital heart disease and pregnancy is a growing field with new challenges for electrophysiologists. ICD and radiofrequency ablation are helping in treating more serious arrhythmia. Fig. 2 summarises some of the features of arrhythmias in pregnancy.

■ References

1. Rosano GM, Rillo M, Leonardo F, Pappone C, Chierchia SL. Palpitations: what is the mechanism, and when should we treat them? *Int J Fertil Womens Med* 1997; **42:** 94–100.

2. Bailey MS, Curtis AB. The effects of hormones on arrhythmias in women. *Curr Womens Health Rep* 2002. **2**: 83–8.

3. Mark S, Harris L. Arrhythmias in pregnancy. In: Wilansky S, ed. *Heart Disease in Women*. Philadelphia: Churchill Livingstone, 2002: 497–514.

4. Shotan A, Ostrzega E, Mehra A, Johnson JV, Elkayam U. Incidence of arrhythmias in normal pregnancy and relation to palpitations, dizziness, and syncope. *Am J Cardiol* 1997. **79**: 1061–4.

5. Tawam M, Levine J, Mendelson M, Goldberger J, Dyer A, Kadish A. Effect of pregnancy on paroxysmal supraventricular tachycardia. *Am J Cardiol* 1993. **72**: 838–40.

6. Rosano GM, Leonardo F, Sarrel PM, Beale CM, De Luca F, Collins P. Cyclical variation in paroxysmal supraventricular tachycardia in women. *Lancet* 1996; **347**: 786–8.

7. Widerhorn J, Widerhorn AL, Rahimtoola SH, Elkayam U. WPW syndrome during pregnancy: increased incidence of supraventricular arrhythmias. *Am Heart J* 1992. **123**: 796–8.

8. Lee SH, Chen SA, Wu TJ, *et al.* Effects of pregnancy on first onset and symptoms of paroxysmal supraventricular tachycardia. *Am J Cardiol* 1995. **76**: 675–8.

9. Blomstrom-Lundqvist C, Scheinman MM, Aliot EM, *et al.* ACC/AHA/ESC guidelines for the management of patients with supraventricular arrhythmias – executive summary. A report of the American College of Cardiology/American Heart Association task force on practice guidelines and the European society of cardiology committee for practice guidelines (writing committee to develop guidelines for the management of patients with supraventricular arrhythmias) developed in collaboration with NASPE-Heart Rhythm Society. *J Am Coll Cardiol* 2003; **42**: 1493–531.

10. Elkayam U, Goodwin TM. Adenosine therapy for supraventricular tachycardia during pregnancy. *Am J Cardiol* 1995; **75**: 521–3.

11. Schroeder JS, Harrison DC. Repeated cardioversion during pregnancy. Treatment of refractory paroxysmal atrial tachycardia during 3 successive pregnancies. *Am J Cardiol* 1971; **27**: 445–6.

12. Pauli RM, Hall JG, Wilson KM. Risks of anticoagulation during pregnancy. *Am Heart J* 1980; **100**: 761–2.

13. Tan HL, Lie KI. Treatment of tachyarrhythmias during pregnancy and lactation. *Eur Heart J* 2001; **22**: 458–64.

14. Rashba EJ, Zareba W, Moss AJ, *et al.* Influence of pregnancy on the risk for cardiac events in patients with hereditary long QT syndrome. LQTS Investigators. *Circulation* 1998. **97**: 451–6.

15. Belhassen B, Shapira I, Pelleg A, Copperman I, Kauli N, Laniado S. Idiopathic recurrent sustained ventricular tachycardia responsive to verapamil: an ECG-electrophysiologic entity. *Am Heart J* 1984; **108**: 1034–7.

16. Sung RJ, Keung EC, Nguyen NX, Huycke EC. Effects of beta-adrenergic blockade on verapamil-responsive and verapamil-irresponsive sustained ventricular tachycardias. *J Clin Invest* 1988; **81**: 688–99.

17. Natale A, Davidson T, Geiger MJ, Newby K. Implantable cardioverter-defibrillators and pregnancy: a safe combination? *Circulation* 1997. **96**: 2808–12.

18. Wolbrette D. Arrhythmias during pregnancy –a therapeutic challenge. *Business Briefing: Women's Healthcare* 2005: 51–5.

19. Lee MS, Evans SJ, Blumberg S, Bodenheimer MM, Roth SL. Echocardiographically guided electrophysiologic testing in pregnancy. *J Am Soc Echocardiogr* 1994; **7**: 182–6.

20. Tateno S, Niwa K, Nakazawa M, *et al.* Arrhythmia and conduction disturbances in patients with congenital heart disease during pregnancy: multicenter study. *Circ J* 2003; **67:** 992–7.

21. Hidaka Y, Akagi T, Himeno W, Ishii M, Matsuishi T. Left ventricular performance during pregnancy in patients with repaired tetralogy of Fallot: prospective evaluation using the Tei index. *Circ J* 2003; **67:** 682–6.

PELVIC PAIN

Cynthia Farquhar

All women at some time experience pelvic pain associated with events such as menstruation, ovulation or sexual intercourse. Although only a few women seek medical advice for such pain, it is the commonest reason for laparoscopy examination in the UK. Visceral pain in the abdominal and pelvic organs is transmitted by the autonomic nervous system in the T10–L1 distribution. The viscera are not very sensitive to thermal or tactile sensation, and they are poorly localised in the cerebral cortex. Stimuli that do produce pain are as follows:

- distension and/or contraction of a hollow organ;
- rapid stretching of the capsule of a solid organ;
- any irritation of the parietal peritoneum, e.g. blood or pus;
- tissue ischaemia or necrosis, as may happen in torsion of an ovarian cyst;
- neuritis secondary to any inflammatory, neoplastic or fibrotic processes in adjacent organs.

The differential diagnosis of pain in the pelvis can be subdivided as follows.

- *Acute*, when the patient is ill and requires resuscitation with intravenous fluids for hypovolaemia, sepsis or dehydration. There may be a need for urgent surgery.
- *Subacute*: the onset of the pain is sudden but does not cause the patient to be severely ill. The diagnosis may need to be established, although the patient may just require observation over 24–48 hours. If the pain does not improve or the diagnosis is in doubt, then laparoscopy may be warranted.
- *Chronic* in nature and may be the result of long-standing pathology. Symptoms, clinical findings and findings at laparoscopy show poor correlation with up to 50 per cent of patients who undergo laparoscopy showing no abnormality.

■ Acute and subacute pain

The differential diagnosis for this type of pain can be classified in the following way. Investigations and treatment may be similar, but severity can vary and the necessity to any surgical intervention will be a clinical decision. In all these cases, it is important to consider a possible physiological cause or a pregnancy-related condition.

- *Physiological*: menstruation or ovulation. Some women habitually experience some dull pain in the midline or in one or other iliac fossa at the time of ovulation usually 14 days before the next period (Mittelschmerz). Occasionally slight vaginal bleeding accompanies the pain. The timing of the pain and the absence of any abnormal pelvic findings usually make the diagnosis clear. Pain is not an unusual feature with menstruation and usually implies that the woman is ovulating and there is an increase in local prostaglandins within the uterus at that time.
- *Pregnancy related*: it is always important to remember to consider pregnancy in any woman during her reproductive years when she presents with acute pelvic pain. The severity of pain will dictate the management. Miscarriage may be related with bleeding and pain usually reflects the inevitable nature of the miscarriage, on examination the cervical os will be open. Ectopic pregnancy, which is still a major cause of maternal mortality, may present with varying symptoms depending on the gestation. Although this problem can be treated conservatively with methotrexate, the vast majority of cases will need some form of operative intervention. Other problems in pregnancy include fibroid degeneration, which may be very acute and need hospital admission. Apart from pain, it can also cause the pregnant uterus to become very irritable.

- *Ovarian* causes of acute pain usually reflect cyst accidents in the form of torsion, rupture or haemorrhage (Fig. 1). The degree of peritonism will dictate the management.

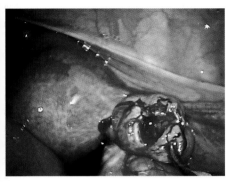

Figure 1 Laparoscopic view of a haemorrhagic ovarian cyst.

- *Infection*: pelvic inflammatory disease (PID) occurs in the sexually active. It is usually bilateral in origin and is associated with a low-grade pyrexia, tachycardia and discharge. If not adequately treated initially, then tubo-ovarian abscesses (Fig. 2) may occur, which may need surgical drainage.

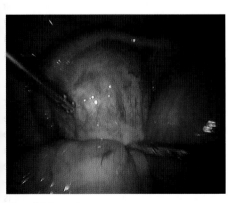

Figure 2 Tubo-ovarian mass.

- *Endometriosis*: this condition may cause both acute and chronic pelvic pain, and diagnosis is usually confirmed by laparoscopy.
- *Neoplasia*: this would include fibroids, ovarian cysts and malignant disease within the genital tract. Apart from the conditions mentioned above, it is unusual for malignancies to give acute pain.

- *Urinary tract*: other non-gynaecological causes include urinary tract infection, retention and renal stones.
- *Gastrointestinal*: the degree of acuteness may vary and the pathology would vary depending on the age of the patient. Diagnoses include appendicitis, gastroenteritis, constipation, diverticular disease, inflammatory bowel disease, acute hernial accidents, volvulus, mesenteric infarction and malignancy.

Routine investigations

These may vary from patient to patient, but full blood count and pregnancy test may be sufficient depending on the history. If infection is considered, then swabs should be taken from the vaginal vault, from the endocervix to exclude *Chlamydia*, and from the urethra and rectum, if gonorrhoea is a possibility. A mid-stream specimen of urine may exclude a urinary infection. Plain abdominal X-rays may be useful, if bowel problems are an option. An intravenous pyelogram may exclude a calculus. The mainstay of investigation is the ultrasound scan of the pelvis and, when in doubt, laparoscopy may be undertaken.

■ Chronic pelvic pain

Any acute cause of pain can lead on to a chronic picture. A history of pelvic pain is associated with an increased number of sexual partners and an increased incidence of psychosexual trauma as a child. The investigations are similar and may lead to laparoscopy and, indeed, in some cases, may result in hysterectomy and pelvic clearance. Whilst there is a place for this with endometriosis and chronic PID, if there is no obvious pathology, then it will not result in cure for all women.

- *Adhesions*: these may be found in up to 20 per cent of patients with chronic pain (Fig. 3), although they may not be the cause of the pain.
- *Residual ovary syndrome* in women who have had a hysterectomy associated with pain and dyspareunia, and a fixed tender ovary at the vaginal vault. Treatment may be by suppression of the ovary or removal.
- *Endometriosis*: in this condition, there is abnormal implantation of endometrium outside the uterine

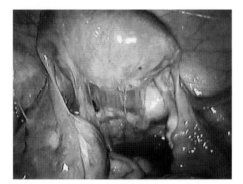

Figure 3 Laparoscopic view of adhesions.

cavity. It may cause dysmenorrhoea, dyspareunia, menstrual upset, pelvic pain and infertility. Diagnosis is usually by laparoscopy. Adenomyosis is a variant of this condition when endometrium invades the myometrium, and this causes pain with the period and a very tender uterus. The surgical option is dependent on symptoms.

- *Chronic PID*: this is a consequence of acute infection, and leads to damage and consequent pain and menstrual upset.
- *Irritable bowel syndrome*: this condition is often confused with a gynaecological cause of lower abdominal pain.
- *Pelvic congestion*: the pain is dull and aching with occasional sharp exacerbations, and is associated with dilated veins in the broad ligament and uterus. There may be local tenderness. The women are usually in their reproductive years and may be nulliparous. Diagnosis can be made by venography, laparoscopy or ultrasound (Fig. 4), and treatment is medically with progestogens.

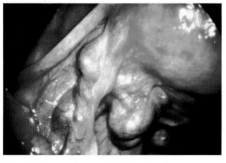

Figure 4 Ultrasound scan of dilated pelvic veins.

PELVIC SWELLINGS

Tony Hollingworth

Swellings that arise from the pelvis can be considered under their anatomical site of origin. A number of structures may appear to be pelvic when their true site of origin is really abdominal. Ultrasound scanning has improved the detection of lesions that are not necessarily palpable without a vaginal or rectal examination. The background to the swellings can be simply described by the 'five Fs':

- fat
- fluid
- faeces
- flatus
- fetus.

Careful history-taking, clinical examination and appropriate imaging should be able to establish the diagnosis. Many of these swellings will be dealt with under individual organ sites. Therefore, this section will provide an overview and reference should be made to those sections in this book. These swellings will be considered anatomically from anterior to posterior, finally dealing with the bony surround of the pelvis (Fig. 1).

■ Bladder

- Simple distension or retention.
- Transitional cell carcinoma (see Haematuria).

The commonest difficulty, which arises in the diagnosis of pelvic swellings, is to differentiate between the distended bladder, pregnant uterus, ovarian cyst and uterine fibromyoma, and the commonest mistakes are made between these swellings. The distended bladder is the easiest to dispose of, the passage of a catheter settling the question; yet neglect of this simple procedure has led to the abdomen being opened.

■ Vagina

- *Haematocolpos.*
- *Hydrocolpos.*

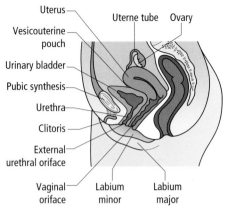

Uterus
Uterne tube   Ovary
Vesicouterine
pouch
Urinary bladder
Pubic synthesis
Urethra
Clitoris
External
urethral oriface
Vaginal   Labium   Labium
oriface   minor   major

Figure 1 Sagittal section diagram of the female pelvis.

Distension of the vagina by menstrual fluid is not likely to be mistaken for anything else, if only on account of the absolute closure of the atretic membrane, which gives rise to it. This condition is often referred to as 'imperforate hymen'; this is not correct because the atresia is at a higher level in the vagina than the hymen, which is always perforate.

Haematocolpos (blood–filled vagina) is practically the only central tumour occurring between the rectum and the bladder reaching from the level of the hymen to the pelvic brim (see Menstrual periods, absent). It presents in girls about the age of 16–17 years, who frequently present with acute retention of urine owing to the fact that the swelling fills the pelvis, and the distended bladder in front is forced upward into the abdomen. Primary amenorrhoea (absent periods) is present, although monthly symptoms without loss of blood may have taken place for some time. Two swellings are present: the tender distended bladder in the lower abdomen, which can reach as high as the umbilicus, and the distended vagina filled with menstrual fluid in the pelvis. The uterus can usually be felt like a cork movable upon its upper extremity. The lower pole of the haematocolpos presents a blue-coloured swelling at the vulva (see Menstrual periods, absent) (Fig. 3).

A similar swelling may be found on rare occasions in newborn girl babies. The vagina is filled with a milky fluid (hydrocolpos).

■ Uterus

- *Pregnancy related*, either normal or abnormal, with or without associated tumours of the uterus or ovary.
- *Non-pregnancy related*.
  - *Benign*: the most common of which are fibroids (leiomyoma). Others causes include haematometra and pyometra (blood or pus in the uterine cavity, respectively), many of which will prove to be benign, but malignancy should be considered and excluded
  - *Malignant*: the most common being endometrial carcinoma, but rarer tumours would include mixed Müllerian tumours, uterine sarcomas and choriocarcinomas.

A comprehensive history is always important and, in the reproductive age group, one should always consider the possibility of pregnancy with uterine swellings. Pregnancy and fibroids are the two most common causes of uterine swelling and, together with other causes, will be dealt with more fully in Uterine swellings.

■ Cervix

The cervix is an integral part of the uterus (womb) and its size will vary depending on the age of the woman. It increases in size with puberty and may continue to do so with pregnancy or the development of cervical fibroids. It will eventually reduce in size with the onset of the menopause. If the woman develops a prolapse, then it can become oedematous, especially if it appears outside the vagina (procidentia). The swellings can again be divided into benign and malignant, and will be covered in Cervical swellings.

■ Ovary

The ovary can be considered as a reproductive organ made up three basic types of cells:

- those that produce the eggs or ova (totipotential cells);

- those cells that produce secretions (sex-hormone secreting);
- the remaining cells that wrap these cells together (epithelial cells).

Each of these types of cells can produce ovarian swellings, the totipotential cells leading to dermoid/germ-cell swellings, and the hormone-secreting sex-cord cells may produce excess amounts of hormone, which can lead to irregular shedding of the endometrium in the case of oestrogen, hirsutism and virilism with an excess of testosterone production. The epithelial cells account for the majority of ovarian swellings. Further classification can be considered as follows.

- *Benign*: includes cysts and fibromas.
- *Malignant*: primary origin in the form of epithelial tumours (85 per cent), sex-cord tumours (6 per cent), germ-cell tumours (2 per cent) and, uncommonly, sarcomas or lymphomas. Secondaries (6 per cent) originate from the gut, breast, lung and thyroid.

The differential diagnosis of ovarian swellings will be considered elsewhere (see Ovarian Swellings). Ovarian cancer is the most frequently occurring genital tract cancer in the UK, although overall is much less common than breast cancer by a factor of 6 to 1. It is estimated that a general practitioner will see one new case of ovarian cancer every five years.

The ovary produces a cyst every month in the form of an ovarian follicle, which will in turn release an egg (ovum). These follicles may reach up to 25 mm in diameter. As a rule of thumb, an ovarian cyst up to 5 cm in diameter may resolve without any action, except for repeating an ultrasound scan after two to three menstrual periods to ensure its resolution. If the cyst grows larger than 5 cm, it is likely to require removal. The main complications of an ovarian cyst include torsion, rupture and haemorrhage. The largest cyst removed in the UK weighed 63 kg; the world's largest was removed in 1905 in the USA and weighed a staggering 145 kg. If the cyst increases to a very large size, it is likely to be benign, or possibly of borderline malignancy. The ovary is not usually

palpable on vaginal examination until it is at least 5 cm in diameter. It should *not* be palpable in a postmenopausal woman and any ovarian cyst in these women should be considered with a high index of suspicion until proved otherwise.

■ Fallopian tubes

- *Pregnancy related*, tubal gestation or progressive extrauterine pregnancy (ectopic).
- *Inflammatory*: salpingitis, which may lead to a hydrosalpinx or pyosalpinx.
- *Malignant*: carcinoma of the Fallopian tube being very uncommon.

With small tumours confined to the pelvis, or rising only a little above the brim, diagnosis is often difficult. In practice, however, extrauterine gestation and its resulting blood tumour stand out pre-eminently as a swelling, which must be recognized at once if treatment is to be successful (Fig. 2).

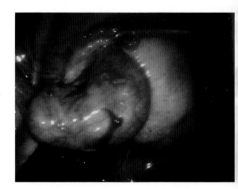

Figure 2 Laparoscopic picture of an ectopic pregnancy.

Before rupture or abortion has occurred, a tubal gestation is essentially a small tumour in one posterolateral corner of the pelvis, attached to the uterus, indefinite in consistency, remarkably tender, and perhaps – although not always – associated with amenorrhoea of short duration and acute attacks of pain in the pelvis. Definite signs of pregnancy may be entirely wanting but a pregnancy test will be positive. It may be mistaken for a chronic salpingo-oophoritis, a small cystic ovary, a small pedunculated fibroid or a small ovarian dermoid.

The differential diagnosis may be difficult, and attacks of pain unassociated with menstruation are not likely to occur in any of the above conditions; the pains are usually the result of overdistension and stretching of the tube from haemorrhage into its wall or lumen around the fertilized ovum. Unless the swelling is tender (often very tender), it is not likely to be due to a tubal pregnancy. When tubal abortion has occurred, or tubal rupture, the signs of internal bleeding accompanied by sudden pain and collapse, with haemorrhage from the uterus or the passage of a decidual cast, usually make the diagnosis obvious. Intraperitoneal haemorrhage is more commonly severe and copious with tubal rupture than with tubal abortion. If the patient recovers from the initial bleeding, the clinical picture may be that of a retrouterine or peritubal haematocele. The uterus is pushed forwards and upwards against the symphysis pubis, and the mass of blood clot can be felt posteriorly causing the posterior fornix and also the anterior wall of the rectum to bulge. Vaginal examination is very tender. Tubal miscarriage is most likely to be mistaken for an ordinary intrauterine miscarriage; but the presence of a tender mass on one side of the uterus, with a closed cervix and a negative ultrasound scan, and the absence of uterine contractions or extrusion of any products of conception, should make the diagnosis clear. Pain is much more severe and external bleeding is much less in extrauterine pregnancy.

The essential point in diagnosing an ectopic pregnancy is to approach every woman of childbearing age who complains of irregular bleeding and abdominal pain with the possibility of pregnancy, and then ask the question where is that pregnancy. No two cases are alike and there are more exceptions to the rule in the symptomatology of this condition than in any other. Risk factors for ectopic pregnancy include history of pelvic inflammatory disease, tubal surgery including sterilisation, progesterone-only contraception and a history of infertility. It must be emphasized that, whilst maternal death is not common in the UK, ectopic pregnancy remains a major cause.

Progressive extrauterine gestation is a rare occurrence, and is the result of continued growth of an embryo after a partial separation from the tube as a result of rupture or extrusion from the fimbriated end (abortion). The continued enlargement of a mass beside the uterus, with amenorrhoea and progressive signs of pregnancy, are the most characteristic points. Abdominal pain in late pregnancy is a characteristic feature. The uterus may be felt in the pelvis separate from the fetal sac. The diagnosis, however, is difficult, because there is always some effused blood, which obscures the outlines of the uterus, and makes it appear to be a part of the pelvic mass. The fetus is often situated high above the pelvis and it tends to lie transversely facing downward. A radiograph reveals the fetus adopting a position that is characteristically odd, the spine hyperextended or acutely flexed, and the head and limbs at unusual angles to the trunk.

If, on a lateral view, radiography shows fetal parts overlapping the maternal spine the pregnancy must be extrauterine. Ultrasonography will establish the absence of an intrauterine gestation and also the size of the uterus, which never exceeds that of 5 months' gestation even in the presence of a full-term extrauterine pregnancy, and the cervix does not soften to the same degree. In those cases where the fetus lies in the front of the false sac, it will feel very superficial owing the absence of uterine wall in front of it, and between it and the examining hand. The fetus is, however, often difficult to palpate, owing, perhaps, to the placenta in front, which may give rise to a loud vascular souffle just medial to the anterior superior iliac spine on the side from which it derives its main blood supply (via the ovarian vessels).

The swellings due to salpingo-oophoritis are usually easy to distinguish. They form fixed tender masses in the pelvis, seldom of any definite shape, but occasionally present with the characteristic retort shape, with its narrow end near the uterus, which the tube assumes when distended with fluid (Fig. 3). The history is usually that of an acute illness at some period, with

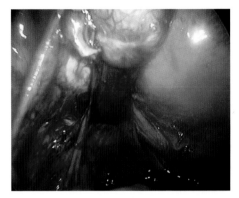

Figure 3 Laparoscopic picture of pelvic inflammatory disease.

usually bilateral pain in the pelvis, rise of temperature and peritoneal irritation. These patients have been sexually active. It is preceded, as a rule, by uterine discharge and heavy vaginal bleeding. This inflammatory disturbance in women can be associated with long periods of infertility, owing to occlusion of the fimbrial ends of the tubes. In the chronic state, pelvic pain, congestive dysmenorrhoea, dyspareunia, vaginal discharge, menorrhagia and infertility occur. The signs of suppuration, pyrexia and leucocytosis, wasting and daily sweating are usually absent, and the pus in the tubes is sterile. Swabs should be taken including from the endocervix for *Chlamydia* and the patient should be referred to the local genitourinary medicine clinic for ongoing/contact tracing management.

A large pelvic abscess may accompany salpingo-oophoritis, or may occur alone without infection of the tubes, as is seen occasionally in puerperal septic infections. When it does occur, it is of course peritoneal. It fixes the uterus in a central position, bulges into the posterior fornix and rectum, and tends to rupture into the rectum, before which occurrence there may be copious mucoid discharge from the anus. It is usually acute in onset and accompanied by signs of local peritonitis. A swinging temperature, leucocytosis, sweats and the symptoms of fever are present, all suddenly improving when the abscess discharges itself. It is likely to be confounded with pelvic cellulitis, in which

the uterus is fixed in a laterally displaced position. This swelling causes one lateral fornix to bulge and extends right out to the lateral pelvic wall, tends to burrow along the round ligament to the groin, and may point there like a psoas abscess. It can be slow in onset, chronic and not accompanied by signs of local peritonitis. It always follows labour, or abortion, whereas pelvic abscess of peritoneal origin may occur with salpingo-oophoritis or appendicitis, quite apart from pregnancy. Pelvic cellulitis never bears any relation to salpingo-oophoritis. It may take many weeks to resolve, which it usually does without pointing.

Malignancy within the Fallopian tube is extremely uncommon and, as a consequence, has no obvious localising signs. It may well behave like an ovarian cancer and the diagnosis may only be confirmed histologically after surgery.

■ Pelvic peritoneum, retroperitoneal swellings and connective tissue

Encysted peritoneal fluid, hydatid cysts and retroperitoneal lipomas are generally diagnosed as ovarian cysts, and their true nature is only discovered at operation. There are no definitive signs by which these conditions may be diagnosed and, as they all require operative treatment, postoperative diagnosis meets their requirements. Encysted peritoneal fluid due to tuberculosis may be suspected, if tuberculous lesions are present elsewhere in the body. They lack the definite outline of an ovarian cyst and are often semi-resonant on percussion.

Urachal cysts occur in front of the uterus and in close relation to the bladder; but in spite of this, they are usually mistaken for ovarian cysts. It is to be remembered, however, that ovarian cysts are only likely to occur in front of the uterus when they are large, but dermoid cysts of the ovary of small size occasionally do so. Urachal cysts are embryological remnants and rarely attain a large size.

The omentum should also be included in this group, which can form a 'cake' as a result of secondary transcoelomic spread from a primary ovarian tumour. Usually they tend to be palpable abdominally and, as the omentum originates from the tranverse colon, it is really an abdominal swelling, although it can become involved with the tumour pelvically.

Bowel

Appendicitis with pregnancy occurs occasionally and may be mistaken for torsion of an ovarian pedicle. The swelling due to appendix inflammation is, however, in close relation to the anterior superior spine of the ilium and the right iliac fossa. The lump is ill defined and rarely fluctuates unless there is a large abscess. The acute onset may be similar to that of torsion of an ovarian pedicle. There is usually a definite fluctuating tumour when an ovarian cyst is present, and some interval between it and the iliac crest can usually be felt. Bowel cancer is more common than the common gynaecological tumours as is diverticulitis. These patients tend to present with a history of altered bowel problems, with or without rectal bleeding.

Bone

Abnormal growth of the pelvic bones is very rare, although any tumours may be either cartilaginous or sarcomatous. Any tumours will be found to be continuous with the bones in the pelvis from which they arise. If it is growing from the sacrum, then it will have the rectum in front of it, unlike all gynaecological swellings in the pelvis, which have the rectum posterior to them. In most cases, the uterus and adnexae can be palpated bimanually, and shown to be free from disease and unconnected with the mass. The only possible gynaecological problem for which it may be mistaken is adherent inflammatory reaction from infection of the tubes and ovaries (salpingo-oophoritis). When complicated by the presence of a pregnant uterus, their true nature may be difficult to determine unless examination reveals that they are absolutely fixed and continuous with the bones of the pelvis.

Radiological imaging followed by biopsy may determine the diagnosis. These are rare problems and unlikely to present to the gynaecologist.

Other structures

Many of these lesions are not primarily pelvic, but they are included in the list because they are liable to be mistaken for pelvic tumours. Thus, renal, splenic or pancreatic tumours may reach the pelvic brim, but the history ought to show that they have grown down from above, not up from below. Renal swellings may be associated with urinary changes, or absence of urinary secretion on the affected side, as detected by the cystoscope or an intravenous pyelogram.

Malformations of the genital tract are associated with developmental abnormalities of the renal tract. It is not uncommon to find a solitary pelvic kidney in patients with congenital absence of the vagina and uterus.

Splenic enlargements may be associated with changes in the blood picture. Pancreatic cysts are the least likely to be mistaken for pelvic swellings, but they have been difficult to distinguish from ovarian tumours with long pedicles.

Diagnosis will be dependent on appropriate imaging.

PREMENSTRUAL SYNDROME

Tony Hollingworth

Premenstrual syndrome (PMS) can be defined as the cyclical recurrence of psychological, behavioural and physical symptoms during the luteal phase of the menstrual cycle. This is essentially the 2 weeks prior to menstruation and the symptoms resolve by the end of menstruation. The woman should then be free of symptoms between the end of menstruation and subsequent ovulation.

Psychological and somatic disturbances are part of the normal physiology of the menstrual cycle; however, when exaggerated, they may lead to severe psychological disturbance and behavioural abnormalities. The symptoms include bloating, cramping, pain and tenderness in the breasts, temporary gain in weight, and some swelling of the hands and feet. They can also include emotional tension, bad-temper, nervousness, irritability, headache, lack of concentration, depression and insomnia, sufficient to interfere with the normal enjoyment of life. The majority of women (95 per cent) will have some premenstrual symptoms, with only a small percentage (5 per cent) being totally symptom-free.

In a small group of women (5 per cent), the symptoms of PMS have a major impact on their lives and have led to suicide, acts of aggression and even cited as defence in murder trials! The American Psychiatric Association has established guidelines for the diagnosis of PMS, which they have designated as premenstrual dysphoric disorder. These criteria are listed in Box 1. There are no diagnostic blood tests for PMS.

The aetiology remains obscure and consequently presents therapeutic difficulties. The underlying cause may be a combination of imbalances/abnormalities of the ovarian steroid production and central nervous transmitters. It has been shown that women with PMS have lowered levels of whole blood serotonin concentrations and platelet serotonin. Several selective serotonin reuptake inhibitors (SSRIs) have now been show to improve PMS symptoms. Elimination of the cyclical ovarian function results in the complete suppression of symptoms. Despite cyclical ovarian steroid function being the trigger for PMS, there is no definitive test to distinguish it from other disorders. The nature of the symptoms is less important than the timing, and keeping a diary of symptoms may be useful to distinguish primary PMS from secondary. The latter are a group of patients who have true PMS with underlying psychopathology. If the symptoms do not follow the pattern described, then an alternative diagnosis needs to be considered.

Treatment depends on the severity of symptoms and may range from a mixture of counselling, education, exercise and reassurance in patients with mild problems. Essential fatty acids and pyridoxine have been used in the past. SSRIs may be used to good effect in moderate cases. In more severe cases, ovulation suppression can be used and this may start with continuous combined oral contraception usage, providing there are no contraindications to its use. Continuous progestogens, danazol and gonadotrophin-releasing hormone analogues can be used. If

---

Box 1 Criteria for premenstrual dysphoric disorder according the American Psychiatric Association

A Symptoms are temporally related to the menstrual cycle during the last 2 weeks of the luteal phase and remitting after the onset of menses

B The diagnosis requires at least five of the following, and one of the symptoms must be one of the first four
- Markedly depressed mood, feelings of hopelessness
- Marked anxiety or tension
- Marked affective lability, e.g. sudden onset of being sad, tearful, irritable or aggressive
- Persistent and marked anger or irritability, or increased interpersonal conflicts
- Decreased interest in usual activities
- Easy fatiguability or marked lack of energy
- Subjective sense of difficulty in concentrating
- Changes in appetite, overeating or food craving
- Hypersomnia or insomnia
- Feeling of being overwhelmed or out of control
- Physical symptoms, such as breast tenderness, headaches, oedema, joint or muscle pain, and weight gain

C The symptoms interfere with work, or usual activities or relationships

D The symptoms are not an exacerbation of another psychiatric disorder; thus, premenstrual syndrome is, in large part, a diagnosis of exclusion

these are unsuccessful, then in severe cases, total abdominal hysterectomy and bilateral salpingo-oophorectomy may need to be considered with subsequent hormone replacement therapy in the form of continuous oestrogen.

■ Useful websites

www.pms.org.uk
www.womenshealth.gov/faq/pms
www.nlm.nih.gov/medlines

PROLAPSE OF UTERUS AND VAGINA

Jai B Sharma

A prolapse is the protrusion of an organ or structure beyond its normal anatomical position. Pelvic organ prolapse, as defined by the International Continence Society, is the descent of one or more of vaginal segments: the anterior, the posterior, the apex of the vagina or, after hysterectomy, the vaginal vault.

■ Aetiology

Pelvic organs are supported by the pelvic floor. The anatomy of the pelvic floor is given in Fig. 1

in Birth injuries, maternal. The vaginal supports have been divided into three levels by De Lancey. Level 1 is provided by the transverse cervical (Mackenrodt's or cardinal) and uterosacral ligaments as the superior attachment; level 2 by the anterior vaginal wall and recto-vaginal fascia as the lateral attachment; and level 3 by the perineal body and perineal membrane as the distal attachment. The supports of the uterus are shown in Fig. 1 and the ligamentous supports of the uterus in Fig. 2.

Uterovaginal prolapse may be due to breaks in the integrity of the uterosacral ligaments, weakness of pelvic floor muscles and/or changes in the normal vaginal axis. It usually results from child birth trauma, further compounded by urogenital atrophy in elderly women owing to lack of oestrogens. It is more common in elderly multiparous women and is more common in Caucasians than in Afro–Caribbeans. Prolapse in nulliparous women is rare. The various predisposing factors of prolapse are shown in Box 1.

■ Classification

The pelvic organ prolapse is divided into following categories depending upon which part is involved.

- *Cystocoele*: prolapse of deeper part of the anterior vaginal wall including the bladder (Fig. 3).

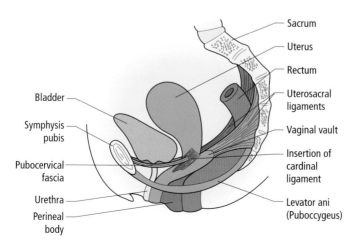

Figure 1 Supports of the uterus.

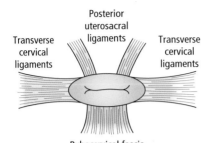

Figure 2 Ligamentous supports of the uterus.

Box 1 Causes of prolapse

- Pregnancy and childbirth trauma
- Ageing and oestrogen withdrawal
- Smoking
- Constipation
- Obesity
- Strenuous exercise
- Excessive and strenuous work in wrong postures
- Pelvic tumours
- Raised intra-abdominal pressure
- Previous surgery:
  - pelvic surgery
  - bladder neck suspension
  - Burch's colposuspension
- Chronic cough

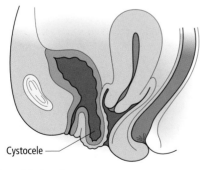

Figure 3 Cystocoele.

- *Urethrocoele*: prolapse of the upper part of the anterior vaginal wall carrying the urethra with it.
- *Cysto-urethrocoele*: the combination of prolapse of both upper and lower part of anterior vaginal wall including the bladder and urethra.

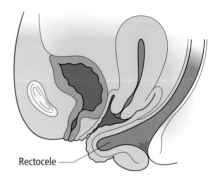

Figure 4 Rectocoele.

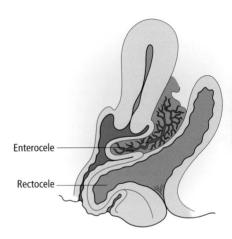

Figure 5 Enterocoele and rectocoele.

- *Rectocoele*: prolapse of the lower part of the vagina including the rectum (Fig. 4).
- *Enterocoele*: prolapse of the posterior fornix with the upper part of vagina; this is related to the pouch of Douglas and may contain loops of small intestines (Fig. 5).
- *Uterine prolapse*: descent of the cervix with the uterus through the introitus. This is classified into the following (Fig. 6):
  - first degree – the cervix descends to the vulva but does not come out through the introitus;
  - second degree – the cervix protrudes through the vulva;
  - third degree – the cervix is below the vulva (Fig. 7);

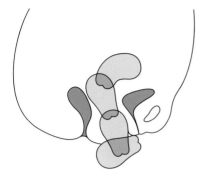

Figure 6 Uterovaginal prolapse, showing the position of the normal uterus and the three degrees of prolapse.

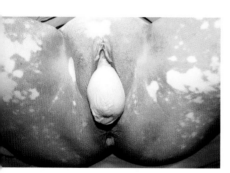

Figure 7 Third-degree prolapse of the uterus.

- fourth degree – the whole of the uterus is outside the vulva (procidentia).
- *Vault prolapse*: prolapse of the vaginal vault after hysterectomy.

Symptomatology

The symptoms of genital prolapse depend upon the part which is prolapsing. Thus women with cystocoele will have more urinary symptoms, while the patients with rectocoele will have more bowel symptoms. However, patients with genital prolapse may not have any symptoms other than prolapse. The various symptoms are shown in Box 2.

POPQ (pelvic organ prolapse quantification) classification of genital prolapse

This objective, site-specific system for describing, quantifying and staging pelvic support was

---

Box 2 Symptoms of prolapse

- Feeling of discomfort
- Heaviness in pelvis
- Lump coming down through introitus
- Worsening of symptoms on standing and at the end of the day
- Dyspareunia
- Difficulty in inserting tampons
- Chronic lower backache
- Vaginal discharge and/or bleeding due to mucosal ulceration and lichenification
- Urgency and frequency of urine (in cystocoele)
- Recurrent urinary tract infections (in cystocoele)
- Incomplete emptying of bowel (in rectocoele)
- Difficulty in moving bowels (in rectocoele)
- Tenesmus (in rectocoele)
- Digital defaecation (in rectocoele)
- Rarely, ureteric obstruction and chronic renal failure

Box 3 Measurements of positions on the vagina and perineal body in relation to the hymen for POPQ (pelvic organ prolapse quantification) classification (see Fig. 8)

Aa 3 cm proximal to urethral meatus on anterior vaginal wall
Ap 3 cm proximal to urethral meatus on posterior vaginal wall
Ba Most distal portion on anterior vaginal wall
Bp Most distal portion on posterior vaginal wall
C   Most distal edge of cervix or vaginal cuff
D   Post vaginal fornix
Gh Genital hiatus – middle of external urethral meatus to post midline hymen
Pb Perineal body – post margin of genital hiatus to mid-anal opening
Tvl Total vaginal length – greatest depth of vagina when points C and D are reduced to normal position

introduced by Bump *et al.* in 1996.[1] It has been approved by the International Continence Society and the American Urogynaecologic Society for the description of female pelvic organ prolapse. It measures positions at nine sites on the vagina and perineal body in relation to the hymen. The details are given in Boxes 3 and 4, and Fig. 8.

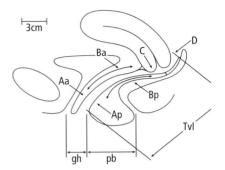

Figure 8 POPQ (pelvic organ prolapse quantification) classification of genital prolapse. Six sites (points Aa, Ba, C, D, Bp, Ap), genital hiatus (gh), perineal body (pb) and total vaginal length (Tvl) used for pelvic organ support quantification. (Reproduced from Bump *et al.*, *Am J Obstet Gynecol* 1996; 175: 10 with permission from Elsevier.)

Box 4 Pelvic organ prolapse staging: POPQ (pelvic organ prolapse quantification) classification (see Fig. 8)

Stage 0: No prolapse
Aa, Ba, Ap, Bp are -3 cm and C or D $\leqslant$ $-(tvl - 2)$ cm

Stage 1: Most distal portion of the prolapse
-1 cm (above the level of hymen)

Stage 2: Most distal portion of the prolapse
$\geqslant -1$ cm but $\leqslant +1$ cm ($\leqslant 1$ cm above or below the hymen)

Stage 3: Most distal portion of the prolapse
$> +1$ cm but $< +(tvl - 2)$ cm (beyond the hymen; protrudes no further than 2 cm less than the total vaginal length)

Stage 4: Complete eversion; most distal portion of the prolapse
$\geqslant + (tvl - 2)$ cm

tvl, total vaginal length.

Box 5 Differential diagnosis of lump at introitus

- Uterine prolapse
- Vaginal prolapse
- Cystocoele
- Urethrocoele
- Rectocoele
- Enterocoele
- Vault prolapse
- Vaginal cyst (Gartner's cyst and others)
- Imperforate hymen with haematocolpos
- Hypertrophy of cervix
- Urethral diverticulum
- Cervical polyp and endometrial polyp
- Chronic inversion of uterus
- Tumours of vulva, vagina and cervix

■ Examination of the patient

After taking a complete history and detailed general physical examination, including heart and chest examination, the abdomen and inguinal regions are examined for any lumps or hernias. Local perineal examination for the prolapse is performed in detail to know which part of the genital tract is affected. Any stress

■ Differential diagnosis

Differential diagnosis of a lump at the vulva and pelvic organ prolapse is shown in Box 5. It requires proper history-taking, examination and investigations to establish a clear diagnosis.

urinary incontinence is checked. The perineum is also examined for its length and integrity of perineal body. Any concomitant rectal prolapse or anal pathology, such as haemorrhoids, are identified. Speculum examination using Sim's speculum can be done in the Sim's lateral position (left lateral position with the left leg being extended and the right leg flexed at the hip and knee). The Sim's speculum can be used to determine which part of the pelvic floor is affected. Bimanual examination is performed to assess the position and size of uterus, and to exclude any adnexal pathology.

Investigations

A mid-stream urine specimen should be sent for culture and sensitivity. A full blood count, blood sugar, blood urea and other renal function test should be performed if considered necessary. Urodynamic studies may be required in the presence of a severe degree of prolapse (procidentia) and urinary stress incontinence. In cases of severe prolapse with ureteric obstruction, renal tract ultrasound or an intravenous urogram should be performed. Cystoscopy is only indicated when bladder stones or other bladder pathologies are suspected.

Management

The treatment for genital prolapse can be either conservative or surgical depending upon the severity of symptoms and prolapse, the patient's age, her willingness for the treatment, as well as her suitability and fitness for surgery.

Conservative treatment

Patients with first- or second-degree uterine prolapse, or with a small cystocoele or rectocoele may not need any surgical treatment. They should be counselled and could be followed up as outpatients. They can be advised about perineal floor exercises in consultation with a physiotherapist who will teach them to contract the correct muscles. Vaginal cones may be used for the same purpose.

Pessary treatment

This is also a type of conservative treatment in which a suitably sized (depending upon the size of introitus) ring pessary (52–102 mm) is put in the vaginal vault, keeping the cervix high up in the vagina. It is used when the patient is awaiting surgery or for women who present a high surgical risk. Appropriate counseling is important. The pessary should be changed every 4–6 months. Follow-up is important as the pessary can cause ulcerations in the vagina or can get embedded in the vagina, and it is important to avoid these complications. The use of ring pessaries has not become popular in developing countries owing to unreliable follow-up. There have been reports of vaginal cancer due to a forgotten pessary, which has become embedded and caused ulceration eventually leading to malignancy. Pessaries can also be used during pregnancy as a temporary measure for prolapse.

Surgical treatment

This is usually the mainstay of treatment for genital prolapse. The type of surgery depends upon the age of the patient, her fertility status, and the severity and type of prolapse. A complete procidentia may need to be reduced by packing the vagina and using local oestrogen cream prior to surgery. This will decrease any local swelling and also help to heal any decubitus ulcer, which is best treated before surgical treatment.

The following procedures are available:

Manchester repair (Fothergill's suture)

This is rarely performed these days. The approach is vaginal and there is conservation of the uterus. The elongated cervix is partially amputated. Cervical amputation is followed by approximating and shortening of the Mackenrodt's ligaments anterior to the cervical stump and elevating the cervix. Any repair of an associated cystocoele or rectocoele is undertaken if necessary at the same time.

Vaginal hysterectomy and repair

This is the mainstay in the treatment of prolapse, especially in women who have completed their family and in elderly fit women. In this operation, the uterus is removed by the vaginal route after dividing and ligating the uterosacral and the cardinal ligaments, followed by the uterine arteries and finally the broad ligament. The uterosacral ligaments should be tied posteriorly to obliterate the potential enterocoele space. An anterior repair (cystocoele repair) is performed for cystocoele and urethrocoele, which are usually present with uterine prolapse. Kelly's repair is performed in cases of stress urinary incontinence. For severe stress urinary incontinence, tension-free vaginal tape should be used with prolapse surgery. Enterocoele and rectocoele repair are usually performed at the same time. if present.

■ Vaginal vault prolapse

This is the prolapse of the vault of vagina, usually after an abdominal or vaginal hysterectomy. Small vault prolapse may be dealt with conservatively by perineal floor exercises. A shelf pessary may be used if surgery is not considered an option. However, large vault prolapses usually require surgical treatment. Vaginal sacrospinous ligament fixation is done by the vaginal route by tying the vaginal vault with the sacrospinous ligament. For more severe vault prolapse, an abdominal sacrocolpopexy (open or laparoscopic) is a better choice of procedure. In this case, a Mersilene tape strip is attached to the vault and the vault is attached to the sacral promontory.

The surgery could be performed under a spinal block and, very occasionally, with local anaesthetic, if the patient is not suitable for a general anaesthetic.

■ Reference

1. Bump RC, Mattiasson A, Bø K, et al. The standardization of terminology of female pelvic organ prolapse and pelvic floor dysfunction. Am J Obstet Gynecol 1996, **175**: 10–17.

PROLONGED PREGNANCY

Dhammike Silva and Dilip Visvanathan

There are many terms that have been used to describe this condition, which include 'post dates', 'post maturity' and 'post term'. A term pregnancy is defined as a pregnancy from 37 to 41 completed weeks of gestation. Therefore, a prolonged pregnancy has been traditionally defined as a 'pregnancy that lasts for more than 294 days'.[1]

Prolonged pregnancy may be associated with the following.

■ *Uteroplacental insufficiency*, which may lead to a higher rate of emergency Caesarean section during labour, intrapartum death and stillbirth. The increased rates of stillbirth with increasing gestation from term are illustrated in Table 1.

Table 1 The increase in rates of stillbirth and infant mortality with advancing gestation from term[4]

	37 weeks	43 weeks
Stillbirth	0.35/1000	2.12/1000 ($\times$6)
Stillbirth + infant mortality	0.7/1000	5.8/1000 ($\times$8)

■ *Macrosomia*: the intrauterine growth continues, leading to an increase in fetal weight. As a result, in a prolonged pregnancy, there is an increased incidence of macrosomia. This leads to problems at the time of delivery, including shoulder dystocia, bone fractures and Erb's palsy in the baby, and cervical and perineal trauma[2] in the mother.

■ *Poor neonatal outcome*: epidemiological studies have also shown an increase in neonatal and infant mortality after a prolonged pregnancy.[3] In a prolonged pregnancy, there is an increase in meconium-stained liquor due to development/-maturation of the vagus nerve, which results in reflex anal tone changes. Even though there is a theoretical increased risk of meconium aspiration syndrome, this has not been borne out by any of these studies.

Interventions in a woman with a prolonged pregnancy include induction of labour and, less frequently, elective Caesarean section in an attempt to reduce these potential complications. Induction of labour has been shown to reduce the perinatal mortality rate without increasing the rate of Caesarean section, especially if the induction is after 41 completed weeks of gestation. It is now routine practice in most units to offer induction of labour after 41 weeks of gestation, which has been supported by Royal College of Obstetricians and Gynaecologists guidelines.[5]

Despite this practice, there is a considerable amount of controversy surrounding the routine induction of labour for prolonged pregnancy. Most of the meta-analyses rely on a single study, which has the largest number of recruits. Repeat analysis of these results indicates that the risks of prolonged pregnancy may not be as high as previously indicated and the risks of emergency Caesarean section have likewise been overestimated. A recent study further confuses the issues, as it suggests that the length of pregnancy may vary between racial groups. Stillbirth rates in certain groups occur earlier in the pregnancy than previous studies have suggested. If the results of this study are confirmed, then it may mean that the timing of induction of labour should be earlier than 41 weeks in these racial groups.[6]

The causes of prolonged pregnancy include incorrect dates, fetoplacental factors and true prolonged pregnancy (Box 1).

Box 1 The causes of prolonged pregnancy

- Incorrect dates
- Fetoplacental causes, e.g. anencephaly
- Maternal causes – previous prolonged pregnancy

■ Incorrect dates

Pregnancy has been dated from the first day of the last regular menstrual period (LMP) using Naegle's rule of adding seven to the date and subtracting three from the month number. This results in an average pregnancy of 280 days. If the date of conception is certain, then it will be approximately 2 weeks less if the menstrual cycle is 28 days. If the pregnancy occurs after *in-vitro* fertilisation, then 16 days must be subtracted from the date of embryo transfer to obtain the LMP.

Dating scans in the first trimester of pregnancy have been shown to reduce the incidence of prolonged pregnancy because of the unreliability of just using the LMP date alone. It is estimated that 10–45 per cent of women do not remember the date of their LMP. Furthermore, the length of gestation is assumed as 266 days, which may have genetic, racial and geographical variation.

If the periods have a 28-day regular cyclicity, the woman has not used any hormonal contraception for 3 months prior to conception and has not had bleeding after the LMP, the accuracy of the LMP to date pregnancy increases.

Ultrasonography is now routinely used to confirm pregnancy that has been dated by the LMP. The crown–rump length (CRL) in early pregnancy (from $6^{1}/_{2}$ to 12 weeks) has been shown to be more accurate than gestational age calculated by LMP.[7] The sex of the fetus or racial characteristics do not seem to influence this accuracy.

Crown–rump length is measured with the fetus in the longitudinal axis and the callipers being placed on the outer margin of the head and the rump. Later on in pregnancy, it becomes more difficult as the fetus curls up. If measured correctly (Fig. 1), it is the most accurate dating measurement with an error margin of ± 5 days. The problems with CRL measurement are that, if there is any degree of fetal flexion, then the CRL will be underestimated (Fig. 2). In very early pregnancy, it is important not to include the fetal limbs or the yolk sac, as this will overestimate the CRL. When dating a twin pregnancy, the CRL of the larger twin is used.

After 12 completed weeks, the fetus tends to curl up even further and it becomes more difficult to measure the CRL accurately. The biparietal

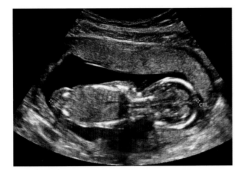

Figure 1 The proper fetal attitude for accurate measurement of crown–rump length.

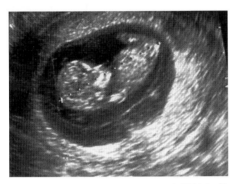

Figure 2 Measurement of crown–rump length (CRL). In this image, there is a certain amount of fetal flexion, which would underestimate the CRL.

diameter (BPD) of the fetal skull then becomes the standard measurement to estimate gestational age. From the 12th week to the 22nd week the relationship of BPD to gestational age is linear.

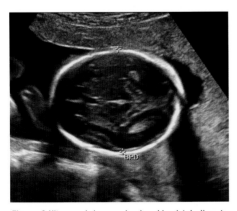

Figure 3 Ultrasound image showing biparietal diameter measurement taken at the optimum section.

The BPD is the maximum diameter of a transverse section of the fetal skull at the level of the biparietal eminences (Fig. 3). An accurate measurement of the BPD has the following characteristics; the section must be ovoid, have a midline echo (falx), have the cavum septum pellucidum visualised at one-third the distance of the fronto-occipital distance and the thalami must be symmetrically positioned on either side of the midline echo.

If the correct section is not taken for the BPD measurement, the potential margin of error can be high. The BPD is difficult to measure, if the head is in an occipito-anterior or posterior position. Tilting the patient or filling the bladder may help in achieving the optimal fetal position. The head can sometimes appear flattened and the BPD is consequently underestimated. This usually occurs when the fetus is in the breech or the transverse position. In these situations, the head circumference is a more accurate measurement. Composite measures for pregnancy dating include the femur length (Fig. 4) and abdominal circumference as well.

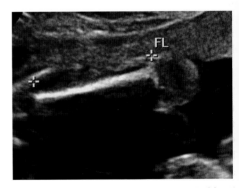

Figure 4 Ultrasound image showing measurement of femur length.

After 24 weeks' gestation, dating becomes less accurate as genetic, racial and individual pregnancy factors may influence the linearity of the measurements. The predicted date may vary from the actual one by 2–3 weeks.[7–9]

Table 2 summarises the ultrasound measurements taken to estimate gestational age and the accuracy of these for redating a pregnancy.

Table 2 The parameters used for gestational age assessment. If the LMP is uncertain, redating may be carried out. If the LMP is certain, a repeat scan is suggested in 2 weeks to exclude growth restriction and aneuploidy as a cause.

Parameter	Gestational age	Accuracy
CRL	6½ to 12 weeks	±5 days
BPD	13–27 weeks	±7 days
BPD/HC	>28 weeks	14–21 days

BPD, biparietal diameter; CRL, crown–rump length; HC, head circumference.

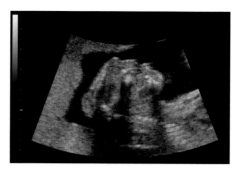

Figure 5 A fetus with anencephaly at ultrasound.

■ Fetoplacental causes

In other mammals, the onset of labour is determined by the fetal hypothalamo–pituitary–adrenal axis. There is a drop in serum progesterone levels associated with a rise in serum oestrogen levels and increased steroid production by the adrenal gland. However, in humans, studies have failed to show a drop in progesterone or change in oestrogen level in maternal plasma before and after the onset of labour. An increase in oestrone levels in the umbilical vein following spontaneous onset of labour has been shown, indicating that these changes may be occurring in the fetoplacental unit. Prolonged pregnancy may be rarely associated with low oestrogen levels,[10] which occurs in the following conditions.

Anencephaly

This occurs when there is a failure of closure of the cranial end of the neural tube at the end of the third to fourth week of gestation. Consequently, there is an absence of the forebrain (cerebrum and cerebellum), skull vault and almost always the covering scalp plus a poorly developed brainstem. The condition is incompatible with extrauterine life.

Anencephaly can now be diagnosed from 11 weeks. In the early stage, there is acrania. Here the vault of the skull is missing but the forebrain is intact. This may progress to exencephaly, which is herniation of the forebrain. Amniotic fluid erodes the forebrain leading to anencephaly. At scan, it will not be possible to obtain a BPD measurement, as the cranial vault is symmetrically absent (Fig. 5). The orbits are more pronounced giving a frog's eye appearance. There is a 50 per cent risk of associated lower spinal cord defect. An omphalocoele may also be present. The liquor volume may be increased and fetal movements may be marked.

In the past, maternal serum alphafetoprotein levels were used to screen for neural tube defects. At 16–18 weeks of pregnancy, a level that was greater than 2.5 multiples of the mean detected 88 per cent of all anencephalic infants.

Absence of a fetal pituitary gland

Absence of a fetal pituitary gland, usually in anencephaly, leads to fetal adrenal cortex atrophy with a consequent reduction in dehydroepiandrosterone sulphate (DHEAS) production. DHEAS is a precursor of serum oestradiol, which, in turn, is reduced. This is thought to be the reason for prolonged labour.

Fetal adrenal hypoplasia

This is a rare inherited disorder where there is atrophy of the adrenal cortex. Consequently, there is deficiency of both mineralocorticoid and glucocorticoid activity. In pregnancy, there are low serum oestriol levels and there is a tendency towards prolonged labour. The importance of this condition is that neonates can present with salt wasting and hyperpigmentation.

Placental sulphatase deficiency

This is a rare condition in which there is a deficiency in one of the enzyme systems required for the synthesis of oestrogen in the human placenta. Most case reports describe prolonged pregnancy with failure of induction of labour. Most of the boys presented with salt wasting and hyperpigmentation during the neonatal period.[11]

Previous prolonged pregnancy

A previous history of prolonged pregnancy increases the risk in a subsequent pregnancy of being prolonged to 20 per cent.[12] This was thought to be due to the influence of parental genes. Initially only maternal genes were thought to be implicated; however, a more recent study has shown that, if a woman changes her partner between pregnancies, her risk of a prolonged pregnancy is significantly reduced. Other factors that also contribute are advancing maternal age and a body mass index (BMI) of $>25\,kg/m^2$. Increases in BMI result in excess fat in the ischiorectal fossae preventing descent of the presenting part of the fetus.

References

1. World Health Organisation. Recommended definitions, terminology and format for statistical tables related to the perinatal period and use of a new certificate for cause of perinatal deaths. Modifications recommended by FIGO as amended October 14, 1976. *Acta Obstet Gynaecol Scand* 1977; **56:** 247–53.
2. Olesen AW, Westergaard JG, Olsen J. Perinatal and maternal complications related to postterm delivery: a national register-based study, 1978–1993. *Am J Obstet Gynecol* 2003; **189:** 222–7.
3. Crowley P. Interventions for preventing or improving the outcome of delivery at or beyond term. *Cochrane Database Syst Rev* 2000; (2): CD000170.
4. Hilder L, Costeloe K, Thilaganathan B. Prolonged pregnancy: evaluating gestation-specific risks of fetal and infant mortality. *Br J Obstet Gynaecol* 1998; **105:** 169–73.
5. Royal College of Obstetricians and Gynaecologists (RCOG). *Induction of Labour*. Evidence based clinical guideline, no. 9, 2001. London: RCOG.
6. Balchin I, Whittaker JC, Patel RR, Lamont RF, Steer PJ. Racial variation in the association between gestational age and perinatal mortality: prospective study. *BMJ* 2007; **334:** 833.
7. Taipale P, Hiilesmaa V. Predicting delivery date by ultrasound and last menstrual period in early gestation. *Obstet Gynecol* 2001; **97:** 189–94.
8. Hadlock FP, Deter RL, Harrist RB, Park SK. Computer assisted analysis of fetal age in the third trimester using multiple fetal growth parameters. *J Clin Ultrasound* 1983; **11:** 313–16.
9. Mongelli M, Chew S, Yuxin NG, Biswas A. Third-trimester ultrasound dating algorithms derived from pregnancies conceived with artificial reproductive techniques. *Ultrasound Obstet Gynecol* 2005; **26:** 129–31.
10. Romero R, Pilu G, Jeanty P, *et al:* *Prenatal Diagnosis of Congenital Anomalies*. Norwalk, CT: Appleton & Lange, 1988: 43–5.
11. Rabe T, Hosch R, Runnebaum B. Sulfatase deficiency in the human placenta: clinical findings. *Biol Res Pregnancy Perinatol* 1983; **4:** 95–102.
12. Olesen AW, Basso O, Olsen J. Risk of recurrence of prolonged pregnancy. *BMJ* 2003; **326:** 476.

PROTEINURIA IN PREGNANCY

Peter Muller

Proteinuria is defined as excessive protein excretion in the urine. There are generally four primary reasons for its development:[1]

- glomerular filtration abnormalities, e.g. pre-eclampsia or glomerulonephritis;
- tubular reabsorption abnormalities, e.g. acute tubular necrosis;
- overload, e.g. multiple myeloma or rhabdomyolysis;
- acute physical stressors, e.g. acute illness or exercise.

■ Measurement of proteinuria

Dipstick urine

The urine should be obtained as a mid-stream specimen and urinalysis performed within 1 hour of sample collection. Urinary protein is increased in urinary tract infections and should be excluded in all cases. The dipstick urine protein level will be recorded as none, trace, 1+, 2+, 3+ or 4+. Generally, 1+, 2+, 3+ and 4+ equate to 30, 100, 300 and 2000 mg/dL, respectively (Multistix 10 SG, Bayer Diagnostics Manufacturing, Bridgend, UK).

The advantage of dipstick testing is the ease of performance and immediate result. Unfortunately, the dipstick urine protein has been shown to correlate poorly with the quantitative 24-hour urine total protein[2,3] and spot urine protein/creatinine ratio.[4] This is due to the variability of the urine protein levels during a 24-hour period,[5] which in turn may be secondary to changes in water intake, rate of diuresis, exercise, diet, recumbency,[6] as well as interobserver variation from the semi-quantitative measurement.[2] Similarly, in pregnant women with hypertension in pregnancy, up to 66 per cent with significant proteinuria by 24-hour urine protein ($\geqslant$300 mg/24 hour) had recordings of negative or trace protein on dipstick urine. Likewise, dipstick values of $\geqslant$3+ protein failed to predict 24-hour protein levels of >5 g/24 hours adequately.[3] Therefore, the clinician should use this semi-quantitative method solely as a screening test.

24-hour urine protein

The 24-hour urinary protein excretion is considered the 'gold standard' for the quantification of urinary protein.[6] It is usually collected starting in the morning after complete emptying of the bladder. The 24-hour urine demands measurement of the full urine output over a 24-hour period up to and including the first void of the following morning. The advantage of this method is that it is the standard for which disease state and progression is measured. The disadvantage is that the test in cumbersome and time-consuming. Results often take a few days to return to the clinician, making immediate management decisions difficult. Patients' privacy is often compromised in the outpatient setting and compliance is commonly in question. One way to estimate the compliance of the 24-hour urine protein is review the total urine volume and to calculate the creatinine excretion.

Spot urine protein/creatinine ratio

When the glomerular filtration rate is relatively constant, the protein and creatinine excretion rates will also be constant. The protein/creatinine ratio will then correct for the normal variation in water excretion over 24 hours. The spot protein/creatinine ratio would have the advantage of having significantly less variability over 24 hours compared to dipstick testing,[7] and will lead to more clinical efficiency than a 24-hour urine protein. A systematic review demonstrates that protein/creatinine ratio does correlate well with actual 24-hour urine protein levels. The greatest benefit demonstrated was of 'ruling out' significant proteinuria.[6] The ability to detect an absence of significant proteinuria, would lead to less 24-hour urine protein collections, fewer hospital admissions, and possibly fewer medical interventions.

■ Evaluations of the kidney

Microscopic urinalysis

Direct microscopic evaluation of the urinary sediment for specific urinary casts will often point to a specific disease process. These would include the following:[1]

- hyaline cast – concentrated urine, after exercise;
- red cell casts – glomerulonephritis;
- white cell cast – pyelonephritis, interstitial nephritis;
- renal tubular casts – acute tubular necrosis, interstitial nephritis.

Fractional excretion of sodium (FENa per cent) and urine osmolality (UOsm)

Urine electrolytes and osmolality may help in distinguishing prerenal azotaemia (the build-up of waste products that accumulate in the blood and body when the kidney fails to function) from other intrinsic renal disease:[1]

- prerenal azotaemia – FENa (per cent) <1 and UOsm >500;
- acute tubular necrosis – FENa >1, UOsm 250–300;
- glomerulonephritis – FENa <1, UOsm variable;
- urinary obstruction – FENa variable, UOsm <400.

Ultrasound

Renal ultrasound is the investigation of choice for the initial evaluation for new-onset renal disease. Although, typical presentations of pre-eclampsia generally do not warrant a renal ultrasound, an atypical presentation of proteinuria in pregnancy may benefit from such an evaluation. This non-invasive approach, which uses no ionising radiation, can identify a distended urinary collecting system, kidney size and echogenicity, renal mass lesions, and evidence of cystic renal disease. Transvaginal ultrasound can be a very successful adjunct in assessing for distal ureteric stones. Most cases of renal colic can be diagnosed with a combination of ultrasound and clinical features, and it is only rarely that other imaging modalities will be required.

Intravenous pyelogram

Intravenous pyelogram (IVP) is used less commonly today to evaluate the renal collecting system and renal stones, unless specific information is required prior to surgical intervention. If an IVP is required as an adjunct to other imaging modalities in pregnancy, the fetal radiation dose can be minimised with limited scans (including a preliminary, plain, abdominal X-ray, early and late postcontrast abdominal films only).

Computerised tomography scan

Non-contrast helical computerised tomography (CT) is 95 per cent sensitive and 98 per cent specific in detecting renal stones and has become the gold standard in investigating renal colic.[1] In pregnancy, however, it delivers a significant radiation dose to the fetus, and alternate imaging modalities are, therefore, preferred. A targeted CT scan can be used as an adjunct to suboptimal renal ultrasound.

Magnetic resonance imaging urography

Recent advances in magnetic resonance imaging (MRI) techniques have enabled MRI urography to be used as an adjunct to ultrasound in the investigation of renal colic/renal tract obstruction in pregnancy. There is no ionising radiation involved and the risks to the fetus are low.

Percutaneous renal biopsy

Renal biopsy is rarely indicated in pregnancy, but may be indicated in unexplained renal failure and/or proteinuria and haematuria, and suspected transplant rejection. Renal biopsy is relatively safe and the risk of significant bleeding requiring transfusion is approximately 0.1–0.3 per cent.[1]

■ Diagnosis

Urinary tract infection

Urinary tract infection can cause mildly elevated proteinuria seen on dipstick or on spot urine protein/creatinine ratio. This generally can be easily differentiated from other causes of proteinuria, by evidence of pyuria and bacteruria with associated urinary symptoms.

Pre-eclampsia

Pre-eclampsia is defined as hypertension occurring after 20 weeks' gestation plus proteinuria,[8] and should be the primary initial diagnosis for new-onset proteinuria after 20 weeks' gestation. A 24-hour urine protein level of 300 mg/24 hours is accepted by international consensus groups for the definition of significant proteinuria.[8,9] Severe pre-eclampsia can be defined by a 24-hour urine protein of greater than 5 g/24 hours. It is important, however, to realize that proteinuria is not seen in all cases of pre-eclampsia and is not mandatory for the clinical diagnosis.[9] Indeed, proteinuria was absent in 14 per cent cases of eclampsia[10] and 13 per cent cases of the HELLP (haemolysis, elevated liver enzymes and low platelets) syndrome.[11] Hypertension and other clinical characteristics that may be used for the clinical diagnosis, in the absence of proteinuria, are the new onset of liver function abnormalities, elevated serum creatinine and platelet count $<100\,000$ with evidence of haemolysis, neurological signs, such as headache or visual disturbances, epigastric pain and fetal growth restriction.[9]

Owing to the discrepancy of random urine dipstick with the other methods, a 24-hour urine protein analysis or protein/creatinine ratio should be performed for all suspected cases of hypertensive disease.[3] However, there is no consensus on the use of spot urine protein/creatinine ratio for defining significant proteinuria. One consensus statement suggests a spot urine protein/creatinine ratio of >30 mg/mmol for the definition.[9] While the 24-hour urinary protein analysis is still seen as the gold standard for the diagnosis of significant proteinuria, spot protein/creatinine ratio has shown reasonable correlation in pregnancy to the 24-hour study,[12,13] and can be used to obtain timely results for the management of newly admitted and day assessment patients.[9] The strength of the spot urine protein/creatinine ratio lies in its ability to exclude the presence of significant proteinuria[6,12,13] and possibly the diagnosis of pre-eclampsia. Although, some authors have failed to find a specific cut-off point to exclude significant proteinuria,[14] others have suggested a reasonable exclusion ratio of 0.2.[12,13,15]

Despite the consensus by many that spot urine protein/creatinine ratio is a reasonable alternative; there are still times where the 24-hour urine protein or serial spot urine protein/creatinine ratio may be recommended. The spot urine protein/creatinine ratio appears to lose its correlation at high levels of proteinuria,[13,16] and the 24-hour urine protein may improve the diagnostic criteria for severe pre-eclampsia (proteinuria >5 g/24 hours.[17] In addition, serial spot urine protein/creatinine ratio or 24-hour urine protein levels may confirm the diagnostic transition from gestational hypertension to mild pre-eclampsia.

Glomerulonephritis

Patients will present with oedema, hypertension and acute renal insufficiency, making this difficult to differentiate from pre-eclampsia. Oedema is often found in periorbital or vulvar regions as well as the extremities. Since the management of pre-eclampsia requires a focused urgent plan, the clinician's primary goal is to exclude this from the differential. Urinalysis will demonstrate haematuria, red-cell cast, white blood cells and mild to moderate proteinuria. Specific aetiologies for glomerulonephritis will require exhaustive serologic examinations and possible renal biopsy. The treatment plan depends solely on the specific disease.

Acute tubular necrosis

The clinical setting for acute tubular necrosis (ATN) is commonly clear, where sudden profound hypotension occurs following hypovolemic or septic shock. However, nephrotoxic agents may precipitate the tubular damage. This may involve an exogenous source, such administration of aminoglycosides or radiographic contrast, or an endogenous source from rhabdomyolysis. Clinical history, 'muddy brown' or renal tubular casts on urinalysis, and an FENa of >1 will assist in differentiating ATN from other intrinsic renal disease.

Treatment consists of strict fluid balance to avoid fluid overload, and supportive care. Although larger doses of frusemide are commonly used to improve urine output, in randomised trials, this has not been shown to affect recovery time.[1]

Prerenal azotaemia

This is the most common type of renal failure outside pregnancy. Prerenal azotaemia in pregnancy can be due to a decrease in intravascular volume or a change in vascular resistance. A decrease in intravascular volume may be attributed to haemorrhage, dehydration, gastrointestinal loss or trauma. An increase in renal vascular resistance may be due to various drugs, such as non-steroidal anti-inflammatory drugs or angiotensin-converting enzyme inhibitors, or the decreased perfusion caused by renal artery stenosis. Urinalysis, FENa and a blood urea nitrogen (BUN)/creatinine ratio (usually >20:1) can assist in differentiating prerenal from intrinsic renal disease. Treatment is generally correcting the volume depletion or removing the inciting agent.

Obstructive uropathy

Obstruction of the genitourinary system can lead to a postrenal azotaemia. This is an uncommon cause of proteinuria in pregnancy; however, it has been seen in multiple pregnancy where complete obstruction of the ureters can occur. The importance of identifying urinary obstruction as the cause of proteinuria is the fact that it is usually a readily correctable problem. Patients generally present with lower abdominal or flank pain. Urinary electrolytes demonstrate a low FENa, high osmolality and a high BUN/creatinine ratio. Ultrasound in pregnancy will generally detect bilateral hydronephrosis or enlarged bladder. The severity of hydronephrosis will differentiate this from physiologic hydronephrosis seen in most pregnancies. Postobstruction diuresis will generally follow the release and fluid balance management is essential to prevent hypovolaemia.

■ Conclusion

New onset of proteinuria in pregnancy should alert the clinician to review for evidence of preeclampsia. The lack of proteinuria does not exclude the disease. However, not all cases of proteinuria in pregnancy are related to hypertensive disease, and the clinician should be familiar with the other causes and the appropriate evaluations.

■ References

1. Tierney LM, McPhee SJ, Papadakis MA. *Current Medical Diagnosis and Treatment*, 45th edn. New York: McGraw-Hill, 2006.
2. Kuo VS, Koumantakis G, Gallery ED. Proteinuria and its assessment in normal and hypertensive pregnancy. *Am J Obstet Gynecol* 1992; **167:** 723–8.
3. Meyer NL, Mercer BM, Friedman SA, Sibai BM. Urinary dipstick protein: a poor predictor of absent or severe proteinuria. *Am J Obstet Gynecol* 1994; **170:** 137–41.
4. Phelan LK, Brown MA, Davis GK, Mangos G. A prospective study of the impact of automated dipstick urinalysis on the diagnosis of preeclampsia. *Hypertens Pregnancy* 2004; **23:** 135–42.
5. Koopman MG, Krediet RT, Koomen GC, Strackee J, Arisz L. Circadian rhythm of proteinuria: consequences of the use of urinary protein:creatinine ratios. *Nephrol Dial Transplant* 1989; **4:** 9–14.
6. Price CP, Newall RG, Boyd JC. Use of protein:creatinine ratio measurements on random urine samples for prediction of significant proteinuria: a systematic review. *Clin Chem* 2005; **51:** 1577–86.
7. Newman DJ, Pugia MJ, Lott JA, Wallace JF, Hiar AM. Urinary protein and albumin excretion corrected by creatinine and specific gravity. *Clin Chim Acta* 2000; **294:** 139–55.
8. Report of the National High Blood Pressure Education Program Working Group on High Blood Pressure in Pregnancy. *Am J Obstet Gynecol* 2000; **183:** S1–S22.
9. Brown MA, Hague WM, Higgins J, *et al.* The detection, investigation and management of hypertension in pregnancy: full consensus statement. *Aust NZ J Obstet Gynaecol* 2000; **40:** 139–55.
10. Mattar F, Sibai BM. Eclampsia. VIII. Risk factors for maternal morbidity. *Am J Obstet Gynecol* 2000; **182:** 307–12.
11. Sibai BM. Diagnosis, controversies, and management of the syndrome of hemolysis, elevated liver enzymes, and low platelet count. *Obstet Gynecol* 2004; **103:** 981–91.
12. Neithardt AB, Dooley SL, Borensztajn J. Prediction of 24-hour protein excretion in pregnancy with a single voided urine protein-to-creatinine ratio. *Am J Obstet Gynecol* 2002; **186:** 883–6.
13. Rodriguez-Thompson D, Lieberman ES. Use of a random urinary protein-to-creatinine ratio for the diagnosis of significant proteinuria during pregnancy. *Am J Obstet Gynecol* 2001; **185:** 808–11.

14. Durnwald C, Mercer B. A prospective comparison of total protein/creatinine ratio versus 24-hour urine protein in women with suspected preeclampsia. *Am J Obstet Gynecol* 2003; **189:** 848–52.
15. Ginsberg JM, Chang BS, Matarese RA, Garella S. Use of single voided urine samples to estimate quantitative proteinuria. *N Engl J Med* 1983; **309:** 1543–6.
16. Quadri KH, Bernardini J, Greenberg A, Laifer S, Syed A, Holley JL. Assessment of renal function during pregnancy using a random urine protein to creatinine ratio and Cockcroft–Gault formula. *Am J Kidney Dis* 1994; **24:** 416–20.
17. ACOG practice bulletin. Diagnosis and management of preeclampsia and eclampsia. Number 33, January 2002. *Obstet Gynecol* 2002; **99:** 159–67

PSYCHOLOGICAL PROBLEMS IN PREGNANCY AND THE POSTNATAL PERIOD

Deborah Chee and Richard Maplethorpe

Psychiatric disorders associated with childbirth are common, both new episodes specifically related to childbirth and recurrences of pre-existing conditions. Pregnancy and childbirth have a combined psychological and physiological effect on a woman's life. Studies have shown that childbearing is associated with a marked increase in incidence and prevalence of psychiatric disorder, although the exact causal mechanisms remain unclear. Postnatal depression is consistently found in 10–15 per cent of mothers.[1] Postpartum psychosis is less common affecting 2 per 1000 deliveries. About 2 per cent of pregnant women using obstetric services have chronic mental health problems.[2]

The majority of women (50–75 per cent) who develop postnatal mental health problems will suffer from mild transitory depressive illnesses, often with accompanying anxiety (the blues). The risk of developing a severe mental illness, either a severe depressive illness or a puerperal psychosis, is substantially increased, particularly in the first 3 months following delivery. These relative risks (RRs) compared to the rest of the female population can be summarized as follows:[3]

- developing a severe depressive illness following childbirth – RR ×5;
- need to see a psychiatrist – RR ×7;
- need for hospital admission due to a psychosis in the first 3 months following childbirth – RR ×324.

The relative risk of developing a new-onset serious psychiatric disorder during pregnancy is lower than at other times; however, obsessive–compulsive disorder becomes worse or can start in pregnancy.

Psychiatric illness leading to suicide is a major cause of maternal death in the UK. Death rates from suicide were very low during pregnancy to within 42 days postpartum but trebled after 6 weeks to 12 months postpartum. However, death rates from suicide within a year after birth are substantially lower than in non-pregnant women (RR 0.09 for pregnancy to within 42 days postpartum group, and 0.31 for 6 weeks postpartum to 1 year postpartum group). The women who commit suicide are more likely to do so in a violent way and not as a 'cry for help'.[3]

■ Postpartum psychiatric illness

Psychiatric disorders in the postpartum period are divided into three categories reflecting severity:

- maternity (baby) blues;
- postpartum depression;
- postpartum psychosis.

Maternity blues

This is a minor transitory mood disturbance occurring in 50–75 per cent of women in the first week following delivery, especially after a first baby. Women in the immediate post-partum period may experience mild 'highs' as well as depressive episodes.[4] The cause of 'blues' remains unknown, with the literature being inconsistent on associated factors, such as hormonal changes and consequently no diagnostic blood tests are indicated.

The 'blues' may cause considerable distress to the mother but usually does not require any specific treatment other than reassurance. Symptoms typically last from a few hours to several days in the immediate postnatal period. These symptoms include tearfulness, sleeplessness, irritability, impairment of concentration, isolation and headache. The maternity blues are not considered a postpartum depressive disorder. It is defined by its brevity; should symptoms persist, then postnatal depression should be considered.

If the symptoms are extreme or prolonged, they must be differentiated from the prodromal features of a puerperal psychosis, which often commences in the same time period. If the symptoms persist over 2 weeks, then a diagnosis of depression should be considered.

Postnatal depression

Postnatal depression is regarded as any non-psychotic depressive illness of mild to moderate severity occurring during the first year following delivery. The peak onset of depression occurs in the first 6 weeks following childbirth. A recent meta-analysis of nearly 60 studies gives a prevalence rate for postnatal depression of 13 per cent.[1] The suffering caused by depression is profound yet often underestimated. Postnatal depression is particularly important because it is so common, and occurs at such a critical time in the lives of the mother, her baby and her family. It is important that the term 'postnatal depression' should not be used as a generic term for all mental illness following delivery.

Psychosocial and biological factors have been postulated (see Box 1). These associations have been used by medical professionals to predict and identify women likely to develop postnatal depression and help them access early assessment and treatment. Each subsequent episode may commence earlier in the postpartum period.

Box 1 Risk factors for postnatal depression

- Depression during pregnancy
- History of previous depression, especially previous postnatal depression
- Discontinuation of antidepressant therapy
- Antenatal anxiety
- Low self-esteem
- Life stress (recent life events, unemployment, moving house)
- Poor family support
- Poor marital relationship
- Childcare stress (including difficulty in breast feeding)
- Infant temperament problems/colic
- Single parent
- Unplanned/unwanted pregnancy
- History of infertility and assisted conception

Earlier onset depression may in part have an endocrine cause. Massive endocrine changes in circulating sex steroids occur at childbirth. The hypothalamic–pituitary axis must adjust to the sudden loss of placenta and re-establish its regulatory functions in relation to ovarian activity as well as starting lactation.[5] Oestrogen may have mood-elevating properties: it has been found to be superior to a placebo in treating postnatal depression[6] and was shown to be an antidepressant in childbearing women.[7] The mechanisms of action, however, remain unclear. Cortisol dysregulation has also been postulated as being causative.[8]

Diagnosis of postnatal depression may be undetected in up to 50 per cent of cases.[9] The clinical picture is similar to other types of depression; however, other symptoms suggestive of postpartum depression include:

- difficulty with practical parenting, including handling or feeding;
- feelings of guilt that she is not coping;
- expressing excessive concern about the baby's health.

Treatment options are no different to depression occurring at other times. Antidepressant medication may be indicated and the criteria for prescribing are the same as for non-puerperal depression. Adequate doses should be used and treatment continued for an appropriate length of time. Breast feeding may usually be continued with caution whilst monitoring the baby.[10]

Postpartum psychosis

For all mothers, the risk of admission to a psychiatric hospital is increased sevenfold in the month following delivery.[11] The peak time of onset of psychosis is within 2 weeks of delivery,[12]

> **Box 2** Summary of puerperal psychotic symptoms
>
> - Women with manic symptoms are excited, overtalkative, euphoric, uninhibited and intensely overactive. 'Patchy perplexity' is common and they may also have grandiose ideas, which may be delusional (e.g. conviction that she is 'chosen' or that the baby has special powers)
> - Postnatally depressed women have more severe symptoms and may exhibit confusion, delusions and stupor. Disorders of perception may be complex, taking the form of visions. Alternatively, these women can present with agitated depression experiencing convictions of hopelessness and uselessness, which sometimes reach suicidal intensity. They become preoccupied with rigid feeding routines or overwhelmed by minor health problems
> - Other symptoms suggesting psychosis include confusion or perplexity, catatonic features, thought disorder, auditory hallucinations and paranoid delusions or ideas of reference such as special messages. The picture may be labile with a mixture of depressive and manic symptoms

---

although there is a small but significantly elevated risk for at least 2 years postpartum, especially in first-time mothers.[11]

Postpartum psychosis affects women in 1–2 per 1000 births. Comparisons of rates across cultures and over time have shown remarkable consistency.[13] This figure has remained consistent in England and Wales over the last 50 years despite improvements in medical care and a reduction in maternal mortality rates.[13]

Presenting symptoms may vary (Box 2), but there is typically an initial 'lucid interval' lasting a few days following delivery and prodromal features may coincide with the onset of the 'blues'. As mothers are now discharged early from maternity wards, initial symptoms may be observed by family members who notice sleeping difficulty, confusion and odd behaviour.

A mother suffering from postpartum psychosis will require admission to a psychiatric unit, preferably a mother and baby unit where available. Pharmacological treatment is dictated by the clinical picture and conventional treatments, including antidepressants, antipsychotics and mood stabilisers, are used in treatment. Child protection issues will arise when the woman may be a danger to the baby.

The short- to medium-term prognosis is good with most patients responding well to treatment and making a complete recovery. The risk of relapse following a subsequent pregnancy, however, remains high from 20 to 50 per cent.[14]

■ Chronic mental illness

Psychotic disorders

Psychosis during pregnancy

Studies have shown a slight but significant reduction in rates of contact with psychiatric services and admissions during pregnancy.[11,15–17] However, discontinuation of antidepressants during pregnancy can precipitate a relapse of depressive symptoms.[18] For bipolar illness, pregnancy is usually a time of remission.[14,19] Pregnancy does not seem to cause a relapse in pre-existing schizophrenia.[20,21]

Psychosis following childbirth (up to 12 months)

A history of bipolar affective disorder, irrespective of whether the previous episode was puerperal or not, confers an extremely high risk of relapse following childbirth. The rate rises from a general population risk of 0.1–0.2 per cent to between 25 and 50 per cent (i.e. up to a 500-fold increase in risk).[14]

Childbearing women with chronic schizophrenia of the disorganised type[22] showed little variation in their symptoms. Women with paranoid psychoses with short episodes of illness or with periods of remission following treatment were at high risk (40 per cent) of recurrence or exacerbation of their illnesses.[21]

Postnatal management will depend on the type of their illness, with a better outcome for women with 'positive' symptoms (Table 1) of schizophrenia both in terms of their response to treatment and their ability to be primary carers for their babies. For mothers with marked negative symptoms, alternative carers will need to be identified as early as possible during the pregnancy, if it is considered that a mother is unlikely to be able to care for the baby.

Table 1 Summary of positive and negative symptoms in schizophrenia

Positive	Negative
Delusions	Emotional apathy
Hallucinations	Slowness of thought and movement
Thought disorder	Underactivity
	Lack of drive
	Poverty of speech
	Social withdrawal

Non-psychotic disorders

Non-psychotic disorders during pregnancy

Studies have been inconclusive with regard to exacerbation of pre-existing mood disorder during pregnancy. Some suggest an increase, especially in the early stages of pregnancy[23,24] but, in a comparison study with non-pregnant women, no such association was found.[25]

Symptomatic psychiatric illnesses have been associated with:

- poor antenatal care;
- inadequate nutrition;
- impulsive behaviour;
- substance abuse.

Depression during pregnancy has been associated with preterm delivery, smaller head circumferences, lower birth weights and poorer Apgar scores.[18] Pregnancy may also trigger the onset of obsessive–compulsive disorder[26,27] or may cause it to worsen,[28] although the data on anxiety disorders is limited.

Non-psychotic disorder following childbirth (up to 12 months)

In women with a history of depression, the likelihood that they will become depressed following childbirth is raised about twofold. Anticipatory support and/or preventive pharmacotherapy are possible options.[29] Other conditions, such as obsessive–compulsive disorders, anxiety and phobic states, and eating disorders may continue unchanged following delivery or may worsen.

In general, childbirth does not improve psychiatric outcomes in women with histories of mental illness. Recent studies have demonstrated adverse effects of postnatal mental illness on the following:

- the mother–infant relationship;[30]
- children's (particularly boys') later cognitive and social development;[31–33]
- attachments and emotional regulation.[31–33]

These effects highlight the need for early detection and effective intervention.

■ Medical conditions presenting as mental health problems

It should be remembered that systemic illnesses can present with psychiatric symptoms, and there is always a need for taking a history and examining the patient. Cerebral thrombosis, meningitis, viral encephalitis and thrombotic thrombocytopenic purpura (TTP) can all present with confusion, delusion and/or depressive symptoms. Cerebral thrombosis and TTP are both more common in pregnancy.[3]

In a woman who presents atypically, i.e. antenatally or with atypical symptoms, or who deteriorates despite treatment, full investigations should be performed. These should include full blood count, urea and electrolytes, liver function tests, coagulation with magnetic resonance angiography or spiral computerised tomography of the skull.

■ Useful organisations/websites

Association for Post-natal Illness – provides information and advice, and a network of local contacts; an information service for partners and families as well as sufferers (www.apni.org).

Meet a Mum Association – provides support for mothers who are or have been suffering from isolation and/or postnatal depression (www.mama.org.uk).

Parentline Plus – provides a free confidential helpline for parents (www.parentlineplus.org.uk).

Newpin – a national organisation running a variety of projects in London, offering help and support to parents and carers of young children (e-mail: newpin@nationalnewpin.freeserve.co.uk)

Other sites
www.cemach.org.uk
www.nice.org.uk/CG45
www.neuroscience.bham.ac.uk/research/app/
www.sign.ac.uk/guidelines/fulltext/60/evidence.html

■ References

1. O'Hara MW, Swain AM. Rates and risk of postpartum depression: a meta-analysis. *Int Rev Psychiatry* 1996; **8**: 37–54.

2. Kumar *et al.* Psychiatric problems in pregnancy and puerperium. In: Barron WM, Lindheimer MD, eds. *Medical Disorders during Pregnancy*, 3rd edn. St Louis, MO: Mosby Inc, 2000.

3. *Confidential Enquiry into Maternal Deaths in UK, 2000–2002.* London: RCOG Press, 2004.

4. Glover V, Liddle P, Taylor A, Adams D, Sandler M. Mild hypomania (the highs) can be a feature of the first post-partum week: association with later depression. *Br J Psychiatry* 1994; **164**: 517–21.

5. Wieck A. Ovarian hormones, mood and neurotransmitters. *Int Rev Psychiatry* 1996; **8**: 17–25.

6. Henderson AF, Gregoire AJ, Kumar RD, Studd JW. Treatment of severe postnatal depression with oestradiol skin patches. *Lancet* 1991; **338**: 816–17.

7. Gregoire AJ, Kumar R, Everitt B, Henderson AF, Studd JW. Transdermal oestrogen for severe postnatal depression. *Lancet* 1996; **347**: 930–3.

8. Checkley S. Neuroendocrine mechanisms and the precipitation of depression by life events. *B J Psychiatry* 1992; **160**(Suppl 15): 7–17.

9. Sharpe D. A prospective longitudinal study of childbirth related emotional disorders in primary care. PhD thesis, University of London, 1992.

10. Yoshida K, Smith B, Kumar R. Psychotropic drugs in mother's milk: a comprehensive review of assay methods, pharmacokinetics and safety of breastfeeding. *J Psychopharmacol* 1999; **1391**: 64–80.

11. Kendell RE, Chalmers JC, Platz C. Epidemiology of puerperal psychosis. *Br J Psychiatry* 1987; **150**: 662–73.

12. Brockington IF, Winokur G, Dean C. Puerperal psychosis. In: Brockington IF, Kumar G, eds. *Motherhood and Mental Illness*. London: Academic Press, 1982: 37–69.

13. Kumar R. Postnatal mental illness: a transcultural perspective. *Soc Psychiatry Psychiatr Epidemiol* 1982; **29**: 250–64.
14. Marks MN, Wieck A, Checkley S, Kumar R. Contribution of psychological and social factors to psychiatric and non-psychiatric relapse after childbirth in women with previous histories of affective disorder. *J Affective Dis* 1992; **29**: 253–64.
15. Paffenburger RS, McCabe LJ. The effect of obstetric and perinatal events on risk of mental illness in women of childbearing age. *Am J Public Health* 1966; **56**: 400–7.
16. PughTF, Jerath BK, Schmidt WM, *et al.* Rates of mental disease related to childbearing. *N Engl J Med* 1963; **268**: 1224–8.
17. Kendell RE, Rennie D, Clarke JA, Dean C. The social and obstetric correlates of psychiatric admission in the puerperium. *Psychol Med* 1981; **11**: 341–50.
18. Nonacs R, Cohen LS Depression during pregnancy: diagnosis and options. *J Clin Psychiatry* 2002; **63**(Suppl 7): 24–30.
19. Viguera AC, Nonacs R, Cohen LS, Tondo L, Murray A, Baldessarini RJ. Risk of recurrence of bipolar disease in pregnant and non-pregnant women after discontinuing lithium maintenance. *Am J Psychiatry* 2000; **1572**: 179–84.
20. McNeil TF. A prospective study of postpartum psychosis in a high risk group. *Acta Psychiatr Scand* 1986; **74**: 204–16.
21. Davies A, McIvor RJ, Kumar RC. Impact of childbirth on a series of schizophrenic mothers: a comment on the possible influence of oestrogen on schizophrenia. *Schizophrenia Res* 1995; **16**: 25–31.
22. DSM IV. *Diagnostic and Statistical Manual,* 4th edn. Washington, DC: American Psychiatric Association, 1994.
23. Kumar R, Robson KM. A prospective study of emotional disorders in childbearing women. *Br J Psychiatry* 1984; **144**: 35–47.
24. Kitamura T, Shima S, Sugawara M, Toda MA. Psychological and social correlates of the onset of affective disorders among pregnant women. *Psychol Med* 1993; **23**: 967–75.
25. O'Hara MW, Zekoski EM, Philipps LH, Wright EJ. Controlled prospective study of mood disorders: a comparison of childbearing and non-childbearing women. *J Abnormal Psychol* 1990; **99**: 3–15.
26. Buttolph ML, Holland DA. Obsessive compulsive disorders in pregnancy and childbirth. In: Jenike MA, Baer L, Minichiello WE, eds. *Obsessive Compulsive Disorders: Theory and Management.* Chicago: Year Book Medical Publishers, 1990.
27. Neziroglu F, Anemone R, Yaryura-Tobias JA. Onset of obsessive compulsive disorder in pregnancy. *Am J Psychiatry* 1992; **149**: 947–50.
28. Shear MK, Mammen O. Anxiety disorders in pregnancy and postpartum. *Psychopharmacol Bull* 1995; **314**: 693–703.
29. Wisner KL, Wheeler SD. Prevention of recurrent postpartum major depression. *Hosp Community Psychiatry* 1994; **45**: 1191–6.
30. Martins C, Gaffan EA. Early effects of maternal depression of infant–mother attachment: a meta-analytic investigation. *J Child Psychol Psychiatry* 2000; **416**: 737–46.
31. Murray L, Cooper PJ. Impact of postpartum depression on child development *Int Rev Psychiatry* 1996; **8**: 55–63.
32. Sharpe D, Hay DF, Pawlby S, Schmücker G, Allen H, Kumar R. The impact of postnatal depression on boys' intellectual development. *J Child Psychol Psychiatry* 1995; **36**: 1315–36
33. Essex MJ, Klein MH, Miech R, Smider NA. Timing of initial exposure to maternal major depression and children's mental health symptoms. *Br J Psychiatry* 2001; **179**: 151–6.

PUBERTY, DELAYED

Kausik Banerjee

The timing of puberty can be quite variable in both boys and girls, and this follows bone maturation more closely than the chronological age of the child.

A testicular volume of 4 mL (as measured by an orchidometer) or a maximal testicular length of 2.5 cm is the first sign of puberty in a boy; 50 per cent of the boys in the UK achieve this by the age of 11 years . Failure to develop a testicular volume of 4 mL by 14 years is regarded as delayed puberty in a boy.

The appearance of breast buds is the first sign of puberty in girls, which happens in 50 per cent of girls in the UK at around 11 years of age. This is usually followed by the appearance of pubic hair within the following 6–12 months. Menstruation starts within 2–2.5 years from the onset of breast budding.

By definition, 3 per cent of children will fall outside the upper end of normal age of onset of puberty. Delayed puberty is more common in boys. Concern is raised either because of the lack of physical changes of puberty or because of short stature. The majority of these children do not have any underlying disorder. They have what is known as 'constitutional delay in growth and/or puberty' with the majority of them achieving their final potential eventually.

Delayed puberty is rare in girls and almost 80 per cent of girls with delayed puberty may have an underlying pathology. Puberty is considered to be delayed in a girl in the following circumstances:

- failure to achieve Tanner stage II breast development (breast bud) by 13 years;
- interruption of the sequence of pubertal development;
- failure to achieve menarche within 5 years of breast budding.

■ Pubertal staging

This is conventionally done according to the clinical staging system proposed by Tanner. In girls, this involves assessment of breast development (in boys, assessment of genital development and testicular volume), and axillary and pubic hair development (in both boys and girls). Male doctors should be accompanied by a female member of staff during assessment of pubertal staging in a girl.

Breast staging

B1: Pre-pubertal.
B2: Breast budding.
B3: Development of breast mound (could be difficult to distinguish between in B1 and B2 in obese girls).
B4: Areola projects at an angle to breast mound giving rise to secondary mound.
B5: Adult configuration.

Pubic hair staging

P1: No pubic hair.
P2: Fine hair over mons pubis and/or labia.
P3: Coarse, curly hair confined to pubis.
P4: Extension to near-adult distribution.
P5: Adult distribution.– covering the medial aspect of thighs.

■ Causes of delayed puberty

The aetiologic classification delayed puberty are listed in Box 1.

Constitutional delay

This is a rare cause in girls. There may be a positive family history and there may be associated concern regarding slow growth. Bone age (as determined from X-ray of the non-dominant hand either by the Tanner–Whitehouse method or Gruelich and Pyle method) is delayed in the majority by more than a year. Investigations are required to exclude chronic diseases. The majority of these girls achieve their final height potential and reach puberty, albeit much later than their peers.

Hypogonadotrophic hypogonadism

There is a low or normal level of serum luteinising hormone/follicle-stimulating hormone (LH/FSH), a low level of gonadotrophin-releasing hormone. The causes can be divided into central or systemic.

Hypothalamic and pituitary causes are responsible for about 30 per cent of cases of pubertal delay. Pubertal delay is also typically seen in chronic diseases, including malignancy, inflammatory bowel disease, coeliac disease, diabetes, asthma, cystic fibrosis, congenital heart disease, chronic infections (including human immunodeficiency virus and tuberculosis).

The onset of anorexia nervosa may result in delayed puberty or halt further progression. Normal activation of the hypothalamo–pituitary–gonadal axis takes place after a variable period of time, once a normal eating pattern is established and weight gain is restored.

Ballet dancers, professional gymnasts and long-distance runners often have pubertal delay secondary to functional hypogonadotrophism.

Hypergonadotrophic hypogonadism

This is associated with elevated LH/FSH and low oestrogen. Feedback to the hypothalamo–pituitary axis is lost. The causes are related to end-organ failure (ovary). These conditions are responsible for nearly 30 per cent of cases of delayed puberty in girls.

The commonest cause of gonadal failure in a girl is Turner's syndrome (present in 1:2000 girls). Short stature is the commonest clinical presentation in childhood; however, some may present with primary amenorrhoea either during pubertal age or even later. The classic chromosome abnormality is 45,XO, which is present in about 50 per cent of cases, but 10–20 per cent of women with this syndrome have a mosaic karyotype with 45,XO/46,XX. The remainder have X isochromosome.

Irradiation and chemotherapy are becoming increasingly common causes of ovarian failure in peripubertal children. Procarbazine, nitrosoureas and etoposide can cause permanent ovarian failure, whereas vincristine is associated with transient ovarian failure.

■ Investigations

Investigations to be considered are:

- exclude systemic disease;
- bone age
- serum LH/FSH, oestradiol;
- brain imaging, if clinically indicated.

■ Treatment

- Treatment of the primary cause.
- Observation and reassurance for majority of patients with constitutional delay.
- Pubertal induction can be undertaken with low-dose oestrogen, which has to be slow and gradual. Low-dose ethinyl oestradiol at a dose of 2 μg/day for a year followed by 4 mcg/day for the second year is a commonly accepted regime. Thereafter, the dose of ethinyloestradiol is increased by 2 μg/day every 3–4 months until a final dose of 20 μg/day is reached. A progestogen in the form of norethistrone (5 mg/day) is usually added for the first 5 days of each calendar month, when the total daily dose of ethinyl oestradiol has reached 20 μg/day.

■ Further reading

Bridges N. Disorders of puberty. In: Brook CGD, Hindmarsh PC, eds. *Clinical Paediatric Endocrinology*, 4th edn. London: Blackwell Science, 2001: 173–5.

Garibaldi L. Disorders of pubertal development. In: Behrman RE, Kliegman RM, Jenson NB, eds. *Nelson Textbook of Pediatrics*, 16th edn. Philadelphia: WB Saunders, 2000: 1687–95.

Rosenfeld R. Puberty in the female and its disorders. In: Sperling MA, ed. *Pediatric Endocrinology*, 2nd edn. Philadelphia: WB Saunders, 2002: 490–8.

Box 1 Aetiologic classification of delayed puberty

1. **Constitutional delay**

2. **Hypogonadotrophic hypogonadism**
   - Hypothalamic/pituitary causes
     i. Syndromic
        1. *Lack of gonadotrophin-releasing hormone: Kallmann syndrome, Laurence Moon–Bardet–Biedl syndrome*

   ii. Destructive lesions of hypothalamus/pituitary
      1. *Craniopharyngioma*
      2. *Hydrocephalus*
      3. *Infiltrative diseases including Langerhans cell histiocytosis*
      4. *Germinoma, glioma*
      5. *Prolactinoma*
      6. *Trauma*
      7. *Tuberculosis*
      8. *Cranial irradiation*
   iii. Isolated gonadotrophin deficiency/ multiple pituitary hormone deficiency
   iv. Gonadotrophin deficiency secondary to transfusion-associated haemochromatosis
- Functional
   i. Chronic diseases
   ii. Poor nutrition
   iii. Psychological deprivation
   iv. Steroid therapy
   v. Hypothyroidism

3. Hypergonadotrophic hypogonadism
- Congenital
   i. Gonadal dysgenesis
      1. *Turner's syndrome*
      2. *XY gonadal dysgenesis*
      3. *Noonan's syndrome[a]*
   ii. Metabolic
      1. *Galactosaemia*
      2. *Disorders of steroid metabolism*
   iii. Intersex disorders, including complete androgen insensitivity syndrome
- Acquired
   i. Surgical removal of gonads
   ii. Infection
      1. Mumps
      2. Rubella
      3. Tuberculosis
   iii. Irradiation
   iv. Chemotherapy
   v. Acquired autoimmune diseases, including autoimmune ovarian failure and autoimmune polyglandular endocrinopathies

---

[a]Noonan's syndrome: an autosomal dominant dysmorphic syndrome characterised by hypertelorism (increased distance between inner canthus of the eyes), downward slanting of eyes, low-set posteriorly rotated ears, short stature and right-sided cardiac anomalies. Incidence is 1:2500 live births.

PUBERTY, PRECOCIOUS

Kausik Banerjee

Attainment of breast development corresponding to Tanner stage II before the age of 8 years in a girl is considered as precocious in the UK, although the cut-off point has been lowered to 7 years in the USA. A boy who has attained a testicular volume of 4 mL before the age of 9 years is considered to be precocious. This is also known as true or central precocious puberty, and is caused by premature activation of hypothalamo–pituitary–gonadal (HPG) axis [gonadotrophin-releasing hormone (GnRH) dependent]. This follows a normal sequence.

In USA 8 per cent of white girls and almost 25 per cent of black girls were noted to have stage II breast development before the age of 8 years. However, a recent European survey did not find any definitive trend of precocious puberty in European girls. Young girls who have migrated from the developing world to the developed world show an increased incidence of precocious puberty.

■ Precocious pseudopuberty

This is sexual precocity caused by excess secretion of sex steroids independent of GnRH/gonadotrophins.

■ Physiological variations of normal puberty

Premature thelarche (breast development)

This is isolated breast development in the absence of other signs of puberty. It is commonly observed in infants and almost always happens before the age of 3 years.

Thelarche variant

In some girls with thelarche, the breast development persists or even progresses slowly. Occasionally, there could be an associated increase in height velocity and bone age. Dynamic tests of the HPG axis show a pre-pubertal response.

Exaggerated adrenarche

Adrenarche is the onset of adrenal puberty and represents a change in the pattern of adrenal secretory response to adrenocorticotrophic hormone. Adrenal 17-ketosteroid production commences around mid-childhood (6–8 years), and dehydroepiandrosterone sulphate becomes the predominant adrenal steroid during this time.

Some individuals produce enough adrenal androgens to cause signs and symptoms of sexual precocity, which is known as *exaggerated*

Box 1 Causes of precocious puberty

I. Causes of central precocious puberty [gonadotrophin-releasing hormone (GnRH) dependent]

1. Constitutional or idiopathic (responsible for about 80% of cases in girls)
2. Central nervous system (CNS) tumours
   i. *Hypothalamic hamartoma*
   ii. *Glioma*
   iii. *Astrocytoma*
   iv. *Germinoma*
3. Hydrocephalus
4. Cranial irradiation
5. Neurofibromatosis, tuberous sclerosis
6. CNS infection, hypoxic insult
7. Head injury
8. Primary severe hypothyroidism

II. Causes of GnRH-independent precocious puberty

1. Ovarian tumour
   i. *Juvenile granulosa cell tumour*
   ii. *Teratoma*
2. Autonomous ovarian cysts
3. Hepatoma, hepatoblastoma
4. Congenital adrenal hyperplasia
5. Adrenal tumour/hyperplasia
6. McCune–Albright syndrome
7. Exposure to exogenous sex steroids

adrenarche. This is a relatively common finding in the African and Afro–Caribbean population, with individuals often presenting with the early appearance of secondary sexual hair.

The term *premature adrenarche* is reserved for those who develop adrenarche before the age of 6 years.

Premature menarche

Very rarely, cyclical uterine bleeding may manifest without any other sign of puberty. An endometrial echo is identified on ultrasound at the time of bleeding.

■ Causes of precocious puberty

The causes of precocious puberty are summarised in Box 1.

■ Clinical evaluation

Points to remember are:

■ the majority of the cases have idiopathic central precocious puberty;

■ precocious pseudopuberty is rare;

■ exaggerated adrenarche is more common in girls from African or Afro–Caribbean races.

■ the underlying cause is usually obvious in secondary sexual precocity.

History and clinical examination should be directed towards identifying signs and symptoms of excess sex steroid production and the aetiology of sexual precocity. Family history of sexual precocity and the possible role of exogenous sex steroids should be sought.

Pubertal development in *idiopathic central precocious puberty* is usually normal both qualitatively and quantitatively except for the premature onset. Most cases are sporadic, although a few are familial. The majority of the cases establish a normal menstrual cycle and pregnancy has been reported as early as 4 years of age.

Maternal uniparental disomy (two chromosomes coming from one parent instead of having equal contribution from both parents) of chromosome 14 is a rare cause of central precocity.

Hypothalamic hamartoma (developmental malformation but not malignant) may cause sexual precocity either by acting as an accessory hypothalamus or by generating transforming growth factor α (TGF-α).

The *Van Wyk–Grumbach syndrome* is an unusual syndrome of sexual precocity associated with *hypothyroidism*. Often this is characterised by galactorrhoea. This is the only form of sexual precocity where linear growth is arrested rather than stimulated.

The McCune–Albright syndrome can lead to incomplete sexual precocity. This is a syndrome of precocious puberty, café-au-lait pigmentation with an irregular border and polyostotic fibrous dysplasia. The condition is caused by a somatic activating mutation of the α subunit of G protein, which couples transmembrane receptors to adenylate cyclase. The sexual precocity is independent of gonadotrophins. Most cases are sporadic but autosomal dominant transmission has been reported.

Congenital adrenal hyperplasia (CAH) is a recognised cause of sexual precocity. Elevated androgen levels secondary to missed diagnosis or poor compliance with treatment can act to 'mature' the hypothalamus, and trigger an early maturation of the HPG axis. Pubertal development does not stop despite subsequent adequate control of CAH and this leads to significantly reduced final adult height.

Benign ovarian follicular cyst is the commonest tumour associated with isosexual precocity. Oestrogen production is modest to marked.

Granulosa cell tumours are usually benign. They are occasionally associated with mesodermal dysplasia and can produce human chorionic gonadotrophin, Müllerian inhibiting hormone and inhibin.

Exogenous steroids are a well-documented cause of sexual precocity. Oestrogen-containing pills and creams are widely available, and soy formulas and ginseng cream are potential sources of phyto-oestrogens.

■ Investigations to consider

■ *Bone age*: in the majority of the cases, bone age is advanced – usually by more than 2 years.

■ An *ultrasound scan of the pelvis* confirms an enlarged uterus with a prominent endometrial echo. The ovaries are usually more than 3 mL in volume.

- *Dynamic test of the HPG axis*: a GnRH stimulation test: shows a pubertal response (luteinising hormone >7 IU/L) in GnRH-dependent sexual precocity and pre-pubertal response in others.
- The *serum oestradiol* is elevated to pubertal level in both GnRH-dependent and GnRH-independent sexual precocity.
- In selected cases, *thyroid function, liver function, adrenal androgens, urinary steroid metabolites* and *alphafetoprotein* measurements should be undertaken.
- *Pituitary imaging*: a magnetic resonance imaging scan of the hypothalamus and pituitary should be performed in confirmed GnRH-dependent/central precocious puberty.

■ Treatment options

Central/GnRH-dependent sexual precocity

Pharmacological doses of GnRH analogues downregulate GnRH receptors and hence inhibit secretion of luteinising hormone and follicle-stimulating hormone. An injectable preparation of triptorelin is the only licensed product for children in the UK. However, leoprorelin and goserelin preparations are also available and used in children. These preparations are given subcutaneously/intramuscularly every 4–12 weeks. Treatment is usually continued up to the age of 10–11 years.

GnRH-independent sexual precocity

- Removal of the primary cause (ovarian cyst/tumour, hepatoma, adrenal tumour, etc.).
- Androgen receptor blockers (cyproterone, flutamide, spironolactone).
- Aromatase inhibitors (testolactone).
- Testosterone biosynthesis inhibitors (ketoconazole).

■ Further reading

Bridges N. Disorders of puberty. In: Brook CGD, Hindmarsh PC, eds. *Clinical Paediatric Endocrinology*, 4th edn. London: Blackwell Science, 2001: 165–72.

Herman-Giddens ME, Slora EJ, Wassermann R, *et al*. Secondary sexual characteristics and menses in young girls seen in office practice: a study from the Pediatric Research in Office Settings network. *Pediatrics* 1997; **99**: 505–12.

Huirne JA, Lambalk CB. Gonadotropin releasing hormone receptor antagonists. *Lancet* 2001; **358**: 1793–803.

Kaplowitz P. Precocious puberty: update on secular trends, definition, diagnosis and treatment: *Adv Pediatr* 2004; **51**: 37–62.

Kaplowitz PB, Oberfield SE. Re-examination of the age limit for defining when puberty is precocious in girls in the United States: implications for evaluation and treatment. Drug and therapeutics and executive committee of the Lawson Wilkins Pediatric Endocrine Society. *Pediatrics* 1999; **104**: 936–41.

Raine JE, Donaldson MDC, Gregory JW, Savage MO, Hintz RL, eds. *Puberty in Practical Endocrinology and Diabetes in Children*, 2nd edn. London: Blackwell Publishing Ltd, 2006: 73–9.

Rosenfeld R. Puberty in the female and its disorders. In: Sperling MA, ed. *Pediatric Endocrinology*, 2nd edn. Philadelphia: Saunders, 2000: 483–90.

■ Useful resources

British Society for Paediatric Endocrinology and Diabetes (www.bsped.org).

Premature Sexual Maturation Group of the Child Growth Foundation (www.heightmatters.org.uk).

For children

Mayle P. *What's Happening to Me*. Secaucus, NJ: Lyle Stuart, Inc., 1973.

For parents

Money J. *Sex Errors of the Body*. Baltimore MD, Paul H Brookes Publishing Co. Inc. 1994.

PUBIC PAIN IN PREGNANCY

Sharmistha Williams

Pubic bone pain is becoming an increasingly common symptom during pregnancy. This may be due to pre-existing disease that has been exacerbated during pregnancy or peculiar to pregnancy itself. There are many physiological changes that occur in the pelvis during pregnancy to account for this symptom, including the following:

- an increase in mechanical stress on the pelvis due to the increasing maternal weight;
- increased laxity of the ligaments and fibrocartilaginous joints as a result of the hormonal changes in pregnancy;
- postural changes associated with advancing pregnancy.

The pain may vary in severity and, in extreme cases, may be so severe and debilitating that difficulty in weight-bearing and walking result. An early diagnosis of the cause of the pubic bone pain is important, as timely intervention has been shown to reduce the morbidity associated with the underlying disease. Difficulties in diagnosis of musculoskeletal disorders in pregnancy result from the limited use of imaging modalities and their potential harmful effects on the unborn fetus.

A classification of the causes of pubic bone pain in pregnancy is given in Box 1.

Musculoskeletal conditions

Diseases involving the pubic rami and/or the symphysis pubis can be classified as follows:

- mechanical (symphysis pubis dysfunction);
- idiopathic (osteitis pubis);
- inflammatory (osteomyelitis); or
- metabolic (osteomalacia).

The commonest condition in pregnancy is symphysis pubis dysfunction.

Symphysis pubis dysfunction

Symphysis pubis dysfunction (SPD) results from instability of the pelvic girdle owing to laxity of and diastasis of the pubic symphysis joint (Figs 1 and 2). The reported incidence of SPD has a wide geographical variation and varies from 1:36 to 1:300 pregnancies within the UK because of the

---

Box 1 A classification of the causes of pubic bone pain in pregnancy

Musculoskeletal conditions
- Disease involving the pubic bones and pubic symphysis
  - symphysis pubic dysfunction
  - osteomyelitis of the pubis
  - osteitis pubis
  - pregnancy-induced osteomalacia
- Referred pain
  - transient osteoporosis of pregnancy affecting the hip joint
  - mechanical back pain and sciatica

Other conditions
- Urinary tract infection

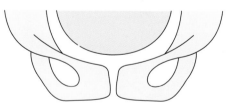

Figure 1 Pubic symphysis diastasis in pregnancy. The normal gap is 6–8 mm in the second half of pregnancy. Diastasis is said to occur if the gap is greater than 10 mm.

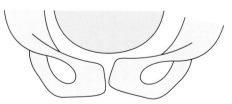

Figure 2 Upward displacement of the pubic rami whenthe patient lifts one leg. It is this instability of the symphysis pubis that results in difficulty in weight-bearing and walking.

lack of objective or subjective diagnostic criteria.[1] While in Scandinavia most women with SPD present in the first trimester of pregnancy, in the UK, presentation is usually in the second half of the pregnancy. Recurrence rates in future pregnancies may be are as high as 85 per cent.[2]

Symptoms include pubic bone pain during the following activities: walking, turning over in bed, climbing stairs, standing on one leg, and lifting or parting the legs. This is due to a loss of abduction of the thigh. Although the pain is commonly localised to the symphysis pubis, it may radiate to the lower abdomen, groin, perineum, thigh, leg and lower back. The pain has been described as shooting, burning, stabbing or grinding in nature.

A waddling gait may be seen in extreme cases. The commonest clinical sign is tenderness over the pubic symphysis or the sacroiliac joint. Active straight leg raising is usually restricted by pain and may cause a palpable displacement of the pubic symphysis. Hip movements, especially abduction and lateral rotation, are also restricted by pain (Fig. 3).

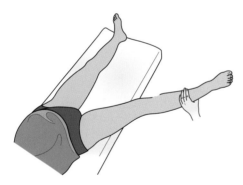

Figure 3 Abduction of the hip.

Clinical tests/examinations are usually carried out by obstetric physiotherapists and include the following.[3]

- *The Trendelenburg sign*: asking the patient to stand on one leg may cause the opposite buttock to sag (normally it should rise),
- *Palpation of the anterior surface of the symphysis pubis* results in pain that persists for more than 5 seconds after palpation.

- *Patrick's fabere sign*: in the supine position, with the anterior superior iliac spine fixed by the examiner, the patient places her opposite heel on the ipsilateral knee with the leg falling passively outwards. Pain in either sacroiliac joint is a positive test. This is illustrated in Fig. 4.

Plain anteroposterior X-ray films of the pelvis may show widening of the symphysis pubis with displacement, when the films are taken with the patient standing on one leg.

Osteomyelitis of the pubis

This low-grade infection of the pubic bone is a rare condition, which usually occurs 2 weeks to 3 months after a urogenital procedure, gynaecological surgery or operative delivery. More uncommonly, it results from spread of bacteria from a distant site in intravenous drug users. The usual symptoms include tenderness over the symphysis pubis or pubic rami, painful reduced hip movements, especially abduction, pain on lateral compression of the pelvis as well as associated systemic features, including a low-grade pyrexia. Blood investigations may show a normocytic normochromic anaemia, leucocytosis plus elevated inflammatory markers (C-reactive protein and erythrocyte sedimentation rate). Blood and urine cultures are positive in about 50 per cent of cases and may be *Staph aureus*, *Enterobacter* species and *Pseudomonas* species. X-rays of the pelvis may show widening and bony erosions of the symphysis pubis (Fig. 5). Radioisotope bone scans would show an increased uptake but are not used in pregnancy.

Osteitis pubis

This is a painful inflammatory condition involving all the structures in the region of the symphysis pubis in a symmetrical pattern. It is most commonly idiopathic but is sometimes associated with pregnancy, seronegative spondyloarthritis, urogenital procedures and trauma.

The symptoms in this condition include pain in the pubis with radiation to the groin, thigh and lower abdomen. The pain is aggravated by climbing stairs, kicking, lying on one side and pivoting on one leg. Coughing and sneezing

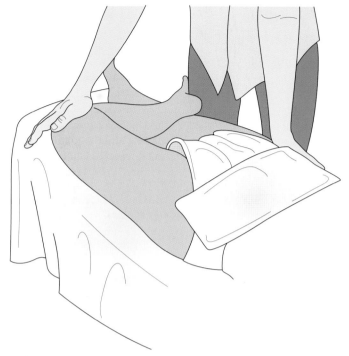

Figure 4 The Patrick's fabere test.

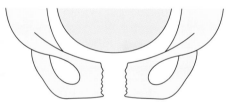

Figure 5 Erosions of the medial margins of the symphysis pubis seen with osteomalacia of the pubis.

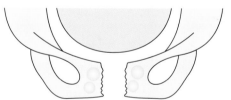

Figure 6 Rarefaction and cyst formation of the pubic rami and erosions of the medial margins of the symphysis pubis. These are characteristic features of osteitis pubis.

may also aggravate the pain. Palpation over the pubic symphysis and bilateral compression of the greater trochanters cause tenderness. Weakness in abduction of the thigh gives rise to a waddling gait. In addition, there may be weakness of the flexors of the hip.

Erosions, cystic changes and rarefaction of the medial margins of the pubic rami are typical on X-ray (Fig. 6). X-rays of the pelvis show diastasis of the pubic symphysis with displacement, when the patient is asked to stand on one leg. Sclerosis of the margins may be a later feature. White cell counts and inflammatory markers are usually not elevated. Bone scans may be negative.

Pregnancy-induced osteomalacia

This is a metabolic disorder of bone due to vitamin D deficiency. Vitamin D requirements are increased in pregnancy and, if these are not met by dietary intake, osteomalacia may result. Vegetarians are particularly at risk of this condition.

Symptoms are vague and, therefore, can often be misdiagnosed. Bone pain usually occurs in the axial skeleton. Localised pain in the pubic area may occur due to pseudofractures (Looser's zones). On X-ray, a thin, translucent band is apparent, about 2 mm in width, which runs perpendicular to the surface of the bone extending from the cortex inwards (Fig. 7). The gait may be

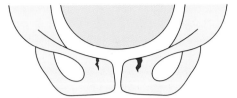

Figure 7 Looser's zones (pseudofractures) in the pubic rami are characteristic of osteomalacia. Vegetarians are at high risk, as they may be unable to compensate for the increased vitamin D requirement of pregnancy.

waddling due to a proximal myopathy. There may be bony tenderness localised to the pubis, but also present over the spine, ribs and sternum.

Diagnosis is usually made by biochemical investigations with low or normal serum calcium, and a raised alkaline phosphatase in nearly all patients. A low serum vitamin D level confirms the diagnosis. X-rays show Looser's zones in the pubic and ischial rami. Biochemistry usually returns to normal with oral vitamin D replacement therapy. If this does not occur, malabsorption needs to be excluded.

A summary of these conditions and differential diagnosis characteristics are given in Table 1. This illustrates the similarities in presentation. Since X-rays are only rarely used in pregnancy, diagnostic confusion may occur. This is why the exact incidence of any of these conditions in pregnancy remains speculative.

Referred pain

Musculoskeletal conditions that affect the spine and the hip joint can sometimes present with pubic bone pain. It is important with all joint problems to look at potential problems in the adjacent joints (above and below). However, there are usually other symptoms and signs that help differentiate them from the conditions that directly affect the pubic bone and symphysis pubis. These conditions are described below.

Transient osteoporosis of pregnancy affecting the hip joint

This is a rare but recognised condition. In pregnant women, the left hip is typically affected, although the right hip and other joints may also be involved.

Symptoms usually include hip pain, either localised to the groin or referred to the anterior aspect of the knee, especially on weight-bearing. The serum white cell count and inflammatory markers are only marginally raised, and may be within the normal range for pregnancy.

X-rays reveal localised osteopenia that may involve the femoral head and acetabulum. Ultrasound may demonstrate an effusion in the hip joint. The condition is usually distinguished from conditions that affect the pubic bone by the lack of localised tenderness when the pubic symphysis is palpated.

Table 1 The characteristics of musculoskeletal diseases of the pubic bone in pregnancy

	Symphysis pubis dysfunction (SPD)	Osteitis pubis	Osteomyelitis	Osteomalacia
Pain over pubis	Yes	Yes	Yes	Yes
Loss of thigh abduction	Yes	Yes	Yes	Yes
High erythrocyte sedimentation rate	No	No	Yes	No
Abnormal biochemistry	No	No	No	Yes
Systemic symptoms	No	No	Yes	Yes
Pubic diastasis	Yes	Yes	No	No
Pubic displacement	Yes	Yes	No	No
Erosions	No	Yes	No	Yes
Cysts/rarefaction	No	No	No	Yes
Looser's zones	No	No	Yes	No

Mechanical back pain and sciatica

The late stages of pregnancy are associated with an increase in lumbar lordosis and angulation of the lumbosacral junction. Up to 50 per cent of women may complain of lumbar backache in the later stages of pregnancy. The pain radiates to the buttocks, and occasionally to the lower limbs and pubic region. This may be sufficiently severe to interfere with sleep. The pain is increased during labour and disappears soon after delivery.

The woman's gait is usually not affected and there is no myopathy. Lumbar movements may provoke the pain. If associated with disc prolapse, straight-leg raising would be affected and localising neurological changes may be seen. There is usually no localised tenderness of the pubic symphysis. The diagnosis is usually made on clinical grounds and imaging of the lumbosacral spine, which is undertaken if the pain is persistent and worsens.

Other conditions

Lower urinary tract infection usually presents with dysuria, frequency and urgency of micturition; however, these symptoms may be less obvious in pregnancy. Women can present with pain behind the symphysis pubis.

Urinary tract infection

A lower urinary tract infection can present with pain behind the pubic bone, which may be confused with the conditions that directly involve the pubic bone. Urinary frequency in the third trimester is common and, therefore, the diagnosis is usually made by routine dipstick of a urine sample that shows proteinuria. A mid-stream specimen of urine would then confirm a urinary tract infection with the growth of 10^5 organisms/mL of urine. Clinical examination usually fails to elicit tenderness over the symphysis pubis. There is no abnormality of gait and abduction of the thigh is normal. Rapid symptomatic relief is obtained with appropriate antibiotic therapy.

References

1. Owens K, Pearson A, Mason G. Symphysis pubis dysfunction – a cause of significant obstetric morbidity. *Eur J Obstet Gynecol Reprod Biol* 2002; **105**: 143–6.
2. Leadbetter RE, Mawer D, Lindow SW. Symphysis pubis dysfunction: a review of the literature. *J Matern Fetal Neonatal Med* 2004; **16**: 349–54.
3. Jain S, Eedarapalli P, Jamjute P, Sawdy R. Symphysis pubic dysfunction: a practical approach to management. *Obstetrician Gynaecologist* 2006; **8**: 153–8.

Useful website

www.pelvicpartnership.org.uk

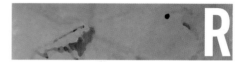

RASHES IN PREGNANCY (SEE ALSO Itching in pregnancy)

Anthony Bewley

Rashes in pregnancy fall into two categories: those directly related to pregnancy and those unrelated to the pregnancy. Rashes unrelated to pregnancy, such as eczema, psoriasis and lichenoid skin disease, are discussed in Itching in pregnancy and Vulval itching.

Rashes directly related to the pregnancy

There are five distinct dermatological conditions that can be induced by pregnancy (Table 1), and all seem to have an abundance of the letter 'P', which combined with the word 'pregnancy' may have the clinician performing a tongue twister just to say the diagnosis. However, once familiar with the conditions (and once seen, they are rarely forgotten), the nomenclature and its potential confusion become clearer. Apart from impetigo herpetiformis, they are all pruritic and it is the itching rather than the appearance that is often most debilitating.

Polymorphic eruption of pregnancy

This intensely itchy condition is thought to be associated with the exposure of skin antigens from the stretched abdominal skin of pregnancy.

Table 1 Rashes directly caused by pregnancy

Condition	Frequency	Distinctive feature	Other features
Polymorphic eruption of pregnancy	Common	Umbilical sparing	3rd trimester
			Polyhydramnios, >1 fetus
Pemphigoid gestationalis	Uncommon	Blisters	2nd/3rd trimester
			Recurs; may affect baby
Prurigo of pregnancy	Common	No urticaria-like lesions	2nd/3rd trimester
Pruritic folliculitis of pregnancy	Uncommon	Folliculitis	2nd/3rd trimester
Impetigo herpetiformis	Very rare	Pustules, scaling	Very serious

Hence it is commoner in the third trimester, multiple pregnancies and polyhydramnios. The rash distinctively appears as urticated (nettle rash-like) lesions in stretch marks and spares the umbilicus (Fig. 1). It is most often primagravidae who are affected. Delivery of the child (which is almost always unaffected by rash) is curative, although the symptoms may persist for a few weeks. Treatment is of the itch (Box 1) and reassurance that the condition is unlikely to recur in subsequent pregnancies.

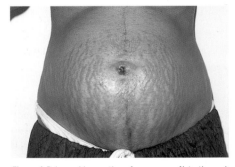

Figure 1 Polymorphic eruption of pregnancy. Note the peri-umbilical sparing.

Pemphigoid gestationalis

Pemphigoid gestationalis, also known (unhelpfully) as herpes gestationalis, is much rarer

Box 1 Management of itching in pregnancy

- Emollients (into the bath or on to the skin)
  - bath additives containing lauromacrogols (e.g. Balneum Plus®) or oat extract (e.g. Aveeno®) may be additionally antipruritic
  - topical emollients range from very watery (e.g. aqueous cream) to very greasy (e.g. white soft paraffin) – let the patient decide which is best
- Avoidance of soaps and detergents – use soap substitutes (e.g. aqueous cream)
- Non-sedating antihistamines (e.g. loratidine) are usually not licensed for pregnancy but are probably safe
- Sedating antihistamines (e.g. chlorpheniramine) have been used safely in pregnancy
- Topical steroid ointments (rather than creams) are probably safe (although not licensed) in pregnancy. Try to keep to the lowest strength possible (usually clobetasone or betamethasone 0.1%) for no longer than 6 weeks
- (Rarely) phototherapy (usually narrow-band ultraviolet B)

than polymorphic eruption of pregnancy. Characteristically, unlike any other pregnancy-related rash, there are true fluid-filled blisters as the pathophysiology is immunobullous, i.e. autoantibodies are formed to the basement membrane of the skin, causing fluid-filled dermoepidermal separation (Figs 2 and 3). It is intensely itchy, may affect the periumbilical skin, and may appear in the second and third trimester. Unfortunately, even though delivery is curative, the child may be born with a similar rash, although this is very rarely dangerous. The mother's rash may persist for several weeks and the condition typically recurs in subsequent pregnancies. Treatment is with systemic steroids – the lowest dose to suppress the condition.

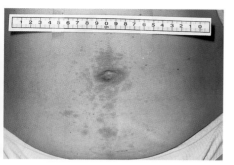

Figure 2 Pemphigoid gestationalis. Note the periumbilical involvement.

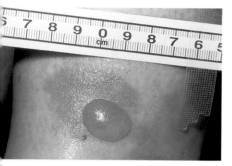

Figure 3 Blistering in pemphigoid gestationalis.

Prurigo of pregnancy

The main differences between this common condition and polymorphic eruption of pregnancy are that it starts earlier, and there are no urticated (hives-like) lesions. In fact, the condition looks like, and is frequently mistaken for, eczema (excoriations, papules and redness, often over the extensors) and scabies. However, the patient does not usually have a history of eczema and it is the extensor surfaces that are affected (rather than the flexures in eczema, and the groin and web spaces in scabies). The child is unaffected but recurrence in subsequent pregnancies is common. Treatment is of the itch (Box 1)

Pruritic folliculitis of pregnancy

Aptly named, this condition causes an intensely itchy sterile folliculitis and looks like a widespread, fine, itchy acne. It often starts in the second trimester and continues to the delivery of the child, which is curative. The child is unaffected, and the condition may or may not recur.

Treatment is of the itch (Box 1), although topical steroids are mostly avoided.

Impetigo herpetiformis

Impetigo herpetiformis looks similar to pustular psoriasis, except it is directly related to the pregnancy. It is the most dangerous of the pregnancy-related rashes and carries a small risk of maternal mortality. Clinically skin lesions are tender, scaly and red, with a broad sheet or surrounding ring of studded pustules (Figs 4 and 5). The lesions may be widespread, but frequently affect flexural (especially the groin) and acral (hands and feet) areas. The patient can be quite unwell with pyrexia, a mild inflammatory hepatitis and general malaise. Treatment is often difficult. Systemic steroids are frequently necessary and, occasionally, other second-line, potentially more toxic preparations (e.g. methotrexate) are required. The fetus may be affected. Once the child is delivered, the rash usually settles. Fortunately, the condition is rare but it can recur in subsequent pregnancies.

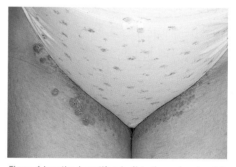

Figure 4 Impetigo herpetiformis. Note the scaly red rash in the groin with a pustular rim.

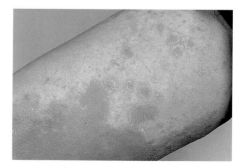

Figure 5 Impetigo herpetiformis: close-up of rash.

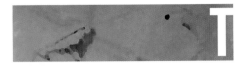

THYROID PROBLEMS IN PREGNANCY

Rina Davison

■ Physiological changes in pregnancy

The structure and function of the thyroid gland alters during pregnancy. In areas of relative iodine deficiency, e.g. Belgium, the thyroid gland often hypertrophies. This is due to increased iodide clearance by the kidney and increased maternal iodine requirements because of active transport to the fetal placental unit. Hence the thyroid gland enlarges in order to trap adequate amounts of iodine.

Thyroid-stimulating hormone (TSH) levels drop in the first trimester corresponding to the peak serum human chorionic gonadotrophin (HCG) during this period. Free thyroxine (FT4) levels may rise and this is attributable to the thyrotrophic action (TSH-like activity) of HCG (usually inconsequential Vomiting in pregnancy).

Hypothyroidism

This can occur in up to 1 per cent of pregnancies and is usually due to autoimmunity (Hashimoto's thyroiditis) or iodine deficiency (see Box 1).

> **Box 1** Causes of hypothyroidism in pregnancy
>
> ■ Autoimmunity
> ■ Iodine deficiency
> ■ Thyroidectomy
> ■ Post radioiodine therapy
> ■ Iatrogenic, e.g. amiodarone, lithium antithyroid drugs

Clinical features

The expression of various clinical features depends on the severity of the condition, and whether this is a new diagnosis or the patient is already on replacement therapy. Symptoms include weight gain, fatigue, forgetfulness myalgia, goitre, dry skin, fluid retention, brady-cardia and cold intolerance (Box 2). The patient may have coexisting autoimmune diseases, e.g. type 1 diabetes.

> **Box 2** Symptoms or signs of hypothyroidism
>
> ■ Goitre
> ■ Carpel tunnel syndrome
> ■ Constipation
> ■ Fluid retention
> ■ Lethargy
> ■ Weight gain

Diagnosis

Elevated TSH and low FT4 makes the diagnosis of primary hypothyroidism. If the TSH is elevated and FT4 normal, the diagnosis is subclinical hypothyroidism. In this case, the patient may or may not have symptoms, but evidence suggests that this group of women should be treated with thyroxine because of the possible deleterious effect on the offspring. Low TSH and low FT4 are found in central hypothyroidism. The patient is likely to have pituitary or hypothalamic dysfunction, and is unlikely to become pregnant owing to impairment of gonadotrophin secretion.

Treatment

Hypothyroidism during pregnancy is treated vigorously with thyroxine in order to achieve a TSH of <2 mU/L. It is recognised that, in established hypothyroidism, a 25–50 per cent increase in thyroxine dosage is required to maintain a FT4 at the higher range of normal. Hence patients need thyroid function tests, with dose adjustments as necessary, at least each trimester. After delivery, the dose of thyroxine returns to pre-pregnancy requirements almost immediately.

Effects on conception, pregnancy and the fetus

Hypothyroidism decreases ovulation and thereby reduces fertility. There is an associated risk of an increased rate of miscarriage, anaemia, hypertension and low birth weight. Fetal thyroid function only begins at 10–12 weeks' gestation and there is increasing evidence that, early in pregnancy, maternal thyroxine crosses the placenta and exerts an effect on brain development. Studies suggest untreated or undertreated maternal hypothyroidism can effect psychomotor development and IQ in offspring. These findings argue strongly for prompt recognition and treatment of hypothyroidism in pregnancy, which will usually lead to good maternal and fetal outcomes.

Hyperthyroidism

The incidence of thyrotoxicosis during pregnancy is lower than the general population; about 1 in 500 pregnancies. Graves' disease is the most common cause (95 per cent), although less commonly, toxic multinodular goitre, toxic adenoma, drugs or, rarely, gestational trophoblastic disease may lead to thyrotoxicosis.

Symptoms and signs

Most cases of hyperthyroidism in pregnancy will have already been diagnosed and will be on maintenance treatment. In cases of poorly controlled or newly diagnosed hyperthyroidism, typical features include heat intolerance, tachycardia, palpitations, goitre, weight loss, tremor and lid retraction (Box 3). Lid lag and exophthalmos indicate Graves' ophthalmopathy.

Diagnosis

Typically there is a raised serum FT4/free tri-iodothyronine (FT3) and suppressed TSH.

Management

Hyperthyroidism may cause maternal heart failure, infertility, miscarriage, intrauterine growth

> **Box 3** Symptoms or signs of hyperthyroidism
>
> - Amenorrhoea
> - Heat intolerance
> - Increased appetite
> - Anxiety
> - Nausea
> - Palpitations
> - Sweating
> - Tachycardia
> - Tremor
> - Vomiting
> - Goitre

retardation (IUGR), premature labour and increased perinatal mortality. Graves' disease after a transient exacerbation of clinical symptoms usually tends to remit in the second half of pregnancy.

The primary therapeutic objective is restoration to maternal euthyroidism using carbimazole or propylthiouracil (PTU) at the lowest dose to maintain the maternal FT4 in the upper normal range through periodic titration. Both drugs cross the placenta and, in high doses, may cause fetal hypothyroidism and goitre. Neither drug is overtly teratogenic but both can rarely cause a skin defect of the child's scalp known as aplasia cutis. Doses of PTU <150 mg per day or carbimazole <15 mg daily are unlikely to cause problems, and breast feeding is safe.

As transplacental transfer of thyroxine (T4) from mother to fetus is only minor, it would be inappropriate to treat the mother with an antithyroid drug/thyroxine combination, i.e. block and replace. Beta-blockers are only used in the short term for the relief of adrenergic symptoms associated with acute thyrotoxicosis. Antithyroid drugs can be withdrawn in the majority of cases after 4–12 weeks of treatment, but thyroid function tests and clinical assessment should still performed each trimester.

Surgery can be performed safely in the second trimester, but is usually reserved for large goitres causing compressive symptoms or suspected carcinoma. Radioiodine scans or therapy is contraindicated in pregnancy and breast feeding.

Neonatal hyperthyroidism

Neonatal hyperthyroidism occurs in 2–10 per cent of babies born to women with active Graves' disease. It can be predicted by determining maternal thyroid receptor antibodies at the beginning of the third trimester. In patients at risk, fetal thyroid status may be assessed through tachycardia, IUGR and thyroid hormone assay through cordocentesis. Treatment is with antithyroid drugs (given to the mother in fetal thyrotoxicosis) or to the neonate. Treatment in the neonate is only needed for a few weeks whilst the antibodies clear from the circulation.

For women with good control on antithyroid drugs, the maternal and fetal outcome is usually good.

Hyperemesis gravidarum

Hyperemesis gravidarum is characterized by prolonged and severe nausea and vomiting in early pregnancy, which can lead to a loss of 5 per cent body weight, dehydration and ketosis, together with electrolyte abnormalities. Management includes hospitalization, intravenous fluids, thiamine and antiemetics. In up to 50 per cent of admissions, disruption of thyroid function occurs. The TSH level is usually low and the FT4 may be increased, although the FT3 is rarely raised. These effects are due to the thyrotrophic action of HCG. Patients may have thyrotoxic symptoms but the thyroid antibodies will be negative. Increased thyroid function of hyperemesis gravidarum is self-limiting and treatment is usually supportive.

■ Postpartum thryoiditis

Postpartum thyroiditis is defined as an exacerbation of autoimmune thyroiditis during the postpartum period. Patients usually suffer from subclinical autoimmune thyroiditis beforehand, which is exacerbated after delivery. However, Graves' disease may also occur or recur in the postpartum period. About 1 in 20 pregnant women develop disordered thyroid function in the postpartum period in the form of persistent or transient thyrotoxicosis, destructive thyrotoxicosis followed by transient hypothyroidism and/or persistent hypothyroidism, but many cases are asymptomatic.

Pathogenesis

There is a destructive autoimmune thyroiditis causing an outpouring of preformed thyroxine from the thyroid gland followed by hypothyroidism owing to depletion of thyroid hormone within the gland.

Clinical features

Thyroid dysfunction is most often subclinical and presentation is usually between 3 and 4 months postpartum. However, in the hyperthyroid state, there may be typical symptoms of thyrotoxicosis and, similarly, in the hypothyroid phase, there may be lethargy, tiredness or depression. Postpartum depression is sometimes found with postpartum thyroid dysfunction and has recently been found to be associated with antithyroid antibodies rather than hypothyroidism itself.

Diagnosis

Diagnosis of postpartum thyroid dysfunction is simple when the patient shows abnormal thyroid function tests and positive thyroid antibodies. In overt thyrotoxicosis, it is essential to differentiate between postpartum Graves' disease and destructive thyrotoxicosis, as the management is different. Radioactive iodine scanning can distinguish the two: showing a low uptake in the thyroid with destructive thyroiditis and a high uptake with Graves' disease. Anti-TSH receptor antibodies are usually absent in postpartum thyroiditis.

Management

In postpartum Graves' disease, treatment options usually begin with antithyroid drugs, but radioactive iodine is an option, if this is a recurrence and the mother is not breast feeding.

In postpartum thyroiditis, the treatment should be symptomatic, namely, with beta-blockers for cardiovascular hyperdynamic symptoms in a thyrotoxic phase, and thyroxine with gradual reduction in dosage, if the patient is symptomatic with hypothyroidism.

Prognosis

In destructive postpartum thyroiditis causing thyrotoxicosis or hypothyroidism, thyroid dysfunction is transient and most patients recover spontaneously to euthyroidism. Only in few cases does hypothyroidism persist and high titres of antibodies are risk factors for persistent hypothyroidism. However, late development (after 5 years or more) of permanent hypothyroidism is found in 25 per cent of patients with postpartum thyroiditis; therefore, these patients should be followed up at appropriate intervals in primary care.

TIREDNESS IN PREGNANCY

Jai B Sharma

Pregnancy is a state in which there are considerable hormonal, physiological and emotional changes, all of which can have profound effects. There are many physiological changes, which can manifest as excessive nausea and vomiting, morning sickness, tiredness, lack of appetite in early pregnancy and excessive appetite in later pregnancy, slight dyspnoea, mild palpitation, constipation (owing to the effects of progesterone) and backache. These occur as a result of hormonal changes, as concentrations of oestrogens, progestogens and other placental hormones (e.g. human chorionic gonadotrophin) increase significantly during pregnancy.

Mild tiredness during pregnancy is a common physiological symptom and may not be of any significance. Apart from physiological changes, increasing fetal movements, Braxton–Hicks contractions as well as urinary frequency can lead to broken sleep, resulting in headaches and tiredness. However, excessive tiredness can be a symptom of abnormal pathology during pregnancy, which must be carefully assessed for any cause, and should be appropriately treated.

■ Causes of tiredness in pregnancy

The various causes of tiredness in pregnancy are given in Box 1. Mild tiredness is almost universal in most pregnant women, possibly owing to hormonal changes. It does not require any specific treatment. However, if the patient is concerned, it is worthwhile examining and investigating her fully to avoid missing any pathological cause of tiredness.

Nutritional causes of tiredness

As shown in Box 1, anaemia owing to iron deficiency, folate deficiency or cyanocobalamin deficiency can cause tiredness in pregnancy. Even protein energy malnutrition during pregnancy can cause tiredness during this period. Deficiencies of various micronutrients and trace elements, such as zinc, selenium, etc., can be other causes. All pregnant women must ensure they consume sufficient calories during pregnancy (2500 kcal/day) and an optimum amount of protein (60 g/day). In developing countries, it is not uncommon to see pregnant women with inadequate calorie and protein intake, which can result in tiredness. Treatment is by advising the women to ensure they have an adequate intake of calories, proteins, trace elements and calcium during pregnancy.

Calcium deficiency is common, especially in developing countries, where most women are vegetarians. They should be advised to take adequate milk and milk products to give them about 1200 mg of calcium/day. If they are unable to take milk and milk products in the desired amount, they should be prescribed calcium tablets at a dose of 1 g/day. The recommended daily dietary allowances of various nutrients are given in Table 1.

Anaemia in pregnancy

Anaemia is an important cause of tiredness during pregnancy, especially in developing countries,

Box 1 Causes of tiredness in pregnancy

Physiological
- Mild tiredness is common in all women

Nutritional causes
- Anaemia
  - Iron-deficiency anaemia
  - Folate deficiency
  - Cyanocobalamin deficiency
- Protein–energy malnutrition
- Micronutrient deficiencies

Infections and infestations
- Upper respiratory tract infections
- Urinary tract infections
- Genital infections
- Malaria
- Typhoid
- Hepatitis A, B, C and E infections
- Tuberculosis
- Worm infestations
- Intestinal infections

Endocrinological causes
- Diabetes mellitus
- Thyroid disorders (hypothyroidism and hyperthyroidism)
- Hyperparathyroidism
- Adrenal insufficiency
- Cushing's syndrome

Systemic diseases
- Heart disease
- Respiratory diseases (asthma, bronchitis, bronchiectasis)
- Rheumatoid arthritis
- Systemic lupus erythematosus and other collagen disorders
- Neuromuscular, including multiple sclerosis

Malignancies
- Leukaemia
- Lymphoma
- Gynaecological malignancies (ovarian, cervical)
- Other malignancies

Miscellaneous causes
- Chronic fatigue syndrome
- Hyperemesis
- Pre-eclampsia and other pregnancy disorders

Table 1 Recommended daily dietary allowances in pregnancy

Nutrients	Requirement
Calories	2500 kcal
Proteins	60 g
Iron	30 mg
Calcium	1200 mg
Folic acid	800 µg
Cyanocobalamin	1–2 µg
Vitamin A	2000 units
Vitamin D	300 units
Vitamin C	40 mg

where its prevalence is very high (up to 80 per cent). Even women with normal haemoglobin but with low iron stores can have excessive tiredness and feel unwell during pregnancy. When given iron supplementation, they experience a dramatic improvement in well-being, and start feeling much better and more energetic owing to the improvement in various iron-dependent enzymes in the body. All types of anaemia-like nutritional deficiency (iron, folate, cyanocobalamin), haemoglobinopathies, and anaemias of chronic disease and inflammation cause tiredness and malaise. For further details, see Anaemia in pregnancy.

Infections and infestations

Various infections (bacterial, viral and others) and infestations (worm) are common and an important cause of tiredness in pregnancy, especially in developing countries (see Box 1). The attending doctors should be aware of this and must take a careful history, perform a detailed examination and investigate properly for appropriate management.

Upper respiratory tract infections

These are common causes of morbidity during pregnancy throughout the world, including the developed nations. In cold countries, flu (viral infection) is common and can happen during pregnancy causing tiredness, fever and malaise. The management is symptomatic by paracetamol, and adequate nutrition and hydration. The management of other respiratory infections, e.g. bronchitis and pharyngitis, is by use of antibiotics, such as erythromycin or azithromycin, and paracetamol with or without cough suppressants. Steam inhalation is useful as an adjunctive therapy.

Urinary tract infections

Urinary tract infections (UTIs) are common during pregnancy owing to the short urethra in women, the proximity of the anus, stasis of urine due to progestogens during pregnancy and compression of the bladder by the enlarging uterus. UTIs present as a burning sensation and frequency of micturition, and are easy to diagnose. However, many women may not have typical symptoms during pregnancy. These may manifest instead as tiredness and other vague symptoms, such as feeling unwell and pain in the abdomen, especially if recurrent. A very high index of suspicion is required on the part of the attending doctor to diagnose and treat UTIs at an early stage, as untreated UTI can cause serious pyelonephritis, intrauterine growth restriction, intrauterine death and preterm labour. The treatment depends upon the culture and sensitivity report, which should always be done on a mid-stream urine specimen.

Genital infections

These are uncommon during pregnancy but can cause tiredness, fever and abdominal and pelvic pain. Pelvic inflammatory disease is usually due to *Chlamydia trachomatis* infection, but can be due to gonorrhoea, *Mycoplasma* or other microorganisms. Treatment is with erythromycin or azithromycin. Tetracycline and doxycycline are contraindicated in pregnancy. Lower genital infections, such as trichomonal and candidal vaginitis, and bacterial vaginosis, usually present as itching with vaginal discharge and have no systematic effects, but rarely may cause tiredness. They can be easily treated using clotrimazole or metronidazole.

Malaria

Malaria is a rare infection in Western countries, but is rampant in many developing countries in Asia and Africa, especially in tribal and rural areas where mosquitoes are in abundance. It causes high-grade remittent fever with rigor and chills with body aches and tiredness. *Falciparum* malaria is particularly hazardous, and can cause abortions, intrauterine growth restriction, intrauterine death and preterm labour. Diagnosis is by peripheral blood film for malaria parasites, and treatment is with chloroquine and other malaricidal drugs.

Typhoid and other intestinal infections

Typhoid is an important cause of fever and morbidity in developing countries. Diagnosis is by blood culture and the Widal test. Treatment is with cephalosporins (cefuroxime) depending upon the culture sensitivity report. Other intestinal infections can present as diarrhoea, fever, pain in the abdomen and tiredness. Oral rehydration therapy with or without antibiotics is required, as the infection often settles down with time.

Hepatitis infections

These are important causes of maternal morbidity in certain geographic areas, such as Asia and Africa, where the prevalence of hepatitis A, B, C and E is high. Hepatitis can be made worse by pregnancy, and some patients can present with jaundice and hepatic coma, which has very high mortality. Mild cases can manifest as tiredness and other vague symptoms; a high index of suspicion is required for timely diagnosis and management. Details of liver disorders during pregnancy are given in Jaundice and liver disease in pregnancy.

Tuberculosis

Tuberculosis can be pulmonary (more common) or extrapulmonary. It is an important and common disease in developing countries in Asia and Africa, but is becoming more common in Western countries owing to infection with the human immunodeficiency virus. It presents with fever, anorexia, loss of weight and cough with expectoration not responding to routine antibiotics. Diagnosis is by sputum examination for acid-fast bacilli on three consecutive days. Treatment is with antituberculous therapy with isoniazid, rifampicin, pyrazinamide and ethambutol, which should be continued in pregnancy for optimum maternal and fetal outcome. As most of these women are anaemic and hypoproteinemic, adequate protein, calories and iron therapy should supplement the antituberculous therapy.

Parasitic infestations

Amoebiasis, giardiasis, hookworm and other worm infestations are rare in Western countries, but are still rampant in developing countries. They are an important cause of malnutrition, anaemia and tiredness during pregnancy in these countries. Diagnosis is by stool examination for ova and cysts on three consecutive days. Treatment is with metronidazole (for amoebiasis and giardiasis) and mebendazole or albendazole (single dose), which can be given safely in the second and third trimester of pregnancy.

Endocrinological causes

Diabetes mellitus

Rarely, diabetes can manifest as tiredness during pregnancy. In the early stages, the typical symptoms – polyuria, polydipsia and polyphagia – may not be apparent. The diagnosis of diabetes should always be kept in mind. Fortunately, most units screen for diabetes in their antenatal protocol, where most patients with high blood sugar are picked up and treated. The details of diabetes in pregnancy are given in Glycosuria in pregnancy.

Thyroid disorders during pregnancy

A severe degree of hypothyroidism often causes infertility and is unlikely to be associated with pregnancy. Thyroid disorders, especially mild to moderate hypothyroidism, are important causes of tiredness during pregnancy, especially in certain geographic areas where iodine deficiency is common. There may be a past history of hypothyroidism before pregnancy in which case the diagnosis is not difficult to make. However, many patients manifest symptoms of hypothyroidism for the first time during pregnancy, making diagnosis difficult and delayed. The attending doctors must keep hypothyroidism in mind in all pregnant women who present with tiredness, feeling unwell, feeling cold and having a lack of energy.

Hyperparathyroidism

Hyperparathyroidism is very rare in pregnancy, but can cause generalised weakness and hyperemesis with renal stones and psychiatric disorders. It needs surgical removal of the parathyroid adenoma.

Adrenal disorders

These disorders are very rare in pregnancy with many patients being infertile. However, mild disorders can be associated with pregnancy and their diagnosis may be missed. Adrenal insufficiency can cause weakness and fatigue. Diagnosis is by blood cortisol levels and treatment is with corticosteroids (hydrocortisone). Cushing's syndrome is excessive production of corticosteroids and can cause tiredness. It needs treatment of the basic condition, such as adrenalectomy.

Systemic diseases

Various systemic diseases, although rarely, can manifest in pregnancy as tiredness, fever and other general symptoms, such as anorexia and weight loss. The attending doctors should always keep a high index of suspicion of these conditions to avoid missing the diagnosis and delaying treatment.

Heart disease

Rheumatic heart disease is very rare in Western countries owing to the more liberal use of antibiotics, but continues to be a major health problem in developing countries. Mitral stenosis is the commonest lesion and can cause severe morbidity and mortality in pregnancy. Many patients conceive after mitral valve replacement and are on anticoagulation therapy. Patients with heart disease present with tiredness, weakness, palpitations and breathlessness in pregnancy. Further details on breathlessness are given in Breathlessness in pregnancy: cardiac causes.

Even patients with congenital heart disease are now venturing into pregnancy after surgical correction of their heart lesion. These patients are at high risk and must be handled in consultation with a dedicated cardiologist, as morbidity and mortality can be very high.

Respiratory diseases (asthma, bronchitis, bronchiectasis)

Asthma is common in the general population and can be associated with pregnancy; it can present as a cough, dyspnoea and tiredness. Treatment is the same as for the non-pregnant state using salbutamol and steroid inhalers. Bronchitis and bronchiectasis and other respiratory diseases are rare, and present with serious illness and tiredness and need treatment in consultation with a chest physician. Further details on breathlessness are given in Breathlessness in pregnancy: respiratory causes.

Rheumatoid arthritis

Rheumatoid arthritis can be associated with pregnancy, causing symptoms of arthritis and tiredness that require medical treatment in consultation with a physician.

Systemic lupus erythematosus and other collagen disorders

Collagen disorders can rarely be associated with pregnancy, causing generalised symptoms of systemic lupus erythematosus, and can lead to abortions, intrauterine growth restriction and intrauterine death. They can be treated with steroids and other specific medicines in consultation with a physician.

Neuromuscular diseases

Various neuromuscular disorders, such as multiple sclerosis and myasthenia gravis, can be associated with pregnancy, causing generalised neuromuscular symptoms and tiredness. They require treatment in consultation with a physician.

Malignancies

Leukaemia, lymphoma, and gynaecological (ovarian, cervical) and other malignancies can very rarely be associated with pregnancy. They can manifest as tiredness, generalised weakness, spongy and bleeding gums, lymph adenopathy, vaginal bleeding and abdominal mass, depending upon the site of malignancy. They need specific surgical and oncological treatment in consultation with a medical oncologist and radiation oncologist, depending on the site of cancer, the gestation of the fetus and maternal expectations.

Miscellaneous conditions
Chronic fatigue syndrome

This is a rare condition during pregnancy, which can present as severe tiredness. It is a syndrome in which patient feels very weak and tired, and usually follows viral illnesses, such as infections with Epstein–Barr virus, Coxsackie virus, cytomegalovirus and other viral infections. The cardinal symptom is fatigue with poor concentration, poor memory, irritability and neuraesthenia. Treatment is by treating the viral infection, general treatment including paracetamol, proper hydration and nutrition, and psychological and psychiatric therapy, usually in consultation with a physician.

Hyperemesis gravidarum

Slight nausea and vomiting are common in pregnancy, but excessive vomiting (hyperemesis) can present as tiredness along with dehydration and weakness, necessitating intravenous hydration and antiemetic therapy. Further details can be seen in Vomiting in pregnancy.

Pre-eclampsia and other pregnancy disorders

Pre-eclampsia presents after 20 weeks of pregnancy with hypertension and proteinuria, and is a cause of significant morbidity and mortality both in the mother and the fetus. It can present as tiredness. The treatment is with antihypertensive drugs, with or without magnesium sulphate, depending upon the severity of hypertension and gestation of the fetus. Further details are given in Blood pressure problems in pregnancy.

■ Conclusion

Tiredness in pregnancy is not an isolated condition, but can be a manifestation of various disorders during pregnancy. It requires careful history-taking and examination, detailed investigations and appropriate treatment of the underlying condition, often in consultation with other specialists for optimum management.

Key points:

1 Tiredness is a common problem in pregnancy and can be physiological.
2 There can be a variety of causes for tiredness, which include anaemia and other nutritional disorders, infections and infestations, diabetes mellitus and other endocrine diseases, systemic diseases, malignancies and miscellaneous causes.
3 The attending doctor must take a detailed history of the patient, should perform a thorough clinical examination and should investigate the patient properly to reach an accurate diagnosis.
4 The management is dependent upon the cause, often in consultation with specialists of other disciplines.
5 General treatment includes adequate nutrition, hydration and symptomatic therapy.

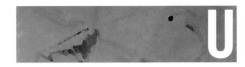

URINARY RETENTION

James Green

Urinary retention is the lack of the ability to urinate. It can occur in the following situations:

- the detrusor muscle in the bladder wall is unable to contract effectively;
- the bladder outlet fails to relax sufficiently;
- contraction of the detrusor and relaxation of the sphincter are uncoordinated, e.g. detrusor sphincter dyssynergia.

The causes for these situations can be divided into two main groups, neurogenic and non-neurogenic.

■ Non-neurogenic causes of urinary retention

There are many non-neurological conditions that should be considered as a cause for urinary retention (see Box 1). These range from obstruction to failure of the ageing detrusor muscle (myopathy).

■ Neurogenic causes of urinary retention

More unusual causes for urinary retention involve the nervous system. In general, the anatomical level of the neurological injury determines the functional effect on the urinary system (Box 2). Spinal lesions may result in dyssynergia, an uncoordinated muscle contraction (see detrusor sphincter dyssynergia above), whereas sacral, cauda equina or other peripheral nerve injuries may produce detrusor areflexia or absence of reflex. However, the situation is often more complex than this as multiple or incomplete injuries can produce mixed patterns. Consequently, the functional result of the injury can often only be

Box 1 Non-neurogenic causes of urinary retention

Obstructive
- Urethral stenosis
- Urethral oedema
- Foreign body (including calculus)
- Post stress incontinence surgery (including sling and injectables)
- Prolapse
- Pelvic mass, e.g. haematocolpos, extroverted gravid uterus, uterine fibroid, ureterocoele, benign and malignant tumours, faecal impaction

Post surgery
- Overdistension leading to detrusor muscle injury

Inflammatory
- Urethritis (infective and chemical)
- Vulvovaginitis (including Herpes)
- Allergy
- Anogenital infection

Pharmacological
- Anticholinergic agents
- Epidural and spinal anaesthetics
- Ganglion-blocking agents
- Alpha-adrenergic agents
- Tricyclic antidepressants

Endocrine
- Hypothyroidism

Other causes
- Iatrogenic
- Urethral sphincter dysfunction/hypertrophy (Fowler)
- Detrusor myopathy
- Psychogenic

Box 2 Neurogenic causes of urinary retention

Conditions affecting the brain
- Cerebrovascular accident
- Parkinson's disease

Conditions affecting the spinal cord
- Spinal cord injury
- Multiple sclerosis
- Intervertebral disc disease (central)
- Ankylosing spondylitis
- Guillain–Barré syndrome
- Tabes dorsalis
- Acquired immunodeficiency syndrome (AIDS)
- Lyme disease
- Tropical spastic paraparesis
- Transverse myelitis
- Herpes zoster
- Poliomyelitis
- Tethered cord syndrome, short filum terminale, spinal dysraphism

Conditions affecting the peripheral nervous system
- Diabetic neuropathy
- Pelvis plexus injury, e.g. after abdominoperineal resection, hysterectomy

determined by video cystometrogram. This has the added bonus of allowing the measurement of the estimated pressure generated by the detrusor muscle during filling and micturition phases. This is important because, if the urinary system is exposed to an abnormally high functioning pressure, then this can damage the upper urinary tract, leading to renal dysfunction and subsequent renal failure.

■ Diagnosis

Urinary retention can be diagnosed clinically or by ultrasound scanning. To identify the cause of retention, a detailed clinical history should be obtained and a clinical examination performed, including the nervous system if a neurological cause is suspected. Infection should be identified by urine culture and serum analysis. Renal dysfunction, although rarer in women, should be excluded.

■ Treatment

The best treatment is to avoid precipitating causes in the first place. Classic examples of this include avoiding faecal impaction or overdistension after surgery.

Once retention has occurred, decompression via a urinary catheter is indicated. An obstructed urinary system that is infected should be treated as an emergency, as septicaemia can result. If the obstructed lower urinary tract has resulted in renal dysfunction, an exact measurement of fluid input and urine output is undertaken to exclude a post obstructive renal diuresis. If the urine output is excessive after catheterisation (i.e. >200 mL/ hour), intravenous fluids (normal saline) should be commenced to stop dehydration occurring, by initially balancing fluid input against the measured output.

In the majority of patients with normal renal function and no urinary infection present, clean intermittent self-catheterisation is the method of choice, providing manual dexterity is adequate. The frequency of catheterisation should be tailored to the individual's bladder capacity. The aim is to avoid overflow incontinence and urinary stasis leading to potential urinary tract infection.

Some conditions, such as overdistension injury to the detrusor muscle, will often recover in a few days, but detrusor areflexia due to incomplete pelvic plexus injury after major pelvic surgery often takes at least 6 weeks to resolve.

Pharmacotherapy, in the form of cholinergics and prostaglandins (PGs), e.g. Bethanechol and PGE2, respectively, occasionally has beneficial results on the detrusor muscle. Surgery has a place in specific patient groups. If urethral stenosis exists, then urethral dilatation can be helpful. Neuromodulation of the S3 nerve root via the S3 foramen has had success in specialist centres in patients with sphincter hypertrophy.

UTERINE SWELLINGS

Karina Reynolds and Nicola Fattizzi

The main function of the uterus (womb) is to contain a developing pregnancy. Its anatomy is, therefore, adapted to fulfil this function and it comprises a cavity encased by involuntary muscle fibres. These are arranged in a herringbone pattern allowing expansion and contraction. When contracting, the fibres act as living ligatures, constricting the blood vessels to the cavity. The uterus is covered by peritoneum and lined by a glandular epithelium, which allows implantation of a fertilised egg.

Swellings of the uterus can be divided into:

■ those that are pregnancy related;
■ those that are non-pregnancy related or anatomically related.

These can essentially be considered benign or malignant, the latter usually being primary tumours, although secondary uterine malignancies do occasionally occur.

■ Pregnancy-related uterine swellings

Normal pregnancy

The most common cause of uterine swelling is pregnancy and this must always be considered during the reproductive years, particularly when associated with a history of amenorrhoea or menstrual upset. The size is dependent on the gestational age, but will usually become palpable abdominally from 12 weeks' gestation.

Molar changes

Gestational trophoblastic disease covers a spectrum of diseases including complete and partial hydatidiform mole, placental-site trophoblastic tumour and choriocarcinoma. The presenting symptoms may include first trimester bleeding, hyperemesis gravidarum or pressure symptoms from a uterus that is large for dates. An excessive amount of beta-human chorionic gonadotrophin (βHCG) is produced providing a 'tumour marker' to monitor regression/progression. Hydatidiform mole precedes choriocarcinoma in 50 per cent of cases. This condition is highly chemosensitive and, when managed appropriately, has an excellent prognosis even in the presence of metastatic disease.

Diagnostic investigations for gestational trophoblastic disease include ultrasound, which shows a typical snowstorm appearance (Fig. 1), and raised urinary/serum levels of βHCG.

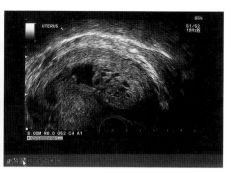

Figure 1 Ultrasound scan of hydatidiform mole showing typical snowstorm appearance.

Clot retention

This can occur following spontaneous miscarriage, termination of pregnancy or delivery, and is due to inadequate uterine contraction that does not cut off the blood supply to the placental bed in the uterine cavity. Bleeding may persist and be either revealed or concealed. Evacuation of the uterus may be required.

Retained products of conception

These are discussed under Bleeding during early pregnancy and Collapse in the puerperium.

■ Non-pregnancy-related uterine swellings

Uterine swellings have varying implications, depending on the age of presentation. The diagnosis is usually made on history and physical examination. Ultrasound scanning is the main imaging modality, although magnetic resonance imaging (MRI) is proving useful in defining the extent of surgery required for management of endometrial malignancies. Hysteroscopy and endometrial sampling are considered when patients present with abnormal vaginal bleeding.

Benign
Müllerian malformations

Adolescent girls, unlike women in other age groups, may present with a uterine mass that is secondary to a Müllerian malformation, such as imperforate hymen, vaginal agenesis with a normal uterus and functioning endometrium, vaginal duplication with obstructing longitudinal septa, and obstructed uterine horns. Cases of outflow obstruction remain asymptomatic until after the menarche. The uterine mass is due to the development of a haematometra (uterus distended with blood) and/or a haematocolpos (vagina distended with blood) owing to accumulating menstrual loss. A frequent presentation of genital obstruction is primary amenorrhoea with normal secondary sexual characteristics plus cyclical abdominal pain. Genital tract abnormalities in general may also present with severe dysmenorrhoea, dyspareunia, infertility, recurrent miscarriage, ectopic pregnancy and obstetric complications if pregnancy occurs.

Investigation of Müllerian anomalies may include assessment of both the internal and external uterine contours with ultrasound and often MRI. Hysterosalpingography, hysteroscopy and even laparoscopy may need to be performed.

In adolescents, pregnancy should always be considered as a cause of uterine mass unlike uterine leiomyomas, which are uncommon in women under 30 years of age, although the youngest patient on record was 13 years old.

Physical examination, pelvic ultrasound and serum βHCG levels clinch the diagnosis if there is any doubt. As in all age groups, the primary diagnostic technique for the assessment of uterine swellings is ultrasonography, followed, if inconclusive, by computerised tomography of the abdomen/pelvis and/or MRI of the pelvis.

Fibroids

Once pregnancy has been excluded in the reproductive age group, the next most common cause of uterine swelling is the presence of fibroids (leiomyomas; Figs 2 and 3). These are the most common form of benign neoplasia of the genital tract. They occur most frequently in middle-aged women of Afro–Caribbean origin and their behaviour is affected by hormonal production, as they have both oestrogen and progesterone receptors. They increase in size during pregnancy and with administration of oestrogen and

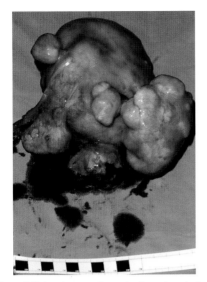

Figure 2 Hysterectomy specimen showing enlarged uterus due to fibroids.

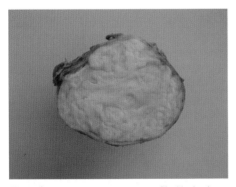

Figure 3 Transverse section across a fibroid showing a whorled appearance.

shrink if gonadotrophin-releasing hormone analogues are given. They present as a spherical nodule characteristically firm to the touch and frequently these are multiple. Their dimensions can range from a few millimetres to several centimetres and they are usually present in the main body of the uterus, occasionally occurring in the cervix or the broad ligament.

The clinical features depend on the size, location and number of the lesions. The most common symptoms and signs include:

- pain;
- awareness of a pelvic/abdominal mass;
- a sensation of pressure;
- abnormal uterine bleeding owing to the increased surface area of overlying endometrium.

Leiomyomas can be divided into four categories based on their position in the myometrium (Fig. 4).

- *Intramural leiomyomas* are the most common and, when large, may modify the uterine outline resulting in a large irregular mass. This type of myoma can give rise to menstrual problems and to complications of pregnancy.
- *Submucosal leiomyomas* can cause bleeding, even when small, secondary to compression of the overlying endometrium and compromise of its vascular supply. As they become larger, they may bulge into the endometrial cavity and increase the surface area of the endometrium. Fertility may be affected. Complications of pregnancy can also occur, including spontaneous abortion, premature rupture of the membranes, dystocia, inversion of the uterus and postpartum haemorrhage. Rarely this kind of myoma can become pedunculated and prolapse through the cervix.
- *Subserosal leiomyomas* develop beneath the peritoneum that covers the external surface of the uterus, and are either sessile or pedunculated. The latter may undergo torsion, infection and even separation from the uterus itself. When separation occurs, attachment to another pelvic structure is possible and results in a 'parasitic leiomyoma'.
- *Intraligamentous leiomyomas* are so called because they develop between the anterior and posterior peritoneal leaves of the broad ligament. These myomas can compress adjacent organs, resulting in intestinal and urinary symptoms. Constipation up to and including bowel obstruction, urinary frequency, urge incontinence, urinary retention and possibly ureteric obstruction may also occur.

All types of myoma can undergo degenerative change. Submucosal myomas are frequently ulcerated and haemorrhagic. Necrosis and haemorrhage can also be found in large fibroids associated with pregnancy or the administration of high-dose progestin therapy. Cystic degeneration occurs and leiomyomas often become extensively

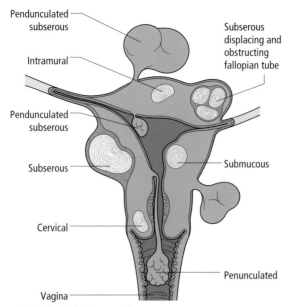

Pendunculated subserous

Intramural

Pendunculated subserous

Subserous

Cervical

Vagina

Subserous displacing and obstructing fallopian tube

Submucous

Penunculated

Figure 4 Diagram of the position of fibroids in the myometrium.

calcified as identified on plain abdominal X-ray. Malignant change of fibroids is reported to occur in 0.1 per cent of cases. Confirmation of diagnosis is generally straightforward with physical examination and pelvic ultrasonography.

Adenomyomas (circumscribed nodular aggregates of smooth muscle, endometrial glands and endometrial stroma, located within the myometrium) can mimic uterine leiomyomas. Adenomyosis is a condition characterised by the presence of endometrial glands and stroma within the endometrium, and can result in a bulky uterus that is tender on bimanual examination. These conditions (adenomyosis and adenomyomas) may be difficult to differentiate from leiomyomas clinically, but ultrasound and MRI are useful in making the diagnosis pre-operatively. The final diagnosis is made on histology.

Other benign causes.

Among the infective causes of uterine swelling, tuberculous endometritis deserves mention. It is secondary to a systemic infection by *Mycobacterium tuberculosis*, generally presenting in women of reproductive age. The endometrium

is the second most commonly infected site in the female genital tract after the Fallopian tubes. Infection develops by haematogenous spread from a primary focus in the lungs or gastrointestinal tract, and uterine infection is usually by direct transmission from the Fallopian tubes. Presentation is usually with lower abdominal pain and an associated uterine mass. However, this infection may mimic ovarian malignancy.

In older women, cervical stenosis secondary to atrophy may occur. This is usually asymptomatic but may result in a distended uterine cavity on imaging. In this age group, the presence of a haematometra (cavity containing blood) or pyometra (cavity containing pus) requires further investigation (usually dilatation of the cervix, drainage and cervical/endometrial biopsy), as the presence of a malignancy must be excluded. In these cases, the distended uterus may present with pain and may be palpable on physical examination.

Cervical stenosis may occur in younger patients. Causes include cervical scarring secondary to trauma (lacerations following parturition or abortion), surgery (cone biopsy, cryotherapy, cervical cauterization) and radiotherapy for primary cervical cancer.

Benign endometrial polyps may also result in an enlarged uterus and should be included in this section (Fig. 5).

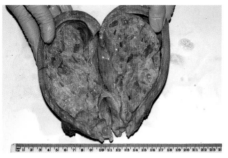

Figure 5 Benign asymptomatic polyp presenting as a pelvic mass.

Malignant (primary and secondary)

Endometrial malignancy frequently results in uterine swelling. The most common primary tumour of the uterus is a carcinoma and overall the prognosis is excellent (Fig. 6). However, uterine sarcoma also occurs and has a less favourable prognosis. The commonest carcinoma is endometrioid but serous carcinomas comprise approximately 10 per cent of all adenocarcinomas. However, the latter accounts for 50 per cent of recurrences and has a poor prognosis similar to high-grade endometrioid cases. Uterine sarcomas, including leiomyosarcomas, endometrial stromal sarcomas and carcinosarcomas (or mixed Müllerian tumours) are more

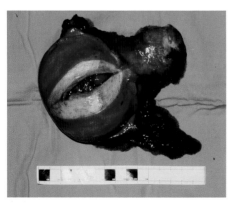

Figure 6 Hysterectomy specimen showing an endometrial cancer.

likely than endometrial carcinoma to give rise to a large mass. In sarcomatous cases, the tumours often fill the uterine cavity and may prolapse through the cervical os.

Uterine malignancy usually presents with abnormal uterine bleeding most commonly in postmenopausal women. Lower abdominal pain or discomfort may also occur. Investigations include endometrial thickness assessment on ultrasound and endometrial biopsy/cytology. Hysteroscopically directed biopsy may be required and the hysteroscopy provides further information on tumour size and location. Ultrasound may provide information on the depth of invasion to assist surgical planning, as can MRI (Fig. 7). The latter can also assess pelvic and para-aortic nodal status.

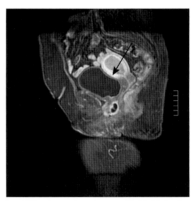

Figure 7 Magnetic resonance image of the pelvis showing an endometrial cancer infiltrating the myometrium.

The cornerstone of treatment is total hysterectomy and bilateral salpingoophorectomy. The role of more extensive surgery and of adjuvant treatment is controversial, and the subject of multicentre randomised controlled trials.

Secondary malignancies of the uterus are less common than primary uterine tumours. The commonest sources of metastatic disease at this site include direct extension from cervical malignancies and, less commonly, other genital tract cancer primaries. Haematogenous spread from the breast and involvement due to lymphoma are also high on the list.

VAGINAL DISCHARGE

Tony Hollingworth

Discharge from the vagina can be classified in the following way:

- physiological, which varies with age and the time of the menstrual cycle;
- pathological
  - pre-pubertal
  - during reproductive age
  - postmenopausal.

■ Physiological discharge

The normal discharge from the vagina is a mixture of secretions from the uterine body, the cervix and the vaginal wall, the bulk of which originates from the cervix as there are more glands there than in any other part of the genital tract. There are no glands in the vagina and, as such, is not mucosa but skin (non-keratinized stratified squamous epithelium).

The secretions vary throughout the menstrual cycle, being abundant, clear and almost free from leucocytes at the time of ovulation. At this time, the elasticity of the secretions is at its greatest (Spinnbarkeit), which allows easier penetration by the spermatozoa. At other times of the month, the cervical mucus is scanty, opaque and tenacious. The secretion from Bartholin's gland, which is thin and mucoid, may be copious under sexual excitement, but under normal conditions it is scanty, and so does not contribute significantly to vaginal discharge.

The vaginal mixed secretion is acid in reaction, owing to the presence of lactic acid produced by the action of Doderlein's bacillus on the glycogen in the basal cells of the vaginal epithelium. This bacillus is normally found in the vagina from puberty to the menopause. The pH of the vagina is 4.5, the vaginal acidity being a bar to vaginal infection; unmixed uterine secretion is alkaline.

Normally, the amount of mixed vaginal discharge should do no more than just moisten the vaginal orifice; however, it may be increased with the presence of an ectropion, where there is eversion of the columnar epithelium towards the vagina (Fig. 1). Ectropion is more common in the reproductive age group, with oral contraceptive usage and after delivery. If excessive, the ectropion may require cautery or cryotherapy. Girls before puberty and women after the menopause do not have the protection of an acid secretion in the vagina.

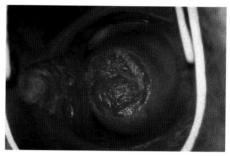

Figure 1 Cervical ectropion.

In pregnancy, the physiological white discharge usually increases owing to the increased shedding of epithelial cells and an increased vascularity of the cervix, which in turn leads to an increase in secretion production.

■ Pathological discharge

Pre-pubertal

The main causes of discharge in a pre-pubertal girl include:

- poor hygiene;
- foreign body;
- threadworms;
- sexual abuse;
- sarcoma botryoides.

In young girls presenting with vaginal discharge, the most common diagnosis is a foreign body that may necessitate ultrasound scanning or an examination under anaesthetic (EUA).

At the time of EUA, a small hysteroscope can be inserted into the vagina, and the irrigating fluid used may flush the foreign body out and so treat the problem. Poor hygiene again is not uncommon and appropriate advice should be given to the mother. Threadworms may give intense itching, especially at night. One needs to be cautious if sexual abuse is considered and the paediatric lead for child protection should be consulted. Each hospital in the UK should now have a named professional for child protection following the recent Climbié report.[1] Sarcoma botryoides is a rare tumour that may present with discharge or bleeding in young girls and would need referral to a cancer centre for further management.

Reproductive age

Vaginal discharge in women of reproductive age is most likely to be caused by infection. However, cervical polyps and malignancy may present with excess discharge or mucus production, and these conditions will be covered in the relevant chapters. The common causes of vaginal discharge to be discussed include:

- *Candida*;
- trichomoniasis;
- gonorrhoea;
- *Chlamydia*;
- pelvic inflammatory disease;
- bacterial vaginosis;
- retained tampon.

In all cases, a relevant history should be obtained followed by any appropriate physical examination plus a vaginal speculum examination in order to take the relevant swabs, as discussed below.

Candida

This is a common infection in women and gives rise to characteristic white patches of thrush on the vagina walls and cervix (Fig. 2). It causes itching, discomfort and redness. It can occur as a complication of diabetes, during pregnancy, following the use of antibiotics and also in women using the combined oral contraceptive

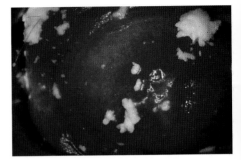

Figure 2 Vaginal Candida.

pill. A swab may be taken for recognition of the mycelium and spores of *Candida albicans* in stained smears and for culture. Treatment may be topical or systemic azoles, e.g. econazole and fluconazole.

Trichomonas vaginalis

This flagellate parasite produces a frothy purulent discharge causing local pain and soreness that is extremely irritating to the external genitalia (Fig. 3). The discharge is green or greenish yellow with small bubbles of gas and has a characteristic odour. The protozoon can be identified on microscopy. *Trichomonas* lives in the vagina in symbiosis with the micrococcus *Aerogenes alcaligenes*, which forms the froth or bubbles so characteristic of the discharge. It is a Gram-negative organism and causes the vaginal walls to have a typical red-stippled (strawberry) appearance). Treatment is with metronidazole and should also include the partner.

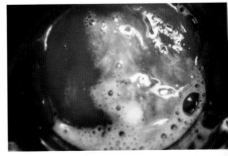

Figure 3 Trichomonal infection of the cervix.

Neisseria gonorrhoeae

Gonorrhoea causes the cervix to be red, swollen and oedematous, being bathed in pus (Fig. 4). There is nothing characteristic of gonorrhoeal discharge visible to the naked eye. The detection of the gonococcus can alone decide the diagnosis. This is often a matter of difficulty because it is only in the few days immediately after infection that the organism can be found in the discharge. In chronic cases, the gonococcus must be looked for in one of three places–in the endocervical canal, in the urethra or in discharge squeezed from the orifices of Bartholin's glands. Gram's method stains the discharge and the organisms are Gram-negative diplococci. Appropriate treatment may be given in the form of spectinomycin depending on the organism's sensitivity, which may vary from one locality to the next. Contact tracing via the local sexually transmitted diseases service is essential.

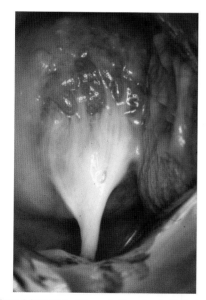

Figure 4 Gonorrhoea of the cervix. Reproduced with kind permission from Peter Greenhouse.

Bacterial vaginosis

This is characterised by a copious whitish discharge, which may be offensive or have a fishy smell (Fig. 5), and is caused by *Gardnerella*, *Mycoplasma* and anaerobes. The vaginal pH is

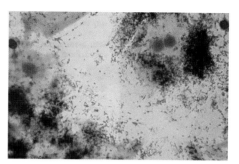

Figure 5 Slide showing 'clue cells' diagnostic of bacterial vaginosis.

>5 and the vagina is not inflamed. Diagnosis can be made using the amine test, in which some of the discharge is placed on a slide and potassium hydroxide is added to it; a typical fishy odour confirms the diagnosis. Treatment involves either metronidazole or local clindamycin cream.

Chlamydia trachomatis

This is an obligate intracellular parasite, which lives in the columnar cells in the endocervical canal (Fig. 6). It may cause discharge, or may be asymptomatic and only detected on screening for fertility problems or prior to a termination

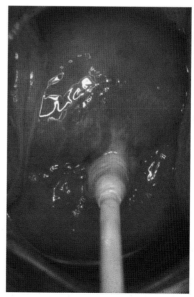

Figure 6 *Chlamydia trachomatis* infection of the cervix. Reproduced with kind permission from Peter Greenhouse.

of pregnancy. An endocervical swab is needed for culture. Treatment involves doxycycline, which should also include the partner plus referral to a Genito-Urinary Medicine clinic.

Pelvic inflammatory disease

This condition presents with bilateral lower abdominal pain, discharge, low-grade pyrexia, tachycardia, bilateral adnexal tenderness and cervical excitation. These women will have a history of sexual activity. The organisms involved include *Chlamydia trachomatis, Neisseria gonorrhoeae, Mycoplasma hominis* and anaerobes. It is treated with broad-spectrum antibiotics, including doxycycline and metronidazole. Effective treatment on the first occasion is important, as successive bouts of pelvic inflammatory disease (PID) may lead to infertility, tubal pregnancy, chronic lower abdominal pain and menstrual problems. Local protocols should be available that will take into account the severity of the symptoms and local antibiotic sensitivities.

It is important to emphasize, once again, that contact tracing of a partner should ideally be undertaken for *Chlamydia*, gonorrhoea and PID.

Retained tampons/foreign bodies

Any retained foreign body will start to cause discharge, which may be offensive after 24 hours. Removal will result in the discharge settling very quickly. If the woman needs a ring pessary to be inserted for prolapse, then it should be changed regularly otherwise discharge may develop.

Postmenopausal

There are essentially two diagnoses:

- atrophic changes; and
- malignancy.

In postmenopausal women, the amount of vaginal discharge produced is reduced, unless they are receiving hormone replacement therapy, and the squamocolumnar junction retreats along the endocervical canal. If the woman develops vaginal discharge, especially if it is offensive in nature, then a malignancy needs to be excluded. She is extremely unlikely to have the infections that occur during reproductive age, with the exception of *Candida*. One would need to exclude either an endometrial or cervical lesion.

In elderly women, a foul discharge may originate from the uterine cavity – a pyometra. The pus can be released by dilating the cervical os, which will usually require a general anaesthetic. It is usually due to senile endometritis, although it can be associated with carcinoma of the uterine body or cervix.

Fistulae may develop as a late manifestation of malignant disease, although this is not common. They can also occur in bowel tumours, Crohn's disease or after radiotherapy.

The majority of the postmenopausal women will have atrophic changes but usually present with postmenopausal bleeding rather than discharge.

■ Reference

The Victoria Climbié Inquiry, by Lord Laming. London: HMSO, 2003.

VAGINAL SWELLINGS

Tony Hollingworth

Generalised swelling and oedema within the vagina may occur due to infection, which may be primary (e.g. *Candida*) or secondary (e.g. infected herpetic lesions). Condylomata (warts) may occur with a frond-like surface. Biopsy may be useful before instituting treatment. Otherwise there are few structures that present as swellings within the vagina. If they do occur, then they may be incidental findings during pregnancy or when taking a cervical smear. They may cause discomfort on intercourse or tampon insertion, or may be found on self-examination. Patients may present with a lump in the vagina; the vast majority will be due to some form of prolapse (see Prolapse of uterus and vagina).

■ Benign swellings

Simple mesonephric (Gartner's) or *paramesonephric cysts* may be seen high up in the vagina in the fornices. They are embryological remnants, which have failed to be obliterated

They may be small, asymptomatic and found incidentally on vaginal examination. Occasionally, they can grow and give some degree of dyspareunia. The characteristic position and cystic 'feel' serve to differentiate them from the various types of vaginal prolapse (Fig. 1). They can be treated by excision or marsupialisation, if necessary.

Small implantation cysts may be seen at the vaginal orifice posteriorly. They are small and may

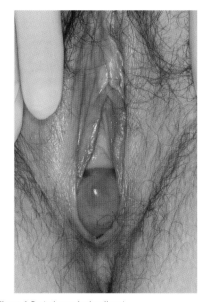

Figure 1 Posterior vaginal wall cyst.

follow operations on the perineum, or lacerations at childbirth. They may cause dyspareunia and occasionally the scarring from removal means that there is no improvement of the symptoms.

Occasionally, an *endometrioma* may burrow through into the posterior vaginal fornix from the floor of the pouch of Douglas into the rectovaginal septum, forming nodular growths, which tend to bleed at the time of menstruation. This condition may be confused with a primary carcinoma of the vagina, although it is not friable. Biopsy and microscopic examination will confirm the diagnosis. It can also cause dyspareunia and may require surgery to resolve it, in some cases involving a general surgeon.

Benign tumours: sessile and pedunculated swellings arise in the vaginal wall, which on histology are found to be papilloma, fibroma or lipoma. They are uncommon and excision may be necessary if they interfere with intercourse.

■ Malignant swellings

As with any type of malignancy, there is always the possibility of primary or secondary tumours. Primary tumours of the vagina are rare and management needs to be undertaken at a gynaecological cancer centre. By and large the prognosis from these tumours is poor despite radical surgery, radiotherapy and chemotherapy. The types of tumour are as follows.

- *Squamous lesions* – the vast majority, usually occur in the upper vagina.
- *Clear cell carcinomas:* these were thought at one time to be related to exposure to diethylstilboestrol whilst *in utero*;
- *Malignant melanomas:* these may present with bleeding rather than swelling. The prognosis is very poor.
- *Endodermal sinus tumour:* this is a very rare type of adenocarcinoma.
- *Rhabdomyosarcoma* (sarcoma botryoides): this is a rare tumour in girls <5 years, which usually presents as vaginal bleeding. It has a characteristic appearance, like a bunch of grapes, and microscopic section proves its nature.
- *Secondary tumours* usually originate from the local organs, namely the cervix and uterus, although there have been reports of secondaries from primary tumours in the ovary, colon and hypernephroma.

Diagnosis is made by biopsy or excision biopsy, depending on the size of the lesion, followed by magnetic resonance imaging of the pelvis and referral to a Gynaecological Cancer Centre.

VOMITING IN PREGNANCY

Mala Arora

Vomiting and nausea are closely related and mediated by the same neural pathways:

- *vomiting* or *emesis* is forceful expulsion of gastric contents;

- *nausea* is the imminent desire to vomit;
- *retching* is the rhythmic contractions of abdominal and chest musculature that precedes or accompanies vomiting.

These often occur together and may be accompanied by hypersalivation (ptyalism).

Vomiting and nausea are physiological during pregnancy, and are the most common symptoms of early pregnancy second only to amenorrhoea. However, when vomiting starts after the 14th week of pregnancy or is excessive, it may be a manifestation of an underlying disorder. Hence vomiting in pregnancy may be physiological or pathological.

Box 1 Causes of hyperemesis gravidarum

Gastrointestinal

Oesophageal

- Gastro-oesophageal reflux disease
- Hiatus hernia
- Achalasia cardia

Gastric
- Gastritis
- Peptic ulcers due to *Helicobacter pylori*
- Disordered gastrointestinal motility seen in diabetes or idiopathic gastroparesis
- Pyloric stenosis – partial or complete
- Fundoplication for obesity
- Aerophagia syndrome
- Gastric carcinoma[9]

Intestinal
- Enteritis
- Intestinal inflammation as in ulcerative colitis or Crohn's disease
- Intestinal obstruction due to adhesions, hernia, mesenteric lymphadenitis, adenomatous polyps, stricture, volvulus, Hirchsprung's disease
- Food poisoning
  - bacterial due to *Shigella*, *Salmonella*, *Staphylococcus*, *Clostridium*
  - viral due to rotavirus
  - toxins, such as *Clostridium botulinum*
  - allergy to foods, such as eggs, nuts or mushrooms
- Intestinal ischaemia, as in mesenteric vein thrombosis, Henoch–Schönlein purpura

Gastrointestinal accessory gland disease
- Hepatitis viral hepatitis A, B, C, D and E, Epstein–Barr virus, cytomegalovirus, leptospirosis
- Pancreatitis due to a calculus in the common bile duct, viral or alcohol induced
- Gallstones

Pregnancy-related
- Multifetal pregnancy – includes twins, triplets and higher-order births
- Gestational trophoblastic disease – includes hydatidiform mole
- Trisomy 21 (Down's syndrome), hydrops fetalis, triploidies
- Ovarian torsion
- Degenerating fibroids
- Pre-eclampsia
- Obstetric cholestasis
- Acute fatty liver of pregnancy

Acute systemic infections
- For example, chorioamnionitis, and viral infections, such as influenza, encephalitis, meningitis, hepatitis, pancreatitis or generalized peritonitis

Central nervous system
- Raised intracranial tension, as in benign intracranial hypertension, neoplasms, meningitis and encephalitis
- Raised intracranial pressure can sometimes occur with pre-eclampsia and eclampsia owing to cerebral oedema, which can cause vomiting in the third trimester

Middle ear
- Ménière's disease
- Acute viral labyrinthitis
- Migraine
- Motion sickness

Cardiological
- Congestive cardiac failure
- Acute myocardial infarction, especially posterior wall and transmural

Endocrinal
- Diabetic ketoacidosis
- Uraemia
- Hyperthyroidism[10–12]
- Hyperparathyroidism[13]
- Adrenal insufficiency or Addison's disease
- Zollinger–Ellison syndrome

Psychological[14,15]
- Anorexia nervosa
- Bulimia
- Psychological or emotional disturbance

Iatrogenic, medication or drug-induced

Surgical
- Ovarian torsion, degenerating fibroids
- Inflammations, such as appendicitis, diverticulitis, cholecystitis
- Renal and biliary colic
- Intestinal obstruction (refer to section on intestinal causes)

Physiological vomiting

Physiological vomiting of pregnancy has been described by the Egyptians as early as 2000 BC. It is most common in the first trimester and may recur in the third trimester in a milder form. Historically, Fairweather proposed in the 1960s that nausea and vomiting of pregnancy was an allergic reaction to pregnancy,[1] which today would be labelled as an immunological response. However, there has been no substantiation of this theory. There are several reasons proposed for physiological vomiting in the first trimester of pregnancy as outlined below.

- Rising progesterone and beta-human chorionic gonadotrophin (βHCG) levels cause delayed intestinal motility and gastric stasis. Physiological vomiting is exaggerated in cases of multiple pregnancy and hydatidiform mole owing to higher βHCG levels.
- High levels of oestrogen and progesterone, which accompany pregnancy, are potential mediators of gastric slow-wave dysrhythmias in nausea of pregnancy.[2]
- Vitamin B6 deficiency, which occurs owing to a change in protein metabolism in pregnancy, hence vitamin B6 is used for its treatment.
- Relaxation of the gastro-oesophageal sphincter and hyperacidity also contribute.
- Few studies found a correlation between female fetal sex and hyperemesis gravidarum.[3]
- During the third trimester of pregnancy, the gravid uterus can mechanically reduce the distensibility of the stomach as well as change the contour of the cardiac sphincter, leading to an increased incidence of vomiting.

Pathological or hyperemesis gravidarum

If vomiting is excessive, develops or persists after 14 weeks of gestation and leads to dehydration and/or ketosis, it is called hyperemesis gravidarum. It affects 1 in 200 pregnant women.[1,4] If vomiting is sustained over a period of time, it will lead to maternal weight loss, oliguria, hypokalaemic alkalosis and constipation. Fetal intrauterine growth restriction is also reported.

In such cases, a pathological cause should be excluded.

The causes of hyperemesis gravidarum are elaborated in Box 1. In a recent study, chronic infection with *Helicobacter pylori* was present in 61.8 per cent of pregnant patients with hyperemesis in comparison with 27.6 per cent of pregnant patients without hyperemesis.[5] Other studies have confirmed this correlation.[6,7] A recent study from Turkey has shown higher levels of the hormone leptin in 18 patients with hyperemesis compared to an equal number of healthy pregnant women.[8]

Differential diagnosis

Although the potential causes of hyperemesis are many, the most common causes are elaborated below.

Gastrointestinal causes

The most frequently encountered causes in clinical practice are gastrointestinal in nature. Exclusion of *Helicobacter pylori* infection is important. In this infection, vomiting may be spontaneous or self-induced for relief of symptoms, as in peptic ulcer.

Gastroenteritis or food poisoning is common. A variety of pathogens can be involved. The onset of vomiting is abrupt and related to the ingestion of food. Other cases may also be reported after ingestion of the same food. Pre-existing allergies to food products, such as eggs or nuts, can cause intractable vomiting after inadvertent ingestion.

Gallstones may be commonly associated with pregnancy, and can cause both hyperacidity and vomiting. They are easily diagnosed on upper abdominal ultrasound scan. If complicated with cholecystitis, the vomiting will be accompanied with right upper quadrant pain and/or fever.

Inflammation of any part of the gastrointestinal tract will manifest with vomiting. The most common example is acute appendicitis, when vomiting is accompanied with right iliac fossa pain. Diverticulitis and cholecystitis will also present with vomiting. Acute pancreatitis can be precipitated by alcohol or may be a compli-cation of underlying gallstones.

Vomiting may be the first symptom in hepa-titis and can precede the appearance of jaundice by a few days. Liver function tests will show ele-vated liver enzymes and hepatitis markers will clinch the diagnosis.

For the other gastrointestinal causes listed in Box 1, there may be a past history of the disease.

Pregnancy-related causes

Multifetal pregnancy (Fig. 1) and hydatidiform mole cause hyperemesis in the first trimester and are easily diagnosed on a first trimester scan. Degeneration of coexistent fibroids (Fig. 2) with pregnancy will present with vomiting and lower abdominal pain. Ultrasound scans show an increase in size of the fibroid. Management is conservative with rest and analgesics.

Ovarian torsion (Fig. 3) can occur with the presence of dermoid cysts of the ovary that can coexist with pregnancy. There is accompanying lower abdominal pain and tenderness. Ultrasound scan will show the cyst, while Doppler signals of the ovarian vessels will show impaired flow. Management is surgical with laparoscopic untwisting of the cyst, if diagnosed early. In late cases where gangrene has set in, the ovary may have to be sacrificed.

Pre-eclampsia and the HELLP (haemolysis, elevated liver enzymes and low platelets) syn-drome occur in the third trimester of pregnancy and are accompanied with raised blood pres-sure and albuminuria. Vomiting may occur because of raised intracranial tension and/or raised liver enzymes, as in the HELLP syndrome.

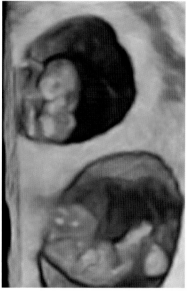

Figure 1 Twin pregnancy on 3-D ultrasound scan.

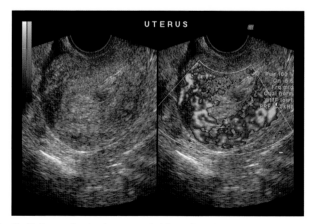

Figure 2 Degenerating fibroid. No vascular signals are present at the centre.

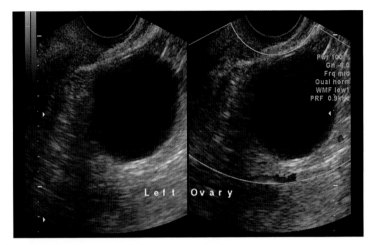

Figure 3 Ovarian torsion. Reduced ovarian perfusion is seen on power Doppler.

Obstetric cholestasis presents with itching, raised levels of alkaline phosphatase and bile acid concentration. Ursodeoxycholic acid, a bile acid itself, is used to treat the condition.

Acute fatty liver of pregnancy is rare but potentially lethal. Liver enzymes are raised with jaundice. There is hypoglycaemia, hyperuricaemia, renal impairment, coagulopathy and encephalopathy may ensue.

Acute systemic infections

As part of generalised viraemia or bacteraemia, all acute systemic infections can be accompanied with vomiting. In these cases, there are coexistent symptoms of infection, such as fever, body ache, malaise and a raised white cell count. In chorioamnionitis, uterine contractions accompany vomiting, which is aggravated due to cervical dilatation.

Central nervous system causes

Raised intracranial tension can be accompanied with vomiting. Benign intracranial hypertension is common in obese young women. It can present for the first time in pregnancy (in the second trimester) or may worsen if existing prior to pregnancy. Headache and papilloedema are present without computerised tomography evidence of a space-occupying lesion.

Neoplasms can occur rarely in association with pregnancy.

Middle ear disease

Middle ear disease can cause vomiting owing to stimulation of the labyrinth. There is often a past history, which is then aggravated in pregnancy. Motion sickness is common in pregnancy, while Ménière's disease generally presents in the fourth decade of life and rarely will coexist with pregnancy. Migraine is often aggravated in pregnancy.

Cardiological causes

Congestive cardiac failure will cause congestion of the liver and hence lead to nausea. In patients with hyperhomocysteinaemia, myocardial infarction may occur at a younger age. If the ischaemia/infarct involves the posterior wall, it irritates the oesophagus and can cause vomiting.

Endocrinal causes

Diabetic ketoacidosis may present for the first time in pregnancy with intractable hyperemesis. Blood sugar and urine ketone estimation will clinch the diagnosis. Uraemia, hyperthyroidism and hyperparathyroidism have all been reported. Addison's disease will cause infertility in the first instance but *de novo* deficiency can develop during pregnancy in cases of tuberculosis of the adrenal gland. Zollinger–Ellison syndrome leads to increased gastric acid production and vomiting.

Psychological disorders

Both anorexia nervosa and bulimia are commonly encountered in young girls and pregnancy often aggravates the conditions. Vomiting in these cases may be spontaneous but is often self-induced. Weight loss is usually significant as are nutritional deficiencies. Treatment is by psychological counselling and antidepressants.

Drug-induced/iatrogenic causes

Drugs are mostly avoided during pregnancy; however, some drugs prescribed in pregnancy can cause gastric irritation, e.g. low-dose aspirin prescribed for patients with antiphospholipid syndrome. Non-steroidal anti-inflammatory drugs may also be prescribed for chronic painful conditions such as arthritis. Steroids and aminophylline may be used for coexisting medical disorders and can lead to vomiting. Accidental poisoning with plant derivatives such as ipecac is a rare cause.

Surgical causes

The most common surgical emergency in pregnancy is acute appendicitis; however, both diverticulitis and cholecystitis will present with vomiting. Patients with acute renal or biliary colic vomit as a general response to pain. Intestinal obstruction due to any cause will present with vomiting.

Types of vomiting

The most important clues to diagnosis lie in the history of vomiting and its accompanying symptoms.

- Vomiting occurring only in the early morning occurs in pregnancy, hyperacidity and uraemia.
- Vomiting occurring after food is more likely to point to peptic ulcer, gastroparesis, pyloric obstruction and food poisoning.
- Projectile vomiting without nausea occurs in raised intracranial tension. Silent regurgitation of food occurs in oesophageal diverticuli.
- Vomiting accompanied by tinnitus and/or giddiness is seen in middle ear disease.

- Vomiting accompanied with diarrhoea occurs in enteritis and food poisoning.
- Vomiting with chest pain signifies myocardial infarction and, when accompanied with abdominal pain, could signify appendicitis.

Gastrointestinal reflux disease is characterised by reflux of gastric contents during gastric peristalsis owing to incompetence of the oesophageal sphincter. In the first trimester, the cause is impaired forward gastric peristalsis, while in the third trimester, the cause could be purely mechanical owing to the gravid uterus pushing up on the stomach. If this becomes a chronic condition, this type of regurgitation will cause damage to the oesophageal lining because of the acidic nature of the contents. In the long run, there is a risk of stricture formation.

■ Investigations

These should include the following.

- *Urine analysis*: urine should be checked for specific gravity and the presence of glucose and ketones. It may occasionally show the presence of bile pigments.
- *Complete blood count*: this will show a rise in haematocrit and haemoglobin percentage. There may be slight leucocytosis.
- *Serum electrolytes*, such as sodium and potassium: this will show hyponatraemia, hypokalaemia and, in severe cases, hypokalaemic metabolic acidosis.
- *Blood sugar*: hyperglycaemia may be present in diabetes, while hypoglycaemia may be present in persistent vomiting, which requires correction with intravenous fluids.
- *Liver function tests*: 20–30 per cent of women show mild elevation of liver enzymes in hyperemesis. In cases of hepatitis, the enzymes are markedly raised and it may be of value to check the hepatitis markers. Serum amylase and/or lipase will be raised in pancreatitis. Liver function tests also provide an opportunity to look at serum protein levels, an indication of the nutritional status of the mother.
- *Renal function tests*, as renal failure is a complication of severe dehydration.
- *Thyroid function tests*: 50–70 per cent of women have transient hyperthyroidism. This is usually a self-limiting condition and does not require antithyroid therapy.[4,12]

- *Parathyroid hormone*, if clinically indicated: hyperparathyroidism is a rare cause of hyperemesis, which may be intractable. High serum calcium levels will point to the diagnosis. Both maternal and fetal morbidity is high and surgery is the definitive cure.[13]
- An *electrocardiogram* will show widened QRS complexes and U waves in hypokalaemia.
- An *ultrasound scan* to confirm intrauterine pregnancy, to exclude multiple pregnancy or hydatidiform mole. It will also show the presence of gallstones, mesenteric adenitis, dilated loops of bowel in intestinal obstruction, the presence of an appendicular lump and small contracted kidneys in uraemia.

■ Complications of vomiting

The most obvious complications are dehydration and malnutrition. Loss of gastric fluid leads to dehydration, metabolic alkalosis and hypokalaemia. The patient will need fluid replacement to treat the dehydration. A general examination will give some idea of the severity of dehydration. The presence of ketones in the urine and a raised haematocrit will confirm the severity of dehydration. The patient then needs to be admitted to hospital.[16]

The fluid replacement regimen should include fluids, such as normal saline or Hartmann's solution. Infusion can be started at the rate of 100 mL/hour. Potassium chloride should be added to the intravenous infusion according to serum potassium levels. Potassium replacement should be carefully titrated.

Nutritional deficiency should be corrected in consultation with a dietician. Vitamin B1, B6 and B12 deficiency is common and may require supplementation. In cases of weight loss and muscle wasting, total parenteral nutrition may be necessary. Poor fetal outcomes have been reported if maternal weight loss is >5 per cent in pregnancy.[17] These include fetal intrauterine growth retardation and even fetal death in severe cases.

Other complications of vomiting include the following.

- Patients may complain of muscular aches and pains in the intercostal and upper abdominal region due to the accompanying retching.
- Constipation, which is common in pregnancy, is aggravated in hyperemesis.
- Thrombosis can be precipitated in susceptible patients due to dehydration.
- Vomiting may cause tears in the oesophageal epithelium, known as the Mallory–Weiss syndrome, which may result in haematemesis.
- Rarely, forceful vomiting will lead to pressure rupture of the oesophagus, termed Boerhaave's syndrome, where the patient will complain of acute severe retrosternal chest pain.
- Vomiting during childbirth or under anaesthesia may result in regurgitation of stomach contents into the respiratory passages leading to Mendelson's syndrome, which requires management in an intensive care unit. Subconjunctival haemorrhages may occur, which are inconsequential, but retinal detachment can be a serious complication.
- Wernicke's encephalopathy has also been reported in continued vomiting and dehydration.[18,19] This is due to thiamine (vitamin B1) deficiency, and is characterised by diplopia, nystagmus, ataxia and confusion. It can be precipitated by infusion of dextrose-containing fluids. In the presence of Wernicke's encephalopathy, the incidence of fetal loss is higher.
- Erosion of the dental enamel is seen in the repeated vomiting of bulimia.

■ Acknowledgements

Acknowledgements are due to Dr Ashok Khurana of the Ultrasound Laboratory, New Delhi, for providing the ultrasound pictures and Miss Subhikha Kakkar for her help in typing the manuscript.

■ References

1. Fairweather DV. Nausea and vomiting of pregnancy. *Am J Physiol* 1968; **102**: 135–75.
2. Walsh JW, Hassler WL, Nugent CE, Owyang C. Progesterone and estrogens are potential mediators in gastric slow wave dysrhythmias in nausea of pregnancy *Am J Physiol* 1996; **270**: G506–14.
3. Tan PC, Jacob R, Quek KF, Omar SZ. The fetal sex ratio and metabolic, haematological and clinical indicators of

severity of hyperemsis gravidarum. *BJOG* 2006; **113:** 733–7.

4. Goodwin TM. Hyperemesis gravidarum. *Clin Obstet Gynecol* 1998; **41:** 597–605.

5. Hayakawa S, Nakajima N, Karasaki-Suzuki M, *et al.* Frequent presence of *Helicobacter pylori* genome in the saliva of patients with hyperemesis gravidarum. *Am J Perinatol* 2000; **17:** 243–7.

6. Lee RH, Pan VL, Wing DA. The prevalence of *Helicobacter pylori* in the Hispanic population affected by hyperemesis gravidarum. *Am J Obstet Gynecol* 2005; **193:** 1024–7.

7. Penney DS. *Helicobacter pylori* and severe nausea vomiting during pregnancy. *J Midwifery Women's Health* 2005; **50:** 418–22.

8. Aka N, Atalay S, Sayharman S, Kilic D, Kose G, Kucukozkan T. Leptin and leptin receptor levels in pregnant women with hyperemesis gravidarum. *Aust NZ Obstet Gynaecol* 2006; **46:** 274–7.

9. Bruggmann D, Bohlmann MK, Bohle RM, Tinneberg HR. Gastric cancer in pregnancy – a case report. *Zentralbl Gynakol* 2006; **128:** 224–8.

10. Panesar NS, Chan KW, Li CY, Rogers MS. Status of antithyroid peroxidase during normal pregnancy and in patients with hyperemesis gravidarum. *Thyroid* 2006; **16:** 481–4.

11. Panesar NS, Li CY, Rogers MS. Are thyroid hormones or HCG responsible for hyperemesis gravidarum? A matched paired study in pregnant Chinese women. *Acta Obstet Gynecol Scand* 2001; **80:** 519–24.

12. Goodwin TM, Montoro M, Mestman JH, Transient hyperthyroidism and hyperemesis gravidarum. Clinical aspects. *Am J Obstet Gynecol* 1992; **167:** 648–52.

13. Kort KC, Schiller HJ, Numann PJ. Hyperparathyroidism and pregnancy. *Am J Surg* 1999; **177:** 66–8.

14. Gadsby R, Barnie-Adshead AM, Jagger C Pregnancy nausea related to women's obstetric and personal histories. *Gynecol Obstet Invest* 1997; **43:** 108–11.

15. Deuchar N. Nausea and vomiting in pregnancy. A review of the problem with particular regard to psychological and social aspects. *Br J Obstet Gynecol* 1995; **102:** 6–10.

16. Jewell D, Yong G. Interventions for nausea and vomiting in early pregnancy. In: *Cochrane Library* 2003: issue 4. Chichester: John Wiley.

17. Gross S, Librach C, Cecutti A. Maternal weight loss associated with hyperemesis gravidarum: a predictor of fetal outcome. *Am J Obstet Gynecol* 1989; **160:** 906–9.

18. Wood P, Murray A, Sinha B, Godly M, Goldsmith HJ. Wernicke's encephalopathy induced by hyperemesis gravidarum. Case reports. *Br J Obstet Gynecol* 1983; **90:** 583–6.

19. Spruill SC, Kuller JA. Hyperemesis gravidarum complicated with Wernicke's encephalopathy. *Obstet Gynecol* 2002; **99:** 875–7.

VULVAL ITCHING

Anthony Bewley

Vulval itching (pruritus vulvae) may be due to generalised or localised disease (Box 1). The sensation of itch is generated by unmyelinated C-nerve fibres distinct from, but similar to, pain nerve fibres. As a consequence, the sensation of itch may not be entirely accurate, and some women describe burning, tingling and even pain (vulvodynia) as part of the same symptomatology. Vulval itch, then, is an entirely unpleasant, intense, unsocial, embarrassing and debilitating sensation that must not be underestimated.

■ Generalised disease (see also Itching in pregnancy)

Dermatological conditions can affect the vulval skin either in isolation or as part of a generalised skin disease. Inflammatory dermatoses are

Box 1 Causes of vulval itching

Generalised disease

Inflammatory skin disease[a]
Atopic eczema
Eczema (other causes, e.g. contact)
Psoriasis
Lichen planus
Pityriasis rosea
Urticaria

Generalised pruritus[a]
Xerosis (dry skin)
Hyper/hypothyroid disease
Liver disease
Chronic renal failure
Haematological malignancy
Drug rashes
Occult malignancy
Iron deficiency
Psychogenic causes

Infections and infestations[a]
Scabies
HIV-related skin disease
Tinea (fungal skin disease)
Body and pubic lice

Localised (vulval) disease

Inflammatory vulval disease
Lichen sclerosus
Lichen planus
Lichen simplex chronicus
Eczema
Psoriasis
Vulvodynia
Plasma-cell vulvitis

Localised pruritus
Overwashing/detergents (irritant vulvitis)
Atrophic vulvitis
Psychogenic
Vulval-intraepithelial neoplasia

Sexually transmitted disease
Vulval warts
Candida
Pubic lice

---

[a]See Itching in pregnancy. HIV, human immunodeficiency virus.

common, so they often affect the vulva. Patients with generalised inflammatory dermatoses may not disclose vulval disease unless specifically asked (usually through fear of a sexually transmitted disease).

■ Localised vulval disease

Perhaps the commonest cause of vulval itch is an *irritant vulvitis* through overwashing. Soaps, shampoos and shower gels often contain detergents, which strip the delicate vulval skin of its natural oily barrier. Soap substitutes (e.g. aqueous cream) are essential in the management of irritant vulvitis, but sometimes a short pulse of moderately potent (e.g. clobetasone butyrate

0.05 per cent) steroid ointment may be necessary. In irritant vulval disease, there are no architectural changes to the vulval anatomy (see Lichenoid vulval disease below), but rather clinical manifestations of localised vulval eczema (redness, excoriation, oozing, scaling).

Lichen sclerosus (Figs 1 and 2) is a well-recognised vulval dermatosis, which affects any age group, but usually middle-aged and older women. Itch is usually the presenting symptom. Vulval examination reveals erythema (early); atrophy, porcelain-white scarring, purpurae and architectural vulval damage (late). Unfortunately, the physical signs are often all too obvious (especially before the advent of combined

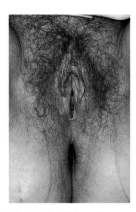

Figure 1 Vulval and perianal lichen sclerosus.

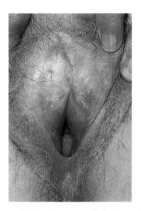

Figure 2 Severe lichen sclerosus with fusion and resorption of the labia minora together with scarring of the clitoral hood.

gynaecology/dermatology vulvoscopy clinics), as women may present quite late in the progression of their disease. Treatment with potent (despite the drug package inserts) topical steroid ointments (e.g. clobetasol proprionate) is essential, although with time and improvement, lower dose topical steroids replace the more potent topical steroids. Emollient soap-substitution is also important as the barrier function of the vulval skin is often compromised. The condition has a 1–4 per cent risk of neoplastic change and so must be monitored carefully.

Lichen planus (Figs 3 and 4) may affect the vulva in isolation and, like lichen sclerosus, may be destructive and is intensely itchy. Differentiating between lichen sclerosus and lichen planus can sometimes be difficult, but checking the rest of the body, particularly the oral cavity, may help with the diagnosis (30 per cent of patients with lichen planus have buccal mucosal involvement). Epithelial surfaces of the vulva may demonstrate the lacy white hyperkeratosis similar to oral lichen planus, and the inflammation may have a more purplish (violaceous) appearance. The signs of late lichen sclerosus (porcelain-white, cigarette-paper scarring, purpurae) are absent. Even so, it may be necessary to take a vulval biopsy to differentiate between lichen sclerosus and lichen planus, and histology is usually fairly distinctive. Classical lichen planus, as part of a widespread papular rash, is usually self-limiting. For recalcitrant and isolated vulval lichen planus,

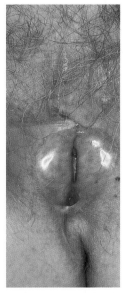

Figure 3 Severe lichen planus with extensive architectural change. Note violaceous inflammation with lacy hyperkeratosis superior to the clitoral hood. (Courtesy of Dr K Gibbon, Whipps Cross University Hospital, London, UK)

treatment is similar to lichen sclerosus, but neoplastic change in lichen planus is very rare.

The habit of scratching the vulval skin (maybe through stress or following eczema) may lead to *lichen simplex chronicus* (LSC; Fig. 5). In LSC neoneuronal growth with opioid-producing nerve fibres may lead to the 'stress-busting' habit of genital scratching. Clinical features are those of persistent vulval eczema. Treatment with topical

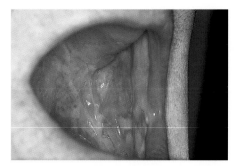

Figure 4 Oral lichen planus. Note the lacy hyperkeratosis of the buccal mucosa.

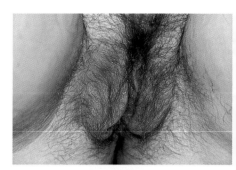

Figure 5 Lichen simplex chronicus affecting the vulva. Note the unilateral eczematous rash.

steroids and emollients is often all that is necessary, but recalcitrant LSC may respond to tricyclics, cognitive behavioural habit-reversal therapy, and opioid antagonists.

Vulval *atopic eczema* is more commonly associated with generalised disease. Excoriation, lichenification (skin thickening), scaling, oozing and pigmentation change are all common. Treatment is primarily with emollients and soap-substitution, but judicious use of topical steroid (e.g. clobetasone butyrate 0.05 per cent) is also important. Sometimes infected eczema may require treatment with topical steroid/antibiotic combination or even systemic antibiotics. Persistent eczema may be driven by specific contact allergens (e.g. clothing dyes) and patch testing may be necessary to identify causative chemicals.

Genital psoriasis is not only itchy, but also sore. *Vulval psoriasis* is scaly, red and well demarcated (unlike poorly demarcated and excoriated eczema). Treatment with moderately potent topical steroids and emollients are very helpful. Sometimes second-line agents (phototherapy, methotrexate, ciclosporin) for difficult disease are used under careful supervision, especially if the patient is pregnant or trying to conceive.

Vulvodynia is persistent vulval pain, often with periposterior fourchette point tenderness, which leads to superficial dyspareunia. Vulvodynia is not always painful, however, and mixed sensations of itch, burning and pain are common. Apart from point tenderness, there is frequently little to see on examination. However, patients with vulvodynia are greatly incapacitated by their disease and the life-impact of their condition must not be dismissed. Consequently, patient education and advocacy is of the essence (Box 2), as is treatment with topical local anaesthetics (2–5 per cent lignocaine gel), emollients, topical and systemic tricyclics.

> ### Box 2 Patient advocate groups (websites)
>
> - *Candida*: www.candida-society.org.uk
> - Eczema: www.eczema.org
> - Herpes: www.herpes.org.uk
> - Human immunodeficiency virus: www.tht.org.uk
> - Lichen sclerosus: www.lichensclerosus.org
> - Psoriasis: www.psoriasis-association.org.uk
> - Vulvodynia: www.vulvalpainsociety.org

Plasma-cell vulvitis is rarer in women than Zoon's balanitis in men, but the conditions are analogous. Aetiology is thought to be relatively long-term poor personal hygiene but this is contentious. Treatment with emollients and topical steroids is usually all that is necessary.

■ Sexually transmitted diseases and other infections

Scabies and pubic lice, of course, cause intractable pruritus vulvae. Specific treatments are available. It is important to remember that 33 per cent of patients with one sexually transmitted disease (STD) may have another concomitant STD. Referral to the local STD clinic is, therefore, essential for diagnosis and management of concomitant disease, and for contact tracing.

Candida is not necessarily sexually transmitted and may be associated with diabetes, antibiotic, oral contraceptive usage and pregnancy. Vulvovaginal disease typically causes a curdish-white discharge, which leads to pruritus and soreness. Treatment with topical imidazole creams and/or systemic imidazoles is usually curative. Recrudescence is common and some advocate complementary medicine and yeast-free diets.

Other causes of vaginal discharge (see Vaginal discharge), such as *Gardnerella*, *Trichomonas vaginalis* and urinary tract infections, may cause pruritus vulvae and soreness.

■ Neoplastic disease

Finally, vulval intraepithelial neoplasia (VIN; often related to previous human papilloma virus infection especially HPV types 16 and 18) may be itchy, especially in the early stages. VIN typically presents with leucoplakia, persistent erosions and plaques, and (later) frank masses. Biopsy is

fundamental followed by appropriate topical (5-fluorouracil, cryotherapy, photodynamic therapy and/or imiquimod) or surgical intervention.

VULVAL SWELLINGS

Tony Hollingworth

The differential diagnosis of vulval swellings includes not only tumours of the vulva itself, but also swellings that appear at the vulva as a result of the displacement of other structures as in cases of uterine prolapse and cystocoele (see Prolapse of uterus and vagina). Hernias into this region can occur and no further discussion is included in this section. Inflammatory lesions and ulceration of the vulva may be accompanied by swelling of the vulva owing to oedema. These conditions are considered under Vulval ulceration. Conditions presenting with itching of the vulva as the main complaint are described under Vulval itching.

Vulval swellings may be specific to the vulva anatomy or dermatological in origin (Box 1). They may be benign or malignant, which can be further divided into primary and secondary. These conditions will be diagnosed either

Box 1 Classification of vulval swellings

Infective	Cystic	Benign	Malignant
Bartholin's abscess	Bartholin's cyst	Fibroma	Squamous cell
Warts	Sebaceous cyst	Lipoma	carcinoma
(condyloma	Mucous cyst	Fibromyoma	Rodent ulcer – basal
acuminatum)	Implantation cyst	Hidradenoma	cell carcinoma
	Dermoid cyst	Papilloma	Adenocarcinoma
	Hydrocoele of the	Lymphangioma	Sarcoma
	canal of Nuck	Myxoma	Melanoma malignant
	vestigial cyst	Angioma	Choriocarcinoma
		Melanoma benign	
		Neuroma	
		Caruncle	

clinically related to their anatomical site or histologically by excision biopsy.

Cystic swellings

- Bartholin's cyst
- Sebaceous cyst
- Mucous cyst
- Implantation cyst
- Dermoid cyst
- Hydrocoele of the canal of Nuck vestigial cyst

The commonest one is a Bartholin's cyst (Fig. 1). This is due to the duct opening of the Bartholin's gland becoming blocked thus producing a swelling in the posterior third of the labium majus. This projects medially so as to encroach on the vaginal entrance and may cause dyspareunia. It is not particularly tender unless it becomes infected, forming an abscess. The cyst tends gradually to increase in size, causing local discomfort until marsupialization is performed. This results in a new duct being formed.

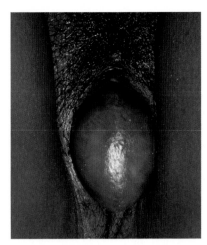

Figure 2 Vulval cyst following female circumcision; the contents were old blood.

to a persistent processus vaginalis. It is essentially a type of hernia and needs to be treated accordingly.

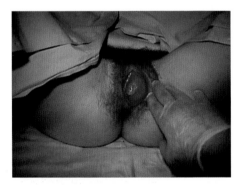

Figure 1 Bartholin's cyst.

Sebaceous cysts are fairly common, affecting the labia majora as a rule. They may occur in groups. Mucous, inclusion, implantation (Fig. 2) and dermoid cysts also occur. The true nature of these cysts is not usually known without histological examination. A very uncommon swelling in the vulva is a cyst in the canal of Nuck. This is a peritoneal diverticulum that passes through the inguinal canal and swelling occurs in the labium major owing

Infective swellings

- Bartholin's abscess
- Warts (condyloma acuminatum)

Bartholin's abscess presents as an extremely painful swelling in the region of Bartholin's gland, which occurs at the entrance to the vagina. Pressure on the gland causes much pain and the area appears reddened. The duct of the gland has become blocked and the secretions within the gland infected. It may discharge by itself but treatment is surgical in the form of marsupialisation to create a new duct. Recurrence may occur.

Warts on the vulva are usually multiple (Fig. 3). They are caused by the human papillomavirus types 6 and 11, and are almost invariably transmitted sexually. They may spread throughout the lower genital tract and anal region. They have been associated with premalignant disease of the cervix. Vulval warts may proliferate and coalesce in which case they are referred to as condyloma acuminata. This situation can be

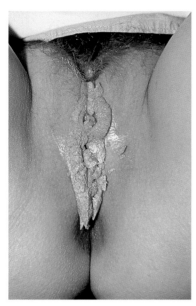

Figure 3 Vulval warts.

problematic in pregnancy and in patients who are immunocompromised (e.g. human immunodeficiency virus or patients with systemic lupus erythematosus on long-term steroids).

■ Blood cysts

- Varicocoele
- Traumatic haematoma
- Endometrioma

Varicocoele of the vulva occurs mainly in pregnancy and can become worse with successive pregnancies. They give a typical varicose appearance in the labia majora and the patient can become conscious of an uncomfortable swelling on standing. The veins seldom rupture during delivery. Varicocoele must be differentiated from an inguinal hernia extending into the labium majus and from a cyst of the canal of Nuck (the processus vaginalis, which has failed to become completely obliterated). Both the latter tend to involve only the anterior parts of the labium majus, but all these conditions extend to the groin. Whereas a hernia is reducible as a rule, a cyst of the canal of Nuck is not. Inguinal hernias

usually disappear as pregnancy progresses, but varicocoeles become worse. If a hernia contains bowel, it is resonant to percussion. A strangulated hernia will not be reducible, but the accompanying acute symptoms and the history should make the diagnosis clear.

A haematoma of the vulva may follow delivery or occur as the result of direct trauma. It is recognized as a bluish swelling, which is painful and tender, and spreads up into the pelvis by the side of the vagina. The appearance is characteristic and the diagnosis is made on the history. An endometrioma is a rare cause of a blood-containing cyst on the vulva and is seldom seen as an isolated finding.

■ Benign new growths

- Fibroma
- Fibromyoma
- Lipoma
- Hidradenoma
- Papilloma
- Lymphangioma
- Myxoma
- Angioma
- Melanoma
- Neuroma
- Caruncle

As the vulva comprises skin, any swelling that can occur in a skin appendage can be found in the vulval region. Both fibroma and lipoma are seen in the vulva, and may become pedunculated. They may occur at any age, are soft, oval or rounded, and covered by vulval skin. They may grow slowly to reach the size of a fist. A lipoma is usually broader based than a fibroma. Several other benign swellings are found on the vulva. They are usually solitary and small (about 1 cm or so in diameter) and their nature is confirmed by histology. A papilloma is a sessile benign tumour of the skin of the labia in women of middle or old age. A hidradenoma is a tumour of sweat gland origin, which may be solid or cystic, and which may ulcerate to allow a red papillomatous growth to be extruded. When ulcerated, it may suggest the diagnosis of carcinoma clinically. Biopsy resolves the problem. Less commonly, fibromyoma, myxoma, angioma, lymphangioma, benign melanoma and neuroma are found, each distinguished by microscopic examination of the excised lesions.

■ Tumours at the urethral meatus

Urethral caruncles are frequent, especially in older women. A caruncle appears as a small, reddish, sessile growth arising from the posterior wall of the urethral meatus causing bleeding and painful micturition. It is often very tender but may be symptomless. It is usually granulomatous, but may be polypoidal and papillomatous. It has to be distinguished from prolapse of the urethral mucosa in which there is a ring of protruding red tissue all round the urethral opening.

■ Malignant new growths

- Squamous cell carcinoma
- Rodent ulcer – basal cell carcinoma
- Adenocarcinoma
- Sarcoma
- Melanoma
- Choriocarcinoma

It must be emphasized that cancer within the vulva is a very uncommon condition and any tumour that occurs in the skin can occur in the vulval region. The commonest type is squamous cell carcinoma, which may have been preceded by pruritus but may be completely asymptomatic (Fig. 4). It occurs mainly in postmenopausal women, usually as a single tumour, although on occasions may present as kissing ulcers. The commonest site is on the labia; it spreads locally in the first instance and then to the inguinal lymph nodes. Squamous lesions account for 85 per cent of vulval cancers, the remainder comprising tumours of the skin and vulval appendages. Other malignant tumours found in the vulva include:

- rodent ulcer (basal-cell carcinoma), forming a flat plaque with its characteristic rolled edge;
- malignant melanoma (pigmented and nonpigmented);

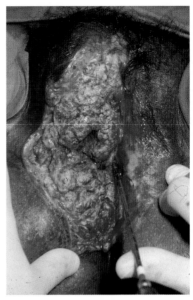

Figure 4 Extensive vulval carcinoma.

- adenocarcinoma arising in Bartholin's gland or in the urethra;
- sarcoma;
- undifferentiated tumours.
- rarely, metastatic tumours from primaries in the cervix, uterine body and ovary can occur;
- choriocarcinoma has also been described.

The diagnosis is dependent on either a biopsy or an excision biopsy. For details of the staging of tumours together with the prognosis for each tumour, see Appendix.

VULVAL ULCERATION

Tony Hollingworth

Ulceration can be defined as a persistent breach in any epithelial surface, in other words, a break in any surface lining. The causes of any ulceration include the following.

- *Physical causes*, including pressure, chemicals, irradiation, etc. In the case of vulval dystrophies (skin conditions), intense itching of a chronic nature may occur in the vulva and the associated

scratching may lead to a breach in the epithelium. These will be considered under Vulval itching.
- *Infection*, which can be divided into sexually or non-sexually transmitted.
- *Vascular insufficiency* or compromise.
- *Sensory loss* allowing ulceration due to trauma as a result of lack of sensation, which usually affects the limbs.
- *Malignancy*, which in the case of the vulva, can produce a localised swelling that becomes ulcerated. The various types of malignancy are summarised under Vulval swellings. Premalignant lesions of the vulva do not usually cause ulceration of the vulva unless there has been intense scratching from pruritic symptoms.

Vulval ulceration (see Fig. 4, *Vulval swellings*) can, therefore, be classified thus:

- infective;
- sexually transmitted;
- non-sexually transmitted;
- systemic-type disease association;
- vulval dystrophies (see above);
- malignancy.

Diagnosis will usually be made from taking a history and examining the patient. The investigations that may be necessary include appropriate microbiology and ultimately a biopsy.

Infective – sexually transmitted

Herpes

Primary infection occurs 2–7 days after inoculation with the Herpes simplex virus (HSV). Prodromal symptoms of tingling or itching are followed by vesicular eruptions, which rapidly erode, resulting in painful shallow ulcers all over the vulva. The patient may develop dysuria and, if secondary infection occurs, the patient may develop retention of urine, bilateral inguinal lymphadenopathy, fever and general malaise. Herpes virus can be obtained from the vesicular fluid in the early stages, 85 per cent being due to the HSV type 2. The lesions, which are very painful, persist for 2–6 weeks before healing occurs and antibody appears in the blood (Fig. 1). The ulcers tend to recur at intervals of weeks or months, and

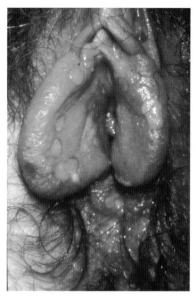

Figure 1 Ulceration due to Herpes.

the virus may be recovered from them. Coitus with a non-immune partner will pass on the infection. The disease is self-limiting in time and the lesions eventually heal spontaneously. During pregnancy, the fetus is at risk, if the episode is the primary infection at the time of delivery.

Diagnosis is usually made on clinical examination and virological swabs. Consideration should be made for other sexually transmitted disease screening involving the local Genitourinary Medicine/Department of Sexual Health services.

Syphilis

Primary syphilis gives rise to an indurated ulcer that characteristically is painless unless it becomes secondarily infected. The incubation period is between 10 and 90 days following contact. Genital lesions in women often escape notice because they are hidden inside the vagina or on the cervix. The lesion has to be differentiated from an epithelioma. If an epithelioma is suspected, the ulcer and swelling should be excised, and examined histologically. The serous fluid from a chancre contains the spirochete *Treponema pallidum*, which can be seen under a microscope with the aid of dark ground illumination.

A chancre will persist for 1–5 weeks, but serological tests for syphilis do not become positive for about 4–6 weeks after the appearance of the chancre. The serological tests most commonly performed are the VDRL (Venereal Disease Research Laboratory) slide test and the FTA–ABS (fluorescent treponemal antibody absorption) test, which have replaced the Wassermann, Kahn and TPI (treponemal immobilization) tests. To exclude primary syphilis, serological tests have to be done every week for 6 weeks after the appearance of the chancre.

Two weeks to 6 months after the chancre has healed, the generalised cutaneous eruption of secondary syphilis appears. Numerous, moist, flat-topped papules occur on the vulva and round the anus. They are known as condyloma latum. In only one-third of untreated cases does tertiary syphilis occur but not until some years after the primary lesion.

Lymphogranuloma venereum

This condition is usually found in the tropical and subtropical regions of Africa, Asia and southeastern USA. It is generally transmitted by sexual contact and is primarily an infection of the lymphatic system by a subtype of *Chlamydia trachomatis*. It has three stages, which are outlined below.

1 From incubation to an initial lesion of a vesico-pustular eruption on the vulva (3–21 days).
2 This disappears to be followed by inflammation and swelling of the regional lymph nodes.
3 Painful suppuration in the inguinal glands with hypertrophy and ulceration of the groins, vulva and perineum then follows.

Later scarring may cause anal stricture and/or severe dyspareunia.

The diagnosis is made in one of three ways:

■ positive serological testing either with complement fixation or microimmunofluorescence;
■ isolation of the chlamydial organisms;
■ histological identification of the chlamydial elementary and/or inclusion bodies in the infected tissue.

The treatment is a course of doxycycline.

Granuloma inguinale

This is a chronic venereal infective condition caused by the organism *Calymmatobacterium granulomatis*. Although it is sexually transmitted, it is not highly contagious. However, once infection has established, it causes destruction of tissue, leading to ulceration and the development of massive granulation tissue affecting the vulva and groins. It is almost non-existent in Great Britain, but is seen in India, Brazil and the West Indies, islands of the South Pacific, Australia, China and Africa. It starts as a raised papilloma, which soon ulcerates, the ulcer having a typical serpiginous (tortuous, serpentine-like) outline. The granuloma in the groin rarely suppurates but much scarring develops.

Diagnosis can be made from identifying Donovan bodies in a smear/scraping or biopsy from the ulcer. These Donovan bodies are calymmotobacteria located within cytoplasmic vacuoles of macrophages and turn blue with Giemsa staining.

Treatment options include a course of trimethoprim or sulfamethoxazole; other appropriate antibiotics include doxycycline, ciprofloxacin and erythromycin.

Chancroid

This is a very common cause of genital ulceration in tropical parts of the world and occurs 2–10 days after coitus, although may in some cases be up to 35 days. It begins as a vesicopustule, which becomes a punched-out ulcer with a red base, or as a saucer-shaped ragged ulcer. The lesion is extremely tender and produces a heavy foul discharge, which is contagious. The lesion may be solitary, or there may be several ulcers and associated painful inguinal adenitis, which may break down and discharge. It contains the causative organism, Ducrey's bacillus (*Haemophilus ducreyi*) a Gram-negative rod, which may be difficult to grow, but can be cultured in Nairobi medium. Appropriate antibiotics include azithromycin, erythromycin, ciprofloxacin.

Yaws

This occurs in tropical countries and produces lesions similar in appearance to the condyloma latum of secondary syphilis. It is a contagious but non-venereal infection that usually affects children. It does spread by direct contact and, in time, can lead to bone, joint and soft-tissue deformities. It is due to a spirochaetal organism, *Treponema pertenue*. The diagnosis can be confirmed with the serological tests for venereal syphilis. First-line treatment is with a penicillin agent and, in allergic patients, tetracyclines can be used.

■ Infective – non-sexual

Aphthous ulcers

These are analogous to the painful small ulcers, which can be found in the mouth. The exact cause is not clearly defined but is thought to arise due to a disturbance in the immune system by some external factor.

Treatment is symptomatic.

Tuberculous

This is a rare cause of vulval ulceration but may be associated with inguinal lymphadenopathy. It usually arises from haematogenous spread from primary tuberculosis. Ascending infection or vertical spread is rare. They are very indolent and can only be diagnosed with certainty on microscopic section of a biopsied part of the lesion.

Furunculosis

These are boils and due to staphylococcal infection of the hair follicles. They are common and affect the labia majora in particular. Shaving the area may predispose to this problem.

Diphtheria

This condition is an upper respiratory tract infection with *Corynebacterium diphtheriae*. It causes a low-grade fever and produces ulceration with membranous exudates. It is highly contagious but vaccination has reduced the incidence very dramatically. It can cause vulval ulceration. The diagnosis is on identifying the organism, and treatment is either with erythromycin or procaine penicillin.

Candidal

Mycotic and diabetic vulvitis due to *Candida* can cause soreness and pruritus of the vulva with redness, excoriation and oedema of the skin and a characteristic, white, curd-like discharge containing the mycelium of *Candida albicans*.

■ Systemic disease

Behçet's syndrome

Behçet's syndrome is a rare autoimmune disorder resulting in blood vessel damage. It can be characterised by oral and vulval ulceration, but these patients may also develop skin and eye problems, including uveitis, retinitis and iritis. It is difficult to diagnose, as there are no specific confirmatory tests. It can be treated with corticosteroids. More information can be obtained from www.behcets.com.

Crohn's disease

The vulva and perineum may be affected in up to 30 per cent of cases of Crohn's disease and this may pre-date gastrointestinal symptoms. The lesions appear like knife cuts in the skin; however, discharging sinuses and irregular ulcers are more common. This problem is infrequently seen by the gynaecologist and the reader may want to access www.crohns.org.uk for further information.

Lipschütz ulcers

These mainly occur on the labia minora, and are of acute onset with an associated fever and lymphadenopathy. It is a very rare cause of genital ulceration and has been reported as associated with typhoid and paratyphoid fever, with *Salmonella* being the causative organism.

■ Malignancy

This has been discussed previously but in summary the types of tumours that arise in this area include:

- squamous carcinomas;
- melanomas;
- sarcomas;
- basal-cell carcinomas;
- Bartholin's glands adenocarcinomas;
- undifferentiated tumours;
- possible secondary tumours

■ Definitions

AC The *abdominal circumference* is the perimeter of the fetal abdomen at the level of the stomach, intrahepatic umbilical vein and the confluence of the right and left portal veins. At 20 weeks' gestation, the average AC is 150 mm and there is usually an increase of 10–12 mm per week.

AFI The *amniotic fluid index* is the sum of the maximum vertical amniotic depth measure in each quadrant (see Amniotic fluid abnormalities) for details and values.

AFP *Alphafetoprotein* is a glycoprotein produced by the fetal yolk sac, fetal gastrointestinal tract and eventually the fetal liver. It is measured in the quadruple test for Down's syndrome, where the serum level is usually low, as well as being used as a marker for hepatocellular carcinoma, endodermal sinus tumours and, more rarely, mixed Müllerian tumours. The maternal serum AFP level rises with gestational age. It is elevated in multiple pregnancies, and in a number of fetal abnormalities, including neural tube defects (spina bifida and anencephaly) and abdominal wall defects.

Asynclitism The posture of the baby's head in which one parietal bone is at a lower level than the other, owing to lateral inclination of the head.

Attitude The relationship of the parts of the baby to itself, e.g. flexed or extended head.

BPD The *biparietal diameter* is an ultrasound measurement of the fetal head from the outer edge of the cranium nearest the transducer to the inner aspect of the cranium furthest away. At 12 weeks' gestation, it measures 20 mm and there is an increase of 3–4 mm every sub-sequent week.

Ca125 This is an abbreviation for cancer antigen 125, which is a mucinous glycoprotein produced by the *MUC16* gene. It is used as a tumour marker for ovarian cancer and, whilst sensitive, it is not specific for this type of tumour, as it is elevated in only 80 per cent of cases. It may also be raised in tumours arising from the endometrium, Fallopian tubes, lungs, breast and gastrointestinal tract. It may also be elevated in benign conditions that cause peritoneal irritation, e.g. endometriosis, tuberculosis of the pelvis, pelvic inflammatory disease, appendicitis and pregnancy. It is especially useful in monitoring response to treatment. The normal range is 0–35 U/mL.

Caput Oedema of the fetal scalp (see Fig. 3 in Labour, prolonged).

CRL *Crown–rump length* is an ultrasound measurement from the apex of the skull to the base of the torso not including the limbs. It is used as an early pregnancy dating measurement, at 6 weeks' gestation it will be 3–4 mm and 9–10 mm by 7 weeks.

Denominator The bony landmark on the presenting part used to define the position. It is usually a midline structure, e.g. occiput for a cephalic presentation, mentum or chin when it is a face presenting, or the sacrum if a breech.

Diathesis A predisposition to a specific problem.

Dysgenesis Abnormal development of tissue especially an epithelium.

Dystocia An abnormal labour.

Effacement The thinning or taking up of the cervix, which in primips usually occurs before dilatation.

Embryo A conceptus between the time of fertilization up to 10 weeks' gestation.

Engagement This occurs when the widest diameter of the presenting part is through the pelvic brim. In the case of a vertex presentation, this is the biparietal diameter; for a breech, it is the bitrochanteric diameter.

Fetal weight The weight of a fetus if it were to be born using the 50th centile measurements. The expected fetal weights per week of gestation are as follows:

28 weeks	1200 g
30 weeks	1500 g
32 weeks	1900 g
34 weeks	2300 g
36 weeks	2800 g
38 weeks	3200 g
40 weeks	3500 g

Fetus The embryo is termed fetus from 10 weeks' gestation until the time of birth.

Gestation sac On ultrasound, this is identified as a fluid collection in the uterus with an embryo present. At 5 weeks' gestation the diameter measures 2 mm and then increases 8–9 mm over the subsequent few weeks.

Gravidity This refers to the number of pregnancies the woman has had, including the current one, irrespective of the outcome (e.g. miscarriage, live birth, etc.).

HC The *head circumference* is an ultrasound measurement of the outer perimeter of the cranium at the level of the thalami and the cavum septum pellucidum. It measures 90 mm at 14 weeks' gestation and then increases by approximately 15 mm per week for the remainder of the pregnancy.

HCG *Human chorionic gonadotrophin* is a peptide hormone made by the embryo and subsequently the syncytiotrophoblast. Its role is to support the corpus luteum, thereby maintaining progesterone production, which in turn maintains the pregnancy. It is used in early pregnancy testing and can be detected before a menstrual period has been missed. It usually measures 1000 mIU/mL by day 32 (28-day cycle) and should reach at least 10 000 mIU/mL by day 40 when the fetal head may be visible. The quantification of HCG is useful during pregnancy as the level should double every 36–48 hours and lack of this doubling may point to either a failing pregnancy or possibly an ectopic pregnancy. It can also be used as a tumour marker for trophoblastic disease including hydatidiform mole and choriocarcinoma as well as islet cell tumours.

Infant A child from birth until 1 year of age.

Intrapartum This is synonymous with labour.

Labour The process by which a baby is born. Labour can be defined as the onset of regular painful contractions with dilatation of the cervix and descent of the presenting part. The mechanism of labour in a cephalic presentation involves descent, flexion of the head, internal rotation of the presenting part, extension or crowning, restitution or external rotation of the head, and internal rotation of the shoulders.

LFTs The *liver function tests* largely remain unaltered during pregnancy except for the alkaline phosphatase level; this is raised owing to an isoenzyme produced by the placenta, which may account for half of that level.

Lie The relationship of the longitudinal axis of the fetus to the longitudinal axis of the mother, e.g. longitudinal, oblique, transverse and unstable.

Maternal mortality The number of deaths of women while pregnant or within 42 days of termination of pregnancy irrespective of duration and site of the pregnancy, from any cause related to or aggravated by the pregnancy or its management (but not from accidental or incidental causes) per 100 000 births (see www.CEMACH.org.uk). They are usually divided into:

- **Direct obstetric deaths** Deaths resulting from obstetric complications of the pregnant state, e.g. amniotic fluid embolism.
- **Indirect obstetric deaths** Deaths resulting from previously existing conditions or those developing during the pregnancy, which were not due to direct obstetric causes but were aggravated by the physiological effects of the pregnancy. An example would be maternal cardiac disease.
- **Late obstetric deaths** Deaths which occur between 42 days and 1 year after delivery owing to direct or indirect maternal causes.

■ **Incidental or accidental deaths** Deaths from a cause completely unrelated to pregnancy in women who happened to be pregnant at the time. Examples would include road traffic accidents or accidental overdoses.

Microangiopathy Disease affecting small blood vessels.

Miscarriage The spontaneous loss of a pregnancy prior to 24 weeks' gestation or expulsion/extraction of a fetus weighing 500 g or less.

Moro reflex A primitive response of newborn, used to assess neurological development.

Moulding This occurs when the bones of the fetal skull slide over one another (see Fig, 3 Prolonged labour). The skull bones do not usually fuse until some time after delivery, the only exception being craniosynostosis.

Multigravida A woman with a history of previous pregnancies, usually with live children; also called a multip.

Neonatal death rate The number of deaths within 28 days of birth of all live born infants (regardless of gestation) per 1000 live births.

Nuchal translucency This is the thickness of the cystic area posterior to the occiput and is measured excluding the skin surface and the occiput. An increase in this measurement is suggestive of a chromosomal disorder especially trisomy 21. The level usually used is below 3 mm.

Odonophagia Painful/difficult swallowing.

Parametrium This is the fibrous tissue that separates the supravaginal portion of the cervix from the bladder and extends on to its sides and laterally between the layers of the broad ligament, and contains the uterine artery.

Parity This refers to the number of pregnancies with a birth beyond 20 weeks' gestation or an infant weighing more than 500 g.

Perinatal death rate The number of stillbirths and first-week neonatal deaths per 1000 total deliveries.

Placenta A temporary organ occurring during pregnancy that allows fetomaternal exchange; also known as the afterbirth. Implantation can be low in the uterus, resulting in a placenta praevia, in which it is below the presenting part. The placenta can become morbidly adherent:

■ **Accreta** Where there is abnormal attachment to the myometrium.
■ **Increta** This occurs when the placenta invades the myometrium.
■ **Percreta** Where the placenta penetrates through the myometrium.

Position The location of the denominator relative to fixed points within the maternal pelvis, e.g. occipitoanterior. It is also a term used to describe the relation of the fetal back to the right or left side of the mother.

Postmature When the infant is born after 41 completed weeks of pregnancy. It carries an increase in the perinatal mortality rate.

Premature When the infant is delivered before 37 completed weeks of pregnancy.

Presentation This refers to the part of the fetal body which is in or over the pelvic brim, e.g. cephalic or breech.

Preterm When the infant is delivered between 24 and 37 weeks' gestation.

Previable When the infant is delivered before 24 weeks' gestation.

Primigravida A woman in her first pregnancy; also called a primip.

Prognosis A forecast for the outcome of a condition.

Puerperium The time from immediately after delivery and extending for 6 weeks. It may also be known as the postnatal or postpartum period.

Quadruple test This involves the measurement of serum AFP, HCG, oestriol and inhibin. It is used to screen for Down's syndrome. The levels will obviously change depending on the length of gestation.

Sclerosis Abnormal hardening of a tissue.

Semen analysis See Infertility for values and comments.

Station This reflects the descent of the presenting part into the pelvis and is measured in relation to the ischial spines in centimetres, with minus being used if above the spines and plus if below.

Stillbirth rate The number of infants born with no signs of life after 24 completed weeks' gestation per 1000 total births.

Term This is considered to be from 37 to 41 completed weeks of pregnancy assuming a 28-day cycle. Term may vary between racial groups (see Prolonged pregnancy) but the average time of a human pregnancy is 280 days.

Trimesters The antenatal period is traditionally divided into trimesters. Usually each trimester is associated with particular problems for that trimester:

- **First trimester** The interval from the first day of the last period to 12 weeks' gestation, assuming a 28-day cycle. It is during this period that most organogenesis occurs.
- **Second trimester** The interval between the 13th and 27th week of pregnancy.
- **Third trimester** This extends from the 28th week of pregnancy until the time of delivery.

Tumour marker A substance produced by a particular tumour, which can be measured in the serum to aid diagnosis and response to treatment of that tumour.

U&E *Urea and electrolytes* are measures of renal function. In pregnancy, there is an increase in the glomerular filtration rate and, as a consequence, the serum urea usually falls. The serum sodium, potassium and chloride remain essentially unchanged.

Urate The serum urate level decreases during the early part of the pregnancy owing to the increase in glomerular filtration rate; however, it rises during the later stages of the pregnancy

and can reach levels at term that are higher than non-pregnant values. It is useful in monitoring a woman with pre-eclampsia.

Vertex A diamond-shaped area between the anterior and posterior fontanelles and the biparietal eminences. This is the area that presents to the pelvis when the head is flexed.

■ Tumour staging

Staging is the means by which the extent of the cancer/tumour is assessed at the time of presentation. The following are the FIGO classifications for the four main gynaecological cancers.

Vulval cancer

Stage 0 Carcinoma *in situ*, VIN3 or severe vulval dysplasia. This would be classed as premalignant

Stage I	Tumour <2 cm and confined to the vulva or perineum
Stage IA	<11 mm invasion below the surface epithelium
Stage IB	>1 mm invasion below the surface epithelium
Stage II	Tumour confined to the vulva and/or perineum larger than 2 cm
Stage III	Tumour spread to the lower urethra, vagina or anus and/or local lymph node involvement on one side
Stage IVA	Tumour spread to the upper urethra, bladder or rectum, or local lymph nodes on both sides
Stage IVB	Tumour spread to the pelvic lymph nodes and/or more distant sites

Endometrial cancer

This is a surgically based system.

Stage I

Stage IA	Tumour is limited to the endometrium
Stage IB	Tumour invades less than halfway through the myometrium
Stage IC	Tumour invades more than halfway through the myometrium

Stage II

Stage IIA Endocervical glandular involvement

Stage IIB Cervical stromal invasion

Stage III

Stage IIIA Tumour invades the serosa or adnexa or malignant peritoneal cytology

Stage IIIB Vaginal metastasis present

Stage IV

Stage IVA Invasion of the bladder or the bowl

Stage IVB Distant metastases, including intra-abdominal or inguinal lymph nodes.

Cervical cancer

This staging is based on clinical examination rather than surgical findings. It does not include lymph node involvement.

Stage 0 Full thickness of the epithelium but no invasion of the stroma – CIN3

Stage I Confined to the cervix

Stage IA Diagnosed microscopically, no visible lesions

Stage IA1 Stromal invasion <3 mm in depth and up to 7 mm horizontal spread

Stage IA2 Stromal invasion between 3 and 5 mm in depth and up to 7 mm horizontal spread

Stage IB Visible lesion or a microscopic lesion with >5 mm of depth or >7 mm horizontal spread

Stage IB1 Visible lesion 4 cm or less in greatest dimension

Stage IB2 Visible lesion >4 cm

Stage II Invades beyond the cervix

Stage IIA Without parametrial invasion but involves the upper two-thirds of the vagina

Stage IIB With parametrial involvement

Stage III Extends to the pelvic side wall or the lower third of the vagina

Stage IIIA Involves the lower third of the vagina

Stage IIIB Extends to the pelvic wall and/or causes hydronephrosis or non-functioning kidney

Stage IV Spread has extended beyond the true pelvis or has involved the mucosa of the rectum or bladder

Stage IVA Invades the mucosa of the bladder or rectum and/or extends beyond the true pelvis

Stage IVB Distant metastases

Ovarian cancer

Para-aortic lymph node involvement is considered as regional lymph nodes (Stage IIIC).

Stage I Limited to one or both ovaries

Stage IA Involves one ovary; capsule intact; no tumour on the ovarian surface; no malignant cells in ascites or peritoneal washings

Stage IB Involves both ovaries; capsule intact; no tumour on the ovarian surface and negative washings

Stage IC Tumour limited to both ovaries with any of the following: ruptured capsule, tumour on the ovarian surface, positive washings

Stage II Pelvic extension or implants

Stage IIA Extension or implants of tumour on to the uterus or Fallopian tumour; negative washings

Stage IIB Extension or implants of tumour on to other pelvic structures; negative washings

Stage IIC Pelvic extensions or implants with positive peritoneal washings

Stage III Microscopic peritoneal implants outside the pelvis; or limited to the pelvis with extension to the small bowel or omentum

Stage IIIA Microscopic peritoneal metastases beyond the pelvis

Stage IIIB Macroscopic peritoneal metastases beyond the pelvis <2 cm in size

Stage IIIC Peritoneal metastases beyond the pelvis >2 cm or lymph node metastases

Stage IV Distant metastases – in the liver parenchyma or outside the peritoneal cavity

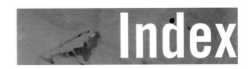